PERSONALITY DEVELOPMENT
THROUGH
POSITIVE DISINTEGRATION

THE WORK OF
KAZIMIERZ DĄBROWSKI

PERSONALITY DEVELOPMENT
THROUGH
POSITIVE DISINTEGRATION

THE WORK OF
KAZIMIERZ DĄBROWSKI

William Tillier, M.Sc. [1]

Foreword by Sal Mendaglio, Ph.D.

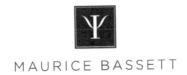

MAURICE BASSETT

Personality Development Through Positive Disintegration: The Work of Kazimierz Dąbrowski

Maurice Bassett
P.O. Box 839
Anna Maria, FL 34216

Contact the Publisher:
MauriceBassett@gmail.com
www.MauriceBassett.com

Cover Design by Tammy Arthur
Editing and interior layout by Chris Nelson

ISBN: 978-1-60025-107-8

Library of Congress Control Number: 2018936896

DEDICATION

This work is respectfully dedicated to Sandra Lee,
my role model of advanced development.

"Oh, how can I forget you?
When there is always something there to remind me
Always something there to remind me
I was born to love you, and I will never be free
You'll always be a part of me."

(Bacharach & David, 1964/1969, A1)

ACKNOWLEDGMENTS

First and foremost, I must acknowledge the faith, support, and patience of my late wife Sandra. I greatly appreciate the ongoing faith and support of Joanna Dąbrowski. I would like to express my appreciation to Maurice Bassett for his support in the publication of this book, and to Chris Nelson for his expertise in guiding its execution. This work benefited greatly from the practical support, encouragement, and friendship of Sal Mendaglio. I also greatly appreciate the review provided by James Duncan and the suggestions of Amanda Harper. I thank Rene, Ziada, Raphael, and Zianne Castaños, Joey Villanueva, Angela Meunier, Jemna Cruz, Angie Saguran, Karen Ziadie, Virginia Larson, Irene Sifrer, and Thaddeus Bear for their unfailing support. Finally, material pertaining to suicide is revised from a previously published paper and is used with kind permission from *Advanced Development* (Tillier, 2017). Dąbrowski's biography is revised from a previously published book chapter and is used with kind permission from Great Potential Press (Tillier, 2008a). Figure 1 is modified from Elizabeth Mika (2015) with her kind permission.

"He shall be found the truly wise.
'Tis Zeus alone who shows the perfect way
Of knowledge: He hath ruled,
Men shall learn wisdom, by affliction schooled."

Aeschylus (525-456 B.C.).
(Eliot, 1909, p. 11).

TABLE OF CONTENTS

EXPANDED TABLE OF CONTENTS

FOREWORD

During Kazimierz Dąbrowski's lifetime, his theory of positive disintegration was virtually unknown outside of Europe. Nevertheless, there were important individual exceptions such as Abraham Maslow and Jason Aronson, luminaries in American psychology and psychiatry, who knew of the theory and appreciated its importance. The situation is very different in the 21st century: positive disintegration is known globally as manifested in publications, research, conferences, and websites throughout the world. Regrettably, Dąbrowski did not live to see the impact his theory has had in education and psychology. The person who contributed most significantly to the growth in popularity of Dąbrowski's theory is the author of this book: William "Bill" Tillier, whom I know affectionately as Tillier.

Tillier was Dąbrowski's student and protégé. To this day, Tillier will say emphatically that knowing the theory and the theorist, was life-changing. Since Dąbrowski's death in 1980, Tillier became not only a proponent of the theory but also its archivist. He maintains a library consisting of Dąbrowski's works and publications regarding positive disintegration. Tillier has worked diligently to disseminate widely the products of his efforts through publications and websites that he has managed over the years. Though his work as archivist is significant, in my view, Tillier's single greatest contribution was making available digital copies of Dąbrowski's English language books, with the Dąbrowski family's permission. No longer are interested parties limited to publications about aspects or parts of the theory: we can read Dąbrowski's articulation of his entire theory. It is important to emphasize that Tillier learned the theory not only from the books, but also from Dąbrowski directly.

My early perusal of Dąbrowski's books proved to be a difficult read. The books revealed an array of assumptions, propositions, and concepts that were alien. Both the juxtaposition of positive and negative to common psychological constructs (e.g., positive disintegration, negative adjustment) and Dąbrowski's reframing of many psychological constructs (e.g., development, personality) were initial barriers to understanding the theory. Through persistence and patience—reading and re-reading the books—I began to gain a better understanding of what I believed Dąbrowski intended. However, it was through my discussions and collaboration with Tillier that my knowledge of the theory deepened.

My growing confidence in understanding the theory led me to publish a number of articles and an edited book (Mendaglio, 2008). Soon after its publication, Tillier proclaimed that the book was the "best secondary source" on the theory of positive disintegration. Though my book contained several chapters on the theory itself (Tillier made a significant contribution to the book), I did not and do not consider my effort as a secondary source. Of course, I felt honored by Tillier's comment and did not complain. However, to me secondary sources are book-length treatments of theories, especially those theories that are difficult reading in the original. My book had some elements of that, but most chapters addressed such matters as application of Dąbrowski's theory to gifted education and comparisons with other theories.

Secondary sources are typically produced by devotees of a theory whose journeys begin by fully appreciating the significance of a theory. Over time, they gain a fulsome understanding of it. Outstanding secondary sources are written by authors who are not only grounded in the theory but who also knew the theorist personally—those who have learned the theory directly from the theorist. Likely the best-known example is the extensive secondary source and biography of Sigmund Freud's theory written by his long-time friend and colleague, Ernest Jones (Jones, 1953). There are lesser known examples in the history of psychology. Heinz Ludwig Ansbacher, a student of Alfred Adler, along with Rowena Ansbacher, produced the definitive book on Adler's individual psychology (Ansbacher & Ansbacher, 1956). Paul Mullahy, Harry Stack Sullivan's student, produced a book on Sullivan's interpersonal theory of psychiatry (Mullahy, 1970). Tillier's book represents the authoritative secondary source for Dąbrowski's theory of positive disintegration. Direct knowledge of the theory and his close relationship with Dąbrowski enable Tillier, more than other any other student of positive disintegration, to communicate not only Dąbrowski's concepts, but also the nuances of their intended meaning.

The book contains numerous concepts that together form the theory of positive disintegration. Tillier intersperses his presentation with many quotations from Dąbrowski's various books. While other authors of secondary sources use fewer quotations, Tillier explains that he does so to prevent the appearance of bias, as the book can only be an interpretation of the original statement of the theory. While the issue of bias cannot be completely avoided by the quotations, they do serve a purpose: they provide readers who are unfamiliar with the original publications a sense of Dąbrowski's writing style. For those of us who have studied the books, the quotations are like old friends. While the quotations are interesting, it is Tillier's profound understanding of the theory that shines through. He makes complex and paradoxical-sounding ideas readily comprehensible and accessible to the reader. To the degree that I understand Dąbrowski's work, Tillier's secondary source is a faithful representation of the original.

When compared to excellent secondary sources of other theories, Tillier's book provides more than simply a faithful rendition of positive disintegration. The book contrasts the ideas inherent in positive disintegration to current scholarly literature. After presentation of the elements of the theory, Tillier interweaves a plethora of citations relating to mainstream psychology, neuropsychology, and genetics, to name a few areas. These citations demonstrate two realizations: Dąbrowski's ideas and their integration into a comprehensive theory were clearly ahead of his time; and, subsequent advances in knowledge confirm his understanding of human functioning. Tillier's integration of literature from related fields also manifests one other matter: Tillier's impressive breadth of knowledge in diverse, but related, fields of study. Tillier's book provides the reader with more than one expects from a secondary source. It is not only an accessible summary of the theory; the book also places Dąbrowski's seminal work in the context of current research and practice.

Sal Mendaglio
Calgary, Alberta
Canada
January, 2018

References

Ansbacher, H. L., & Ansbacher, R. R. (1956). *The individual psychology of Alfred Adler*. New York, NY: Basic.

Jones, E. (1953). *The life and work of Sigmund Freud*. New York, NY: Basic.

Mendaglio, S. (2008). *Dąbrowski's theory of positive disintegration*. Scottsdale, AZ: Great Potential Press.

Mullahy, P. (1970). *The beginnings of modern American psychiatry*. Boston, MA: Houghton Mifflin.

OVERVIEW

WHO WAS KAZIMIERZ DĄBROWSKI?

Kazimierz Dąbrowski (1902-1980) was a Polish psychiatrist and psychologist who devoted his life to the observation and understanding of personality development.[2] Dąbrowski's own life was very challenging, with his later childhood literally spent amid the battlefields of World War I.

Many opportunities followed the First World War, and Dąbrowski was able to study under some of the most prominent figures of the day in Poland, France, and Switzerland, including Jan Mazurkiewicz, Édouard Claparède, Jean Piaget, Wilhelm Stekel, and Pierre Janet. He obtained a master's degree, a medical degree, and a doctorate in psychology. He also embarked on what was to become a prolific writing career. Receiving Rockefeller grants, Dąbrowski first came to America to study at Harvard in the 1930s and then returned to Poland with funding to begin establishing state-wide mental health initiatives.

Sadly, World War II had a major impact on Dąbrowski; his life hung in the balance on many occasions. He was interned several times in the German police prison system. Later, in Stalinist-controlled Poland, he was held again for some 18 months. After his release, severe restrictions were placed on his activities. In typical fashion, Dąbrowski kept working as best he could and published materials that eventually formed the corpus of his work.

As political restrictions on him eased, Dąbrowski was able to return to America in the early 1960s where he met and befriended Jason Aronson and Abraham Maslow. This visit led to the publication of his first major contemporary work in English (Dąbrowski, 1964b). Dąbrowski secured visiting professorships in Alberta and Québec and moved his family to Edmonton in the late 1960s. For the rest of his life he traveled between his homes in Poland and Canada, writing, working with graduate students, and doing what he probably loved most—working with patients in mental health facilities.

Dąbrowski wrote over 20 books and hundreds of articles in Polish. His works were also published in French and Spanish, but unfortunately never received a wide audience in English; his six major English works were out of print for many years. He passed away in Poland in 1980. The last 20 years have witnessed a renewed interest in Dąbrowski's theory. Sal Mendaglio edited a book in 2008 (Mendaglio, 2008a) and two of Dąbrowski's books have reappeared in print (Dąbrowski, 1967/2015; 1964/2016).

WHAT IS IN THIS BOOK?

This work is an introductory survey of Dąbrowski's central ideas. Like many people who read Dąbrowski, I have strong personal reactions to his ideas and naturally resonate to some of his ideas more than others. This makes it challenging to present an objective overview of his theory. Therefore, as I present his ideas, I will liberally quote from Dąbrowski's original materials. It is my hope that this volume will encourage readers to seek out and consult Dąbrowski's primary works. I will clearly identify where I advance neo-Dąbrowskian ideas. I am confident that in the future, subsequent contributions to the literature will further translate, elaborate, and enlarge upon Dąbrowski's ideas.

My goal in writing this book is to introduce Dąbrowski and his theory to a wider audience, primarily within psychology. I will distill and present an integrated and manageable overview of Dąbrowski's theory and place his work into a contemporary context of psychology.

A NOTE ON ORGANIZATION.

This work is presented in 10 chapters. Following this note I present a broad overview of Dąbrowski's personality theory. Chapter

One then introduces Dąbrowski's unique approach to mental health, psychological adjustment, development, and personality. The critical role played by the multidimensional and multilevel worldview is described in Chapter Two, along with details of Dąbrowski's five levels. Chapter Three introduces the role of "the three factors" and of instincts in development. Dąbrowski's important construct[3] of developmental potential is described. The developmental process, the construct of disintegration, and the developmental role played by psychoneuroses are reviewed in Chapter Four. Chapter Five reviews the key psychological structures involved in development, including dynamisms; the inner psychic milieu; and the roles played by emotion, values, and psychological types in development. Chapter Six presents a summary of the philosophical foundations of the theory. Chapter Seven places the theory in a contemporary context with discussions of posttraumatic growth, positive psychology, personality theory, suicide, creativity, and neuropsychology. Self-actualization and the relationship between Dąbrowski's approach and Maslow's are discussed in Chapter Eight. A neo-Dąbrowskian construct of multilevel-actualization is introduced to bridge and advance these two approaches. Educational implications, including applications to gifted education, will be reviewed in Chapter Nine. Chapter Ten offers suggestions for future theory-building and research. Appendix 1 presents a brief biography of Dąbrowski. Appendix 2 presents a bibliography of Dąbrowski-related materials published since 2006 to assist the reader interested in further exploration.

WHAT IS SO SPECIAL ABOUT DĄBROWSKI'S PERSONALITY THEORY?

Why do we need yet another theory accounting for personality? It seems like the personality textbooks are teeming with all varieties of adequate theories already. The simple reasons lie in the unique and unusual approach presented by Dąbrowski's theory. To begin with, let us examine the fundamental aspects of the theory.

The theory encompasses a broad range of human behaviors

Having lived through both great wars, Dąbrowski said he witnessed a vast spectrum of human behavior, ranging from the most primitive, unimaginable acts of violence and cruelty through to the highest and most noble acts of humanity, heroism, and self-sacrifice. Dąbrowski said that he could not find a theory of personality that could satisfactorily explain the lowest actualities of behavior while at the same time accounting for the highest possibilities of human beings. He began studying the life histories and developmental trajectories of eminent individuals and created the *Theory of Positive Disintegration* (TPD) based upon the idea that development involves becoming aware of the many hierarchies, both in life in general and within oneself, and consciously working to advance from lower to higher levels within these different hierarchies.

A positive approach to defining mental health

Dąbrowski rejected traditional definitions that are based on the absence of symptoms. He believed that mental health is reflected by, and should be defined by, the development of a unique and autonomous personality, one that is created based on the ideal of an individual's unique character.

Integration and disintegration

Dąbrowski believed that the average person is characterized by a fairly rigid integration reflecting social indoctrination and incorporating the rules and roles of one's society. He advanced the idea that this integration has to dis–integrate in order to allow an individual to develop autonomy. In his approach, ideally, the disintegrative process will allow for a reorganization and the creation of a new secondary integration reflecting an advanced level of personality development.

Disintegrate and rebuild—not build over

Most theories of development propose that subsequent advances are built "on top of" existing, earlier structures. Dąbrowski rejected this approach, suggesting the unusual alternative that earlier (primary) and lower psychological structures must disintegrate to allow the individual to consciously create new, secondary, and higher integrations. This disintegrative process involves strong anxieties, self-doubts, and depressions that challenge the lower levels and status quo and push the individual to seek autonomy. Dąbrowski coined the term *positive disintegration* to describe the process because, generally, these transformations lead to advanced expressions of development—positive growth. In summary, disintegration—falling apart—is not only positive; in this theory, it is also a necessary prerequisite for advanced psychological development.

Must reinvent the self

As lower psychological integrations break down, one's basic life assumptions and values come under deep introspection. Often, the familiar and rote rationales used in day-to-day life falter, frequently leaving the individual in limbo and crisis. In order to find autonomy, a person has to uncover and discover his or her deep personality characteristics: Who am I? Who do I dream to be? What is my unique idealization of my personality? Why am I here? How do I find meaning in life?

This review of one's character leads to growth and a reformulation and reprioritization of one's values and beliefs. This re-examination brings into focus one's true, authentic personality. With this personality ideal as a guide, one can transform, shape, and re-form the lower aspects of the self, those based on instinct and socialization, to reflect one's unique and autonomous self-defining characteristics—one's essence. These reshaped and newly created psychological structures form "secondary," higher integrations based upon the re-formulation of one's self-construct, value structures, goals in life, perception of reality, and one's personality ideal.

Individuality is not personality

The TPD is unique in its overall approach to personality. Dąbrowski used his own definition of personality and believed that the average person does not have an autonomous personality; rather, the average person shares a "group personality" reflecting his or her culture and social values. Dąbrowski (1967, pp. 4-6) differentiated the terms "individuality" and "personality"; based upon his unique usage, everyone has individuality, but he reserved the term personality for the smaller subset of people who achieve higher development.

Individuality & Unilevelness

Dąbrowski used the term individuality to recognize the uniqueness of people: "We understand the term individuality to mean a distinct human being, differing from other individuals of a given society in such aspects as mental qualities, talents, particular interests, way of behaving, ambition and strength of pursuing his aims" (Dąbrowski, 1967, p. 4). People who fall under the umbrella of individuality generally display a trait Dąbrowski called *unilevelness*. Unilevelness is characterized by a horizontal view of life—people perceive choices that are different but on the same plane—like turning left or turning right. At this, Dąbrowski's first level of development (*primary integration*), the behavior of the average person strongly reflects two aspects: the pursuit of egoistic aims and/or social mores, roles, and expectations. The locus of control of values and behavior is largely external. Reactions tend to be rapid and stereotypic, reflecting social expectations of automatic, stimulus-response reactions with little conscious introspection. This initial, socially-based integration leaves little room for the development of an individualized and autonomous personality.

Personality & Multilevelness

Dąbrowski used the term personality to refer "to an individual fully developed . . . an individual in whom all the aspects form a coherent and harmonized whole and who possesses, in a high degree, the capability for insight into his own self, his own structure, his aspirations and aims (self-consciousness)" (Dąbrowski, 1967, p. 5). Personality is "a self-aware, self-chosen, self-affirmed and self-determined unity of essential individual psychic qualities" (Dąbrowski, 1972b, p. 301). One's values must receive a full and conscious re-examination along with a volitional reconstruction to bring them into harmony with one's emerging personality ideal. Eventually, values are re-incorporated in forming an individually unique hierarchy of values, aims, and goals. This re-formulated value structure allows for the expression of true autonomy and self-determination—the locus of control of behavior becomes internal. Personality is a characteristic of those at advanced developmental levels, a group that consists of individuals who possess a multilevel, vertical view of life. The fully developed and harmonized personality appears at the stage of secondary integration (Dąbrowski, 1970b, p. 174).

Not everyone has the potential to develop

Although I think that folk psychology would like to believe that advanced development is universal, Dąbrowski reflected the conclusions of most established developmental theories when he observed that advanced development is not universally attained. Dąbrowski believed that an individual's developmental trajectory is determined by his or her essence. A component of essence is a constellation of genetic features that Dąbrowski called *developmental potential* (DP). The influence of this potential on development may be positive, equivocal or negative. The exemplars of personality whom Dąbrowski studied led him to conclude that development requires strong positive developmental potential. Developmental factors include a strong innate drive to express one's individuality and the presence of overexcitability. *Overexcitability* (OE) is a description of psychological sensitivity indicated by exaggerated reactions to stimuli in several major areas including physical activity, sensual perception, imagination, intellectual pursuits, and most importantly, emotional sensitivity. Overexcitability involves a lowered threshold and a heightened response to the incoming stimuli of the world as compared with the reactions of the "average" individual. Overexcitability varies between individuals based on both inherited genetics and one's life experiences. People with overexcitability react with unusually strong responses, often to very small or subtle events in the world that the average person might not even notice. When strong positive developmental potential is present—and especially overexcitability—the day-to-day experiences of life create considerable distress and promote the disintegrations needed for development. Experiences of strong OE intensify, deepen and make crises more personal—challenging the fabric of the self. This strong potential will subsequently help the individual to use insights in developing a fundamental appreciation of his or her essence—a description of one's own unique character. Dąbrowski associated strong DP, and especially strong OE, with thriving and positive outcomes to crises that culminate in psychological growth.

Expression of essence shaped through choices—personality shaping

The theory is unusual in emphasizing both essence and existentialism. Although the parameters of development may be constrained by one's essence and genetics, advanced development also relies upon one making day-to-day existential choices that shape and give expression to one's innate essence (Dąbrowski called this *personality shaping*). These choices come to reflect one's personality ideal when aspects that are "less myself" are inhibited or transformed, while aspects that are "more myself" and more in harmony with one's personality ideal are emphasized and enlarged. Thus, development relies on an interaction between one's original genetic essence and the existential choices one makes in day-to-day life; choices guided by one's imagined vision of one's personality ideal.

We must perceive the higher and seek it

An important construct in TPD is *multilevelness*. Dąbrowski (1970b, p. 177) described the structure of reality as "many-sided and multileveled." Individuals with unilevel perception are limited in their potential to develop, in part because they do not perceive the full spectrum of reality. Advanced development is predicated on the ability of an individual to perceive all of the phenomena of life through the lens of multilevelness, revealing "the distinctions of higher and lower functions" (Dąbrowski, 1973, p. ix). This sense of multilevelness also applies to the analysis of oneself: the ability to "look at oneself from above, i.e. from the position of higher processes such as self-awareness, self-control and others" (Dąbrowski, 1972b, p. 23). The individual "starts to feel a difference between what is higher and what is lower, marking the beginning of experience and perception of many levels" leading to "a growing sense of 'what ought to be' as opposed to 'what is' in one's personality structure" (Dąbrowski, 1996, p. 19). Simply, multilevelness is being able to recognize the low road versus the high road.

Authentic development transforms the ego

Paradoxically, the theory suggests that advanced development requires overcoming, transforming, and somewhat destroying one's own ego. Advanced development does not display the ego-driven or selfish motives commonly seen at lower levels. The theory emphasizes development of an individualized personality, but this is achieved by overcoming and transforming one's ego, not strengthening it. The key discovery of authentic development is humility and the realization of one's place, both within society and in the larger cosmos. This "ego deflation" emerges from a new understanding and perspective on the relationship between the self and others. The universe does not revolve around us; this realization comes with our discovery of a deep compassion for and empathy with others. Subsequently, a sign of advanced and authentic development is a deep regard, empathy, and compassion for others, creating a new foundation for "a small e ego" and pro-social behavior.

Emotion must guide cognition

The theory emphases the role of emotion in development and in life. Development is usually seen as driven by cognitive achievements, and cognition is seen as primary throughout life. Decision making is traditionally seen as a rational process generally disrupted by emotions—emotion tosses our thinking to and fro, like a ship in a storm. Dąbrowski expanded conventional views of emotions as approach-avoidance motivations, giving emotion a critical role in helping to guide cognition and to inform our values and choices. A genuine awareness of one's emotions fosters the discovery of one's priorities regarding what is important in life, and this creates and shapes a deep sense of one's unique authenticity. Emotions work with cognition to help one choose behaviors that reflect one's ideal of who one feels one ought to be—one's personality ideal.

Growth as a lifelong process

In biology, growth stops when maturation is reached. Dąbrowski said that where potential for psychological development is strong, maturation takes longer than is usually seen. In ideal development, growth never stops—it is a lifelong process, and psychological maturation is never reached.

Self-perfection trumps self-preservation

Dąbrowski differentiated instincts into higher and lower categories. Lower instincts, including self-preservation, sex, and aggression, are usually controlled and channeled by socialization. In advanced growth, uniquely human instincts transform lower instincts to serve growth and also motivate authentic development. Authentically human instincts include: a broad developmental instinct, self-development, creativity, and, ultimately, the instinct of self-perfection.

Summary

The constructs outlined above give the reader a flavor for the unique way that Dąbrowski framed his understanding of personality and its development. His theory challenges the reader to consider deeper and alternative views of psychology.

DĄBROWSKI'S UNIQUE APPROACH TO MENTAL HEALTH AND DEVELOPMENT

1–1. POSITIVE MENTAL HEALTH

Today, using positive criteria to define mental health is not as revolutionary an idea as it was fifty years ago. Several examples of positive approaches to defining mental health were summarized in "Toward a new definition of mental health" (Galderisi, Heinz, Kastrup, Beezhold, & Sartorius, 2015):

> According to the World Health Organization (WHO), mental health is "a state of well-being in which the individual realizes his or her own abilities, can cope with the normal stresses of life, can work productively and fruitfully, and is able to make a contribution to his or her community." (p. 231)

Dąbrowski's approach to mental health was relatively radical in 1964. It encompassed new definitions of health, methods and interpretations of diagnosis, and new constructs of psychological adjustment and personality. At the center of this approach, a positive definition of mental health laid the foundation for Dąbrowski's unique construct of development and spawned a number of major implications for psychology and psychotherapy.

1–1–1. Marie Jahoda

Dąbrowski was influenced by the work of Marie Jahoda (1907-2001). Jahoda was born in 1907 and grew up in Vienna, where she was "a staunch anti-fascist" and was imprisoned by the Austrian government between 1936 and 1937 ("Marie Jahoda," 2001). She was able to flee to England where, during the war, she operated a secret radio station promoting anti-Nazi propaganda run by the English government ("Marie Jahoda," 2001). She eventually emigrated to the United States where she became a researcher at Columbia University, studying a series of "contentious" topics of the day, including civil rights issues and McCarthyism—the FBI had her under investigation ("Marie Jahoda," 2001).

Jahoda was chosen to survey views on mental health (see Ewalt, 1957) and presented six criteria of positive mental health:

1. One's attitude toward oneself (self-perception).
2. The degree of psychological growth, development and self-actualization seen in one's behavior.
3. The integration of one's psychological functioning including, from above, one's self-perception and behavior.
4. Autonomy as demonstrated by one's degree of independence from social influence.
5. The adequacy of one's perception of reality.
6. The ability to successfully meet life's adversities and master one's environment. (Jahoda, 1958, p. 23)

1–1–2. Positive mental health is not the absence of symptoms

Following Jahoda (1958), Dąbrowski advanced the idea that mental health should not be defined simply by the presence or absence of symptoms. Rather, definitions of mental health must be concerned with constructs of men and women as they ideally ought to be and by the potential of the individual to achieve desirable developmental qualities: "The distinction between mental health and mental illness rests on the presence or absence of the capacity for positive psychological development" (Dąbrowski, 1964b, p. 17). Equating mental health with development, Dąbrowski (1972b) defined mental health as: "Development towards higher levels of mental functions, towards the discovery and realization of higher cognitive, moral, social and aesthetic values and their organization into a hierarchy in accordance with one's own authentic personality ideal" (p. 298). Features reflecting development become the hallmarks representing mental health, chief among them an autonomous, consciously derived hierarchy of values marking the creation of an idealized vision of self—the unique personality of the individual.

Dąbrowski's observations culminated in the conclusion that individual personality is not universally, or even commonly, achieved. Here we see our first indication that socialization and individual development are incompatible—socialization presents strong forces that predispose conformity and that act to squelch and homogenize individual development. In addition, the individual often finds comfort in the group and security in conforming without having to expend a great deal of time or energy on thinking—this conformity is often rote, involving little conscious reflection. In order for a person to create an autonomous self and personality, he or she has to break free from the initial psychological integration based upon socialization and enculturation and embark upon a process of self-discovery and self-creation. Dąbrowski's position was that this developmental breakdown does not occur routinely or easily; thus, the average socialized individual generally does not display advanced individual development or individual personality as Dąbrowski defined it. When combined with Dąbrowski's approach to mental health, this created the unconventional conclusion that the average "well socialized" person lacks a unique individual personality and cannot be considered mentally healthy—the "state of primary integration is a state contrary to mental health" (Dąbrowski, 1964b, p. 121).

1–1–3. Standards of normality

As Dąbrowski pursued these lines of inquiry, psychology was experiencing an emerging emphasis on individual development and autonomy, including the popular work of Carl Rogers (1902-1987), Abraham Maslow (1908-1970), and the rise of the "third force" in psychology (Goble, 1970), forging a new direction that contrasted both psychoanalysis and behaviorism. Yet, there were also appeals from some of the most prominent psychologists of the day for conformity to an external standard. For example, Gordon Allport (1897-1967) suggested that "a normal personality is one whose conduct conforms to an authoritative standard and an abnormal personality is one whose conduct does not do so" (Allport, 1969, p. 1). In this 1957 essay, Allport went on to differentiate normal into statistical (average or usual) and ethical (desirable or valuable) spheres and suggested that we can no longer continue our practice of accepting statistical norms as criteria; psychologists, with the help of philosophers, needed to develop moral guidelines based upon what "is right and good" in order to act as external criteria to guide society. Allport (1969) emphasized the urgent need for such guidelines:

> Our concern for the improvement of average human behavior is deep, for we now seriously doubt that the merely mediocre man can survive. As social anomie spreads, as society itself becomes more and more sick, we doubt that the mediocre man will escape mental disease and delinquency, or that he will keep himself out of the clutch of dictators or succeed in preventing atomic warfare. The normal distribution curve, we see, holds out no hope of salvation. We need citizens who are in a more positive sense normal, healthy and sound. And the world needs them more urgently than it ever did before. (p. 2)

Attempts to define the "normal personality" using statistical methods are also still appearing. For example, Reiss (2008) used surveys to compile sixteen basic desires and values that account for normal motivations characterizing personality types. These desires are genetic in origin and form a hierarchy—different individuals have different desire profiles and will also display differences in the intensity or strength of their various drives. People tend to be intolerant of others who express significantly different values from their own, and this leads to conflicts that are often misinterpreted as personality disorders (Reiss, 2008).

1–1–4. Values and value development

Dąbrowski called for individual growth to be considered as a key index of development and rejected statistical norms as guidelines for defining personality. However, Dąbrowski also rejected social conformity and adjustment to external standards as criteria in defining mental health and rejected suggestions that psychologists (or anyone else) should construct moral guidelines for people to follow. Rejecting any external standard, Dąbrowski believed that the moral guideline that one ought to follow must be of one's own creation, as illustrated in this Friedrich Nietzsche (1844-1900) paraphrase: based upon our unique essence, each of us must create our own values and personality and thus walk our own path in life.

Thus, the construction of an individual idealized personality and personal morality become a central developmental challenge in Dąbrowski's approach.

Dąbrowski (1970b) said:

> In the theory of positive disintegration, we distinguish various levels of development of emotional and instinctive functions. The level of these functions determines the level of values. The construct of hierarchy of values is based on the distinction of levels of emotional and instinctive development of individuals as well as social groups. We hold the opinion that it is possible to obtain in valuation a degree of objectivity comparable to that of scientific theories. It is characteristic that, for instance, moral judgments made by individuals representing a very high level of universal mental development display a very high degree of agreement. (p. 92)

The above quote contains several cardinal ideas:

- Based upon observation, human behavior can be differentiated into several basic and distinct levels reflecting a hierarchy of development. These levels will be readily apparent in the population (see Zafeiris & Vicsek, 2018).

- Levels of *individual function*, *social function* and *development* can be distinguished on the basis of emotional and instinctive factors and by the value structure that characterizes each level. In other words, the characteristic values seen at different levels will be different, allowing each level to be differentiated. Levels of individual function emphasize values putting the self first. Social function highly values mores of one's society, emphasizing both their value and any penalties associated with transgressions against them. Developmental levels can be characterized by autonomously chosen values representing the ideal personality of the individual. Developmental values put others first and subject social values to both rational and emotional scrutiny before they are adopted into one's value hierarchy.

- Homogeneity of values, especially at the lowest and highest levels, can be easily observed, leading to a consensus that represents objective—scientific—evidence of the existence and validity of the levels described.

The presence of values, their nature, and the process by which they are derived all become critical indicators of development and positive mental health. Individuals may exhibit few values, indicating minimal development. Or, individuals may parrot social values out of simple indoctrination or socialization, again signaling minimal development. The critical element that distinguishes greater development is that an individual has come to his or her values through an individual process of self-insight and creation, not simply by indoctrination or by subscription to an external morality or social convention. To paraphrase and anticipate our discussion of Nietzsche, the individual will not be spared the task of developing his or her own values, a process that must take into account and be congruent with the fundamental essence of the individual's idealized self-construct—his or her personality ideal.

In terms of the content or nature of values, we have already seen that Dąbrowski rejected calls for creating and conforming to prescriptive external standards and values. Subsequently, Dąbrowski also clearly rejects any relativistic approach to values. From

Dąbrowski's point of view, the observable convergence of values at the lowest and highest levels is scientific evidence of the fundamental differences between these two levels and of their associated values. It is obvious that both sets of values cannot be equal—both cannot stand. At the end of the day, one level and set of associated values must stand for right—human authenticity—it must be higher—and one must represent egotism, inauthenticity and be lower. However, in contrast to Allport, the details associated with the highest and lowest values are not published and therefore are not prescriptive; it is up to each of us as individuals to observe, discover, discuss, and ultimately decide which values are most compatible with our own character, and to essentially figure out on our own which are higher and which are lower.

It is important to emphasize the critical role played by discussion in this process. Dąbrowski described his approach as *phenomenological hermeneutics*—each individual must describe the phenomenological experience he or she has of the world and then explore this experience through discussion with others. Through this hermeneutic discussion, a consensus can be arrived at, reflecting the commonality of the lowest versus the highest human levels. This process is an important part of development and, as we will see, is related to the important role played by subject-object in development.

Dąbrowski (1970c) believed that the values espoused in connection with the highest levels reflect greater authenticity and greater individuality, yet at the same time greater humanity, humility, and compassion, thus representing ultimate and universal human ideals or values:

> Thus, a theory of more advanced stages of mental development cannot resign itself to just describing what takes place, it must distinguish clearly enough higher levels from lower levels in the sense of being able to say which are more advanced, more "developmental" and therefore, more valuable. (p. 13)

In another passage that defined authentism, Dąbrowski emphasized two fundamental ideas: that, ultimately, individual essence is the nucleus of meaning and that individual essence and the core universal values of humanity develop synergistically:

> Authentism. When individual and common essence is attained at the level of personality, it means that central unrepeatable and experientially unique individual qualities are retained and continue to develop together with universal qualities of humanity. Authentism signifies the realization that the experience of essence, i.e. of the meaning and value of human experience, is more fundamental than the experience of existence. (Dąbrowski, 1996, p. 42)

In summary, Dąbrowski considered the development of an individualized hierarchy of values and a unique idealization of one's personality as critical components that must be present in any construct of mental health. These idealizations serve as an image to guide individual development toward higher levels of converging human authenticity and human values. With appropriate observation and analysis, these values and ideals also serve as an objective, scientifically describable reflection of the levels of both individual and human development.

It is important to emphasize that Dąbrowski did not deny or ignore mental health symptoms; for example, he was not a follower of the sort of anti-diagnostic or anti-psychiatry position espoused by Thomas Szasz (1920-2012), as in, for example, *The Myth of Mental Illness: Foundations of a Theory of Personal Conduct* (1974). However, Dąbrowski was critical of the traditional approach to diagnosis governed by diagnostic manuals, for example, by the *Diagnostic and Statistical Manual of Mental Disorders* (5th ed., American Psychiatric Association, 2013). This approach essentially presents a checklist of symptoms to assist the therapist in making a definite (and billable) diagnosis. Dąbrowski shunned the checklist approach to diagnosis as he felt it was shallow and reductionistic, a criticism also shared by other authors (Kutchins & Kirk, 1997). This was a controversial position given the popularity and wide acceptance of "the DSM way of thinking." From a positive approach, definitions of health or illness based simply upon the presence or absence of symptoms are inadequate to fully capture the subtleties and complexities of psychology and development, thus becoming circular.

For instance, depression is defined by a lack of motivation; a lack of motivation is a symptom of depression. While the positive approach to diagnosis is more challenging for the therapist, it also provides great flexibility, subtlety, and discretion that "checklist psychiatry" removes.

An important antecedent to Dąbrowski's approach to pathology was presented by William James (1842-1910). Eugene Taylor (1984) published James's 1896 Lowell lectures. In the first lecture, James indicated that normal and abnormal mental states exist on a continuum lacking a sharp distinction:

> No one symptom by itself is a morbid one—it depends rather on the part it plays. We speak of melancholy and moral tendencies, but he would be a bold man who should say that melancholy was not an essential part of every character (E. Taylor, 1984, p. 15).

James (1902/1929) explained:

> The normal process of life contains moments as bad as any of those which insane melancholy is filled with, moments in which radical evil gets its innings and takes its solid turn. The lunatic's visions of horror are all drawn from the material of daily fact. Our civilization is founded on the shambles and every individual existence goes out in a lonely spasm of helpless agony. If you protest, my friend, wait till you arrive there yourself! (p. 160)

James subsequently extended the potential for benefits from melancholy to include delusions and hallucinations. In *The Varieties of Religious Experience*, James (1902/1929) emphasized that experiences described in pathological terms might actually lead to "some valued fruits" (Rubin, 2000, p. 215). Rubin continued:

> To James, people confront events daily that create feelings of helplessness, pain, sadness, horror and dread. "Here on our very hearths and in our gardens the infernal cat plays with the panting mouse, or holds the hot bird fluttering in her jaws" (James, 1902/1961, p. 141). James argued that the feelings that

go along with these normal events could lead toward truth. Thus, he counteracts any tendency to assume that those referred to as morbid minded are automatically inferior to those referred to as "mentally healthy." (p. 216)

Echoing James, Dąbrowski (1964b) pointed out that symptoms must be seen in the context of the situation—and the level—at which they appear. For example, depression will be qualitatively different and carry different meanings and implications depending upon the developmental level of the individual. A depression appearing at the lowest level is fundamentally different, and must be seen and managed differently, from a depression occurring at a higher level of development. Thus, when looking at a symptom, it first becomes critical to examine the symptom within the overall context of the individual's level of development.

Second, symptoms must be seen and understood in the context of the history and potentialities of the individual. Reviewing a symptom in context is a critical step to determine the meaning of the symptom and its anticipated impact, and to inform a therapeutic approach. In particular, a judgment must be made as to whether or not a symptom is associated with a developmental transition or crisis and if it is occurring within a general developmental context. For instance, a feature such as anxiety may be considered positive in an individual who has a history of crises having been resolved in personality growth, especially if the individual also exhibits strong potential for future development. This is contrasted by a negative interpretation of the same anxiety in an individual who displays little or no potential for development and who has not demonstrated developmental transitions in the past. This method allowed Dąbrowski to differentiate symptoms into positive and negative forms depending upon their context, again, in historical perspective as well as in relation to the individual's current situation (and current level) and his or her potentialities.

One of the foundations of Dąbrowski's approach is the idea that development must involve the disintegration of earlier forms of psychological integration. Thus, the role played by positive disintegrations in development and the differentiation of negative forms of disintegration that are associated with pathology becomes extremely critical. Dąbrowski's positive construct of mental health is compatible with his observation that certain anxieties, depressions, and disintegrations appear to be cardinal features of healthy development. Dąbrowski and Joshi (1972) linked mental health with the sensitivity to suffering, depression, anxiety, obsessive elements, elements of nervousness (overexcitability), and psychoneurosis which all contribute to the loosening and breaking of primitive human structures. Mental health thus becomes "the capacity for positive disintegration and secondary integration through transgression of the biological life cycle and of one's own psychological type" (Dąbrowski & Joshi, 1972, p. 101).

In summary, the appearance of certain symptoms associated with the potential for development and the process of development become critical features defining mental health in the overall context of the potential for individual growth. As Aronson (1964) observed, "the strength of the theory of positive disintegration is in its integration of psychopathology with personality development" (p. xxviii).

Aronson also went on to point out regarding the theory that "Its weakness is in the looseness in definition of its constructs," an observation we will return to later.

1–2. ADJUSTMENT

If we endorse Dąbrowski's approach to mental health, it becomes obvious that traditional views of adjustment based upon social conformity take on a new and negative interpretation. In addition, as we have seen above, a central theme in Dąbrowski's thinking is that development must reflect a striving for individual goals and ideals and not simply involve acceptance of, nor adjustment to, an external status quo. Thus, development necessarily involves a significant degree of nonconformity and maladjustment.

Dąbrowski used the construct of adjustment in at least three unique ways.

First, he expanded the usage and definitions associated with the term adjustment to include *negative adjustment* and *positive maladjustment.*

Second, he linked the definition of adjustment to hierarchies of values and aims, both in individuals and in groups. Our unique value structures provide criteria by which adjustment and maladjustment can be judged. This creates a developmental evolution or hierarchy of adjustment coinciding with the hierarchy of values.

- At the lowest level, negative maladjustment is an unproductive rebellion from social norms.
- At the next level is the most common type of adjustment— negative adjustment. This is adjustment to what is, the status quo of society.
- The first signs of development are indicated by positive maladjustment to what is.
- This culminates in the highest level, a positive, developmental adjustment to what ought to be.

Adjustment can be used to indicate the relevant level of development, from the indiscriminate and unreflective adjustment to the patterns prevalent in the social environment, to a more considered adjustment to consciously selected values reflecting one's unique personality ideal. Likewise, maladjustment also reflects a developmental continuum, from the pathological and criminal violation of social standards seen in negative maladjustment to the height of rebellion characterizing positive maladjustment, as is seen in the early stages of positive disintegration. For example, thousands of individual Germans publicly opposed Hitler and rejected Nazism (and many were later identified and executed) (Hoffmann, 1996). A more contemporary example would be a student who resists peer pressure to take drugs or participate in bullying.

Third, Dąbrowski conceived of positive maladjustment as a uniquely developmental phenomenon—both a symptom representing potential development and a driving force of development. Positive maladjustment generates conflicts that fuel early disintegrations.

1–2–1. The importance of adjustment and maladjustment

In summary, Dąbrowski emphasized the critical importance of maladjustment by differentiating adjustment into four prototypes: two types of maladjustment and two types of adjustment, as elaborated below.

1–2–1–1. Negative maladjustment

Refers to the traditional constructs of antisocial or criminal behavior. Dąbrowski (1972b) defined negative maladjustment as:

> what we traditionally think of as anti-social or criminal behavior: Rejection of social norms and accepted patterns of behavior because of the controlling power of primitive drives and non-developmental or pathologically deformed structures and functions. In the extreme case, it takes the form of psychosis, psychopathy, or criminal activity. (p. 299)

1–2–1–2. Negative adjustment

Characterized by unthinking, robotic acceptance, and conformity to external values—adjustment to "what is" (traditional socialization). Negative adjustment, or non-developmental adjustment, is the "unqualified conformity to a hierarchy of values prevailing in a person's social environment" (Dąbrowski, 1972b, p. 299). Dąbrowski's concern was that values are accepted without independent or critical evaluation: "It is an acceptance of an external system of values without autonomous choice. An adjustment to 'what is'" (Dąbrowski, 1972b, p. 299). Dąbrowski explained his position on the traditional role of unqualified adjustment as a symptom of health (Dąbrowski, 1970c):

> Adjustment that is a symptom of mental health is, largely speaking, adjustment to what ought to be and not to what is. As no culture is perfect and incapable of further growth and as development results from lack of adjustment rather than from an all-too-perfect adjustment, the idea of simple, unqualified social adjustment as a symptom, or even criterion, of mental health is due to a fundamental error. (p. 11)

Putney and Putney (1964) presented a similar view of negative adjustment when they discussed social conformity and made the point that in a given society, without realizing it, the average person conforms to the unquestioned assumptions of his or her culture. These taken-for-granted assumptions limit an individual's thoughts, actions, and imagination. To overcome this limitation, an individual must become conscious of a given taken-for-granted belief, usually as the result of encountering an opposing or challenging belief. Putney and Putney developed the argument that in America, neurosis is a normal result of social conformity and therefore goes unrecognized—a neurosis is produced by blindly conforming and taking social behaviors for granted, thwarting the genuine satisfaction of an individual's needs. Unrelieved tension is created; the individual does not recognize his or her true motivations and the needs that must be met in order to create satisfaction. The authors concluded that when a countervailing belief is encountered, the aware individual could develop alternative understandings of the world and enlarge his or her repertoire of means to achieve satisfaction. In this way, self-awareness may allow an individual to overcome conformity and to achieve autonomy.

Dąbrowski was unequivocal about the negative connotation of incorporating social values, saying: "It is one of the basic assumptions of the theory of positive disintegration that valuation when it expresses only the point of view of a culture, is unauthentic and unobjective" (Dąbrowski, 1970c, p. 11).

In a contrary view, Viscott (1996) said that to be happy, the individual must accept his or her "as is" self:

In order to live fully, you have to give up your false expectations and accept yourself and the world just as it is. You have to let go of your suffering to see the world clearly. The world makes perfect sense exactly the way it is. When the truth can be told, everything can be understood. What might have been is of no concern to you, it is merely an energy draining diversion that weakens your will. (p. 68)

1–2–1–3. Positive maladjustment

Rejection of external values or mores when in conflict with values representing an individual's hierarchy of values—active rejection of "what is." The construct of positive maladjustment is not new; for example, Robert Lindner (1914-1956) promoted the idea that maturity must be defined by positive rebellion, and the mature person is the positive rebel. In his essay, "Education for Maturity," Lindner (1956) emphasized six key characteristics associated with maturity:

- Developing awareness, especially as it is related to controlling one's own life.
- Developing a unique identity—a deep, integrated sense of individuality.
- Skepticism, a healthy rejection of accepting anything on the basis of faith or conformity and a corresponding inquisitiveness to examine issues independently.
- Personal and social responsibility.
- Employment—as used by Lindner—engaging life with a total commitment to expressing one's personality to the fullest.
- A tension or uneasiness over one's perception of things as they are. (pp. 183-210)

In defining positive maladjustment, Dąbrowski described how an individual's developing sense of internal values and ideals usually comes into conflict with the external world as it is. As one of Dąbrowski's former students, Marlene Rankel (1936-2017) emphasized: "If you can watch the evening news and sleep at night, then there is something wrong with you" (personal communication, 2000). Individuals with strong developmental potential may react to the evening news with strong internal conflict: "Why does it have to be this way?" As the conflicts with one's social environment become more focused, one begins to consciously examine and reject the attitudes and standards that one finds incompatible. The individual's growing sense of autonomous values and personality ideal becomes the basis for this judgment. These conflicts eventually also spill over into a person's internal environment, and positive maladjustment to one's "old" values and habits is a common feature observed in ongoing development. Dąbrowski (1970b) explained:

> positive maladjustment [is] maladjustment to "that which is" and adjustment to "what ought to be;" maladjustment to that which is "less myself" and adjustment to that which is "more myself," maladjustment to that which is negative, nondevelopmental in other people and adjustment to that which is hierarchically higher in them. (pp. 58-59)

Positive maladjustment is a vital process in the development of individuals as well as in social and cultural development. Dąbrowski went so far as to suggest that positive maladjustment creates the foundation of all forms of creative and positive development and is therefore the single most important criteria characterizing the initial stages of development.

This view of positive maladjustment was largely out of sync with American psychology. For example, in describing the forces shaping psychology in the United States after World War II, Herman (1995) noted: "Because adjustment seemed to have such positive civic, as well as personal, overtones, maladjustment was considered a national hazard" (p. 239).

1–2–1–4. Positive adjustment

Conformity to an individually developed and chosen hierarchy of values and ideals—adjustment to "what ought to be." Positive adjustment or developmental adjustment is "conformity to higher levels of a hierarchy of values, self-discovered and consciously followed" (Dąbrowski, 1972b, p. 301). It is an acceptance of a value only after a deliberate, critical examination and an autonomous choice to endorse the value. It is an adjustment to "what ought to be" that emerges from an individual's sense of self, from the sense of who he or she ought to be and how this self ought to interact with the world— the personality ideal. Dąbrowski placed values at the center of personality and linked the criteria of adjustment to the development of an individual hierarchy of values and, in turn, a hierarchy of aims— standards of conduct for development in individuals and in groups. The values that reflect the unique character of the person will constitute his or her criteria of adjustment and maladjustment.

1–2–2. From "what is" to "what ought to be"

In summary, as development proceeds, adjustment changes in character and complexity, from the uncritical negative adjustment to "what is" to a positive adjustment to "what ought to be." This shift involves the intermediary step of positive maladjustment to what is and highlights the inherent crisis associated with the process of adjustment in development. Thus, adjustment reflects one's level of development, from a widespread, indiscriminate adjustment to the social environment through to a deep need to be in adjustment with one's hierarchy of values and personality ideal. Similarly, maladjustment also differentiates lower from higher developmental levels, starting from pathological, psychopathic, and criminal violation of social standards seen in negative maladjustment to positive maladjustments, observable in all mentally developing individuals. From Dąbrowski's perspective, even intense positive maladjustment reflects an awareness of the higher levels of reality and illustrates their impact (Dąbrowski, 1973).

When combined with Dąbrowski's approach to mental health, this reformulation of adjustment becomes a powerful new tool. It is largely this reformulation that allows Dąbrowski to reframe developmental crises and give them a whole new significance in the developmental process. These crises and maladjustments can now be interpreted positively and seen (even encouraged) as a necessary catalyst to development. The further articulation of a new approach to assessment and diagnosis along with a new autopsychotherapeutic methodology provides us with a major new approach to understanding and fostering individual personality development.

1–3. DEVELOPMENT

Traditional approaches to development emphasize ontogeny, usually conceived of as the process of growth and development of an individual organism based upon the biological unfolding of a stepwise series of stages from conception through maturation that gradually lead from simple to more complex levels and forms.[4] For example, in developmental biology many stages are recognized, named, and described between conception and final maturation, including the zygote, morula, blastocyst, embryo, and so forth. The assumption is that in the normal course, development will follow these stages, usually defined in a time-specific manner.

In describing development, Dąbrowski (1970b) distinguished two qualitatively different types of mental life: "the heteronomous, determined by biological or environmental factors and the autonomous, self-conscious, self-determined, and self-controlled" (p. 11). The former type falls within conventional ontogenetic development; however, the latter type involves a more complicated evolutionary process of development. Dąbrowski (1970b) emphasized that advanced development involved a new force of self-determination and autonomy that transcends the normal ontogenetic sequence: "A new quality arises. Things cease to remain under exclusive control of biological and social determinants. Self-conscious, autonomous choice between alternatives becomes real" (p. 12).

The following points from Dąbrowski deserve emphasis:

- Mental development, that is the transition from less refined to more refined functions, is a result of the processes of disintegration.
- There are two, qualitatively different phases of mental development:
  o The lower or heteronomous which is unconscious or only partly conscious and is determined by biological forces or the influences of the external environment.
  o The higher or autonomous, which is self-conscious, self-controlled and depends increasingly on deliberate and authentic acts of choice, that is, acts resulting from increasing and refined understanding of the environment and of oneself.
- The direction and substance of autonomous development can be ascertained:
  o As a continuation of the trends observable at lower stages (e.g., trends towards an increase in consciousness and self-determination, in control over oneself and the environment, in conjunction and codetermination of intellectual and empathic insights and emotional involvement, etc.).
  o As a growth of those qualities which are beneficial for further development. (Dąbrowski, 1970b, pp. 5-6)

Dąbrowski (1996) further differentiated three types of development, again reflecting both ontogenetic and evolutionary processes.

- **Normal development** referred to the most common form and involved the least amount of conflict or psychological transformation. It entails no, or quite limited, developmental potential and overexcitability. This type of development occurs within the framework of the normal (ontogenetic) biological human life cycle (Dąbrowski, 1972b).

- **One-sided development** referred to the situation where an individual has one or two strong individual talents or abilities but lacks global development. These cases do not display advanced integrated personality development and fall within ontogenetic development. Dąbrowski (1996) defined one-sided development:

  > Individuals endowed with special talents but lacking multilevel developmental potential realize their development mainly as a function of their ability and creativity. Such creativity, however, lacks universal components. Only some emotional and intellectual potentials develop very well while the rest remains undeveloped, in fact, it appears lacking. (p. 21)

- **Accelerated** (or **universal**) **development** is the third type of development Dąbrowski described. This type of development is characterized by the strong and relatively equal intensity of forms of developmental potential, overexcitability, and the cognitive and emotional functions. In such cases, development proceeds in a uniform and global fashion. This evolutionary type of development occurs within a framework of the "suprabiological" cycle, with transcendence of the normal biological life cycle (Dąbrowski, 1972b).

Dąbrowski's evolutionary approach to development was partly based on the theory of the nervous system presented by John Hughlings Jackson (1835-1911). In Hughlings Jackson's model, as structures in the nervous system evolve, an increasingly complex coordination occurs that unifies new structures: "As the organism evolves to a higher stage of function, it is not as if something new would be tacked on, which provides new representations. Rather, there is a re-representation" (Meares, 1999, p. 1851). At each higher stage, the "new" structure creates a coordination of earlier structures, with the latest, the cerebral cortex, representing a universal coordination of the brain as a whole. In addition to sophisticated coordination, Hughlings Jackson also said that the development of the self was dependent upon the evolution of new structures, namely the prefrontal cortex. In particular, the prefrontal cortex allowed for a high level of voluntary control over lower and more automatic structures, a fundamental characteristic of higher developmental levels.

This high degree of voluntary control was also linked to a high degree of individual consciousness. The strength of these conscious and volitional elements allowed for transcendence of the normal ontogenetic sequence of development, resulting in developmental achievements not normally seen in the regular course of ontogenetic development. Dąbrowski (1967) said:

> There are people, not few in number, in whom, besides the schematically described cycle of life, there arises a sort of a "side track" which after some time may become the "main track." The various sets of tendencies tear away from the common biological cycle of life. (p. 49)

In these people, the basic drives tend to be transformed or sublimated into higher and more creative forces. For example, the sexual drive is sublimated into lasting emotional bonds with others. The instinct to fight becomes "an attitude of fighting for a good cause and . . . an attitude of sacrifice and love" (Dąbrowski, 1967, p. 49). The transformation of basic instincts in non-ontogenetic development has two impacts. First, the integration of the basic forces and instincts loosens and begins to disintegrate. Second, the developmental instinct rises to the fore and becomes a meta-director of development. The developmental instinct transcends biological influences and opposes biological limitations. As we will subsequently discuss in more detail, this disintegration of primary instincts sets in motion a more widespread disintegration of psychological structures, creating opportunities for subsequent personality shaping and advanced development.

Dąbrowski (1964b) took the further step of suggesting that

development is a function of the level of organization and is not strictly limited to the characteristics and features of the structures that are present. For example, when considering emotional development, we see a "nonontogenetic evolutionary pattern of individual growth" (Dąbrowski, 1996, p. 9). As Dąbrowski (1996) explained: "The *level* of emotional functioning is not produced automatically in the course of ontogenesis but evolves as a function of other conditions" (p. 9).

This sets the stage for several major ideas, including the following:

- An understanding of development must incorporate the impact of factors such as the level of integration present and cannot be solely based upon an analysis of the developmental structures that are present. Much of the theory of positive disintegration is focused upon elaborating these conditions, including the role of instincts in development and those features described by Dąbrowski as developmental potential.

- A key feature of higher growth is the integration of functions, creating a unification of the self. Initially, this integration reflects an early stage of growth characterized by egocentrism, a focus upon achieving one's needs and self-satisfaction, and by a largely unconscious inculcation of the roles, norms, and expectations of society. While this initial integration creates a viable and functional organism, it also impairs any significant and qualitatively different development. At higher levels, integration is characterized by a harmonious expression of the individual's unique perception and formulation of his or her values (emotions) that, in turn, encapsulate the idealization of his or her personality and character.

- Advanced development is largely spawned and governed by the developmental instinct—an instinct reflecting the evolution of our human future. A strong developmental instinct creates the conflicts necessary to precipitate advanced growth. Individuals who do not possess this strong impulse to develop follow the normal course of ontogenetic development and live out their lives at the initial, socially based level of integration.

- Disintegration is a critical mechanism allowing for the reconfiguration of integrating factors. Disintegration creates an opportunity for an individual to become conscious and aware of some aspect of his or her personality. This awareness, combined with the loosening of integration, creates the possibility for the individual to volitionally intervene and consciously rearrange, inhibit, reprioritize or make other changes as required in order to direct his or her development. One uses the benchmark of one's formulation of one's ideal self—the personality ideal. This development can surpass the normal, ontogenetically controlled stages of growth commonly seen in individuals who remain integrated at the first level.

- A critical aspect of higher development is the transformation and transcendence of lower instincts and impulses. What makes us human is our ability to become conscious of, and therefore inhibit, the lower instincts and impulses associated with our animal ancestry. Human behavior becomes a reflection of an organism directed by moral values; lower instincts such as aggression are transformed and sublimated to be reapplied in the quest to achieve a harmony with this new, individualized moral value structure. These new values represent authentically human qualities and characteristics that stand in stark contrast with our animal ancestors.

- Successive integrations and disintegrations, re-evaluations, and changes in the structure of personality lead to new and different unifications, co-ordinations and integrations which eventually reflect qualitatively different and higher levels of function.[5]

- Advanced development depends upon and reflects the conscious and volitional intervention and action of the individual.

- The traditional ontogeny of the lifecycle can be transgressed by "additional factors" such as the impact of autonomous factors, new values, revised goals, and aims; new interests and the inhibition of previous instincts; interests and behaviors; and by the individual.

Dąbrowski was optimistic that his observations reflected a new era in human evolution, portending factors reflecting and predisposing the authentic development of advanced personality.

Aronson (1964) summarized Dąbrowski's approach to development:

> Dąbrowski postulates a developmental instinct: that is, a tendency of man to evolve from lower to higher levels of personality. He regards personality as primarily developing through dissatisfaction with and fragmentation of, the existing psychic structure—a period of disintegration—and finally a secondary integration at a higher level. Dąbrowski feels that no growth takes place without previous disintegration. He regards symptoms of anxiety, psychoneurosis and even some symptoms of psychosis as the signs of the disintegration stage of this evolution and therefore not always pathological. (p. xiv)

Dąbrowski's framework recognized an interaction between the individual's characteristics and, in particular, his or her developmental potential and the environment. This interaction ideally creates optimal levels of anxiety, crises and psychoneuroses—levels intense enough to produce development but not so strong as to overwhelm the individual. Dąbrowski believed that psychology would eventually elaborate on and confirm the positive roles played by these so-called negative symptoms and would eventually include them in an approach to positive mental health. For example, research suggests that anxiety plays an important role in life and that an optimal level of anxiety is desired (Samanez-Larkin, Hollon, Carstensen, & Knutson, 2008). Dąbrowski (1967) presented a succinct summary:

> The author's basic thesis can be stated as follows: Personality development, especially accelerated development, cannot be realized without manifest nervousness and psychoneurosis. It is in this way that such experiences as inner conflict, sadness, anxiety, obsession, depression and psychic tension all cooperate in the promotion of humanistic development. Those especially trying moments of life are indispensable for the shaping of personality. An effort to overcome and transform

psychoneurotic dynamisms reveals the action of self-directing and self-determining dynamisms that make autopsychotherapy possible and successful. (p. vi)

Dąbrowski's unique description of development was presented in a complicated theoretical model reflecting the reality of individual personality development as he observed it. Given Dąbrowski's objectivity and humbleness, he did not simply assume that his observations and subsequent model were correct; rather, he invited the scientific investigation and operationalization of his theory. Advances in our understanding of genetics have challenged the standard model and have necessitated an expanded understanding of development and reproduction, accounting for epigenetic factors influencing development. As our understanding of psychology and development continues to advance, Dąbrowski's "non-ontogenetic, evolutionary approach" will, no-doubt, be further researched, documented and refined. In my opinion, Dąbrowski's theory represents the most sophisticated and satisfying developmental explanation existing in psychology to date.

1–4. PERSONALITY

In both everyday usage and in psychology, the construct of personality is taken to mean some sort of attribute or collection of traits about an individual. It is taken for granted that each of us has a personality. However, Dąbrowski's usage of the construct of personality was unique, and as he defined it, personality was not a universal attribute: "The development of the personality occurs through a disruption of the existing, initially integrated structure, a period of disintegration and finally a renewed, or secondary, integration" (Dąbrowski, 1964b, p. 2). Personality is the "final outcome of painstaking experiences of self-education and autopsychotherapy. It is, at the same time, the highest form of organization of mental functions that can be achieved by man" (Dąbrowski, 1973, p. 108). Rather than viewing personality as an initial given, Dąbrowski reserved the term for individuals who attain advanced levels of autonomy as expressed through authentism and self-determination.

Dąbrowski (1972b) defined personality as: "A self-aware, self-chosen, self-affirmed and self-determined unity of essential individual psychic qualities. Personality as defined here appears at the level of secondary-integration" (p. 301). Dąbrowski (1973) suggested that personality is the aim and outcome of development and is the product of a long and painful process of self-creation, self-education, and autopsychotherapy: "Man becomes more truly himself having passed through a variety of painful experiences, having exercised his own will and having made his own choices" (Dąbrowski, 1970b, p. 78). In this developmental process, Dąbrowski (1973) emphasized the creation of one's inner psychic milieu (environment), including features like a unique sense of self, elaboration of one's values, taking the perspective of the other, and self-control. As these psychological features strengthen and work together, one's energies focus on expression of one's identity and purpose in life. This identity is reflected by the conscious choices one makes, especially in arriving at one's values—a major component in the creation of the ideal personality that eventually forms to uniquely reflect an individual. In turn, this personality ideal shapes and forms the development of one's values.

As we will see, the personality ideal is derived from a combination of one's initial essence—the genetic underpinnings of one's character—and the conscious, volitional day-to-day choices one makes in life.

1–4–1. Personality versus individuality

Dąbrowski differentiated personality from *individuality*. Individuality represents the raw essence, both positive and negative, that makes one unique. On the other hand, through a process of self-awareness and self-choice, one creates personality by the unique shaping, refinement, and idealization of one's essence, in the process inhibiting negative aspects and enhancing positive elements.

In Dąbrowski's approach, the process of development breaks the stereotypic and "routine-ridden" self, allowing for the creation and later implementation of the personality ideal. This is not accomplished until secondary integration and therefore, in Dąbrowski's approach, the term personality was not applied to individuals at prior levels of development. Dąbrowski did not provide an alternative term in his writings, although in conversation he would refer to "group personality" or "herd personality" to emphasize that individuals at the primary stage of development derive their personality identity from identification with their social group.

1–4–2. The achievement of personality

Dąbrowski also linked his definition of mental health to the progress toward the development of the personality: "Mental health is the progressive psychic development of the personality; therefore, progressive psychic development is the movement toward higher and higher levels of personality functions in the direction of the personality ideal" (Dąbrowski, 1964b, p. 112). Dąbrowski felt that his view of personality captured "the two crucial aspects of fundamental human tendencies: the preservation of identity, uniqueness and unrepeatability, on the one hand and the requirement of continuous, incessant development, on the other hand" (Dąbrowski, 1973, p. 112). For Dąbrowski, the process of personality creation is never complete; the individual must pay lifelong attention to the aspects of self-awareness, authenticity, self-education and self-perfection.

Dąbrowski (1967) described achieving personality as a turning point in life:

We have repeatedly emphasized that the "birth" of personality—by which we mean a decisive turning point in one's life—is a drastic experience for an individual. He senses the advent of something "other" in himself, he feels that the hierarchy of values thus far accepted by him undergoes changes and that he is becoming much more sensitive to certain values and less to others. In this period, the individual changes fundamentally and at the same time there comes to power within him a new or a higher type of driving elements, a new system of internal environment arises and he becomes more selective in his attitude toward external contacts. (p. 45)

Dąbrowski was not alone in subscribing to the idea that an individual can generate substantial and authentic changes to his or her personality. For example, DeGrazia (2000) emphasized the aspects of self-creation and "self-shaping" in the process of consciously making changes to one's personality. In a philosophical discussion, Roskies (2012) said that one can utilize self-reflective decision-making, deliberation and choice to purposefully intervene to determine and alter future states of one's self. Roskies (2012) concluded:

> What it is to be self-caused is to use one's own mental states as control variables to affect one's future mental and physical states and to intentionally take steps now to affect one's future self. Self-causation is thus less metaphysically demanding than has been previously noted. In brief, to be a *causa sui* [cause of itself], in any sense that we need it, is to be a self-conscious or deliberate shaper of one's character through time. (p. 339)

The achievement of personality reflects a qualitative developmental advance. This advance is not merely a quantifiable increase in some attribute or another—it represents a qualitatively new view of the world. Once the basic tenets of personality have been "selected," further qualitative changes do not occur; rather, growth becomes quantitative and additive. As Dąbrowski (1973) said:

> We may define personality as an individual, unique, unrepeatable unity of basic mental qualities. Those qualities that were chosen at the time of the "birth of personality" and later, authentically developed as central and most important, do not undergo qualitative changes. They will grow quantitatively and may be supplemented by new qualities. (p. 109)

Dąbrowski made his requirements for personality explicit:

1. Personality is a self-conscious, self-chosen, empirically elaborated, autonomous, authentic, self-confirmed and self-educating unity of basic mental, individual and common qualities. Those qualities undergo quantitative and qualitative changes with the preservation of central elements.
2. Personality is a secondarily integrated set of basic

mental qualities of an individual that undergoes quantitative and qualitative changes with the preservation of central lasting qualities.

3. Personality is the unity of integrated mental qualities of man; that is to say, personality is the final and highest effect of the process of positive disintegration, empirically and intuitively elaborated. (Dąbrowski, 1973, p. 111)

Dąbrowski's theory requires that at least some individuals demonstrate considerable change throughout their lives. The amount personality can change in an individual's lifetime has been the subject of considerable theoretical debate and research in psychology (e.g., Harris, Brett, Johnson, & Deary, 2016; Heatherton & Nichols, 1994; Heatherton & Weinberger, 1994; Srivastava, Oliver, Gosling, & Potter, 2003; Tickle, Heatherton, & Wittenberg, 2001; Worchel & Byrne, 1964). The general issue of personality change is an interesting and complicated one that appears to call for more research (Caspi, Roberts, & Shiner, 2005). Srivastava et al. (2003) noted that approaches to personality change commonly fall into two categories.

The first category represents biologically-based approaches that generally see the traits of personality as genetic attributes that develop according to a developmental stage process model and that are essentially in place and unmodifiable after about the age of 30. This viewpoint was first expressed by William James, who said: "It is well for the world that in most of us, by the age of thirty, the character has set like plaster and will never soften again" (James, 1890/1950, p. 121). Clark (2007) suggested that a modification of this position was called for, saying: "It isn't until past the age of 50 that character may set like plaster; before then, it's more like being set in clay—change can occur, but gradually and with effort" (p. 242). An example of a contemporary personality theory espousing the biological approach is Eysenck's (1996) three-factor model.

The other common contemporary approach to personality change is the contextual/social trait view which suggests that traits are multifactorial and are influenced by ongoing exposure to the social environment, and therefore ongoing, lifelong personality change is expected (Haan, Millsap, & Hartka, 1986). In support of this view,

Roberts et al. (2017) found that personality traits show major changes across the life course and also meaningful changes in response to experiences, including therapeutic interventions.

In conversation, Dąbrowski commented upon the anecdotal observation that it is common for people to meet friends from childhood after many years and comment, "You haven't changed a bit." On the other hand, every so often, we meet an old friend who seems quite different than we remember. Dąbrowski encompassed views from both theoretical models: He endorsed biological and genetic aspects as the underpinnings of personality but also emphasized the vital importance of the individual's role in making day-to-day choices that create ongoing opportunities to shape and change one's personality throughout the course of one's life.

1–5. A SYNOPSIS OF DĄBROWSKI'S APPROACH

As this book unfolds, Dąbrowski's constructs will be elaborated in detail. For now, here is a synopsis of the main points of Dąbrowski's theory, many of which make his approach unique:

- Five levels of function account for the broad spectrum of human behavior observed.
- Definitions of mental health based upon quantifications of adjustment to social norms are rejected; to be adjusted to a sick society is to also be sick.[6]
- The absence of symptoms alone is not enough to define mental health. Positive mental health is defined by the presence of desirable and developmental traits.
- The average person exhibits socialized behavior (Level I) emphasizing the acceptance of externalized values and roles (social norms) with little conscious evaluation. The adoption of social roles and mores provides a sense of internal harmony; however, these same forces discourage the development of an individualized and autonomous personality.
- The average socialized person is largely unconscious or semiconscious of his or her unique self and potentialities.
- Developmental potential describes a constellation of genetic

features that promote opportunities for disintegration of lower levels and that spur advanced growth. Developmental potential varies among the population and is not a universal feature.

- A critical role is given to "nervousness," an aspect of developmental potential that Dąbrowski referred to as overexcitability—the observation that some people display a heightened response to stimuli and a lowered threshold to stimuli. This heightened reactivity contributes to positive disintegration and to the development of multilevelness.
- The theory assigns a prominent developmental role to the genetic instinct or drive to develop and express one's unique self-autonomy (the third factor).
- Development is based upon the disintegration and replacement of lower levels and the creation of new levels based upon autonomous values and ideals. Lower levels do not form the foundation of, nor are they largely incorporated into, higher levels.
- Crisis, internal conflicts, anxiety, and depressions (psychoneurosis) are necessary features of the developmental process. "Symptoms" must be considered from a developmental perspective; when occurring in a developmental context, symptoms traditionally linked to psychopathology are seen as vital components of personality development.
- Three levels describe a process of disintegration and psychoneuroses involving crises, anxieties, self-doubts and depressions that drive the process of self-examination and that set the stage for self-improvement.
- A qualitative shift in one's perception of reality characterizes the second, higher phase of development and integration. This shift—multilevelness—involves comparisons of lower realities versus higher possibilities. When higher possibilities are perceived but lower ones are acted upon, vertical conflicts arise.
- Advanced development (Level V, secondary integration) is characterized by a return to harmony based on the realization

and implementation of internalized values reflecting an individual's unique personality ideal.

- Character emerges from one's essence (genetics) but is shaped by conscious and volitional existential choices to create an autonomous personality.
- Emotion plays a critical role in developing one's individual hierarchy of values; emotions guide one's reactions and direct one's cognitive endeavors.
- The theory promotes a balanced approach to development; strong intellectual development must be guided and controlled by a corresponding level of emotional development, awareness and sensitivity.
- An internalized and organized approach to development is emphasized. One's inner psychic milieu becomes the locus and engine of development.
- Dąbrowski reserves the term *personality*, defining it as the highest level of development: The conscious, self-determined, and self-created idealized self at the center of advanced development.
- Human authenticity reflects individual awareness, qualities, personality and internally chosen values, not adopted social influences and mores nor rote social conformity.
- The focus of valuation/behavioral choices shifts from rote, external, environmental influences to fully conscious, volitional choices based upon individualized criteria (a unique hierarchy of values and one's personality ideal).
- Four types of human adjustment are differentiated, including a positive form of maladjustment; to be maladjusted to a sick society is generally a positive feature.
- A more subtle and refined approach to diagnosis and treatment is presented.
- The theory advances a system of psychotherapy emphasizing the client's role as self-educator (synomous terms: education-of-oneself, self-education) and acting as his or her own therapist (autopsychotherapy).
- Internal harmony and peace of mind characterize the lowest

level (follow the rules, don't think outside the box and you'll be happy), and the highest levels of development (following one's heart and values creates inner harmony). Maximum internal conflict (positive disintegration) characterizes the active process of development—dis-ease spurs growth, not homeostasis.

- The theory utilizes many passé terms and uniquely defines a number of constructs; Dąbrowski's two main books contained glossaries (Dąbrowski, 1970b, 1972b), and another book was devoted to describing constructs (Dąbrowski, 1973).

1–6. WHAT DĄBROWSKI SHARES IN COMMON WITH OTHER APPROACHES TO DEVELOPMENT

Dąbrowski's theory also shares specific characteristics with other scientific approaches to development. Namely, it:

- Is based upon a sound foundation and incorporates a number of well-established ideas and approaches from traditional neurology, psychiatry, psychology, and philosophy.
- Reflects most other developmental approaches in utilizing a hierarchical, level-based model of human development.
- Incorporates traditional cognitive approaches to psychology, but in contrast with most approaches, Dąbrowski advocates placing cognition in the service of one's emotions.
- Concurs with the majority viewpoint that advanced development is rare within the general population.
- Recognizes a strong role for environmental influences when genetic factors are equivocal.

1-7. CHAPTER SUMMARY

By embracing a positive definition of mental health and by reconceptualizing adjustment, Dąbrowski sets the stage for a radical new approach to development. As we will see, this approach allowed Dąbrowski to elaborate the key characteristics of advanced human development and create the foundation for his description of positive disintegration, the critical process at the heart of development. Dąbrowski utilized various traditional constructs but integrated them into a unique new approach to development. He also introduced several important new constructs, such as multilevelness, developmental potential (including the important ideas encapsulated by overexcitability and third factor), positive disintegration as the key process of development, and the role played by psychoneuroses in development. Dąbrowski also included a unique formulation of the authentic and autonomous personality. Dąbrowski described traditional ontogenetic development as occurring in a quantifiable, stepwise manner. He also described evolutionary development as characterized by qualitative advances leading to advanced levels of function.

MULTILEVELNESS, MULTIDIMENSIONALITY AND DĄBROWSKI'S FIVE LEVELS

2–1. MULTILEVELNESS

The basic differentiation between the lower, unilevel experiences of life, versus the higher experience of multilevelness, is fundamental to Dąbrowski's approach. Dąbrowski said that he felt his revival of a multilevel approach based upon the schema presented by Plato (circa 428-347 BC), as we will elaborate in Chapter Six, was one of his most important accomplishments (K. Dąbrowski, personal communication, ca. 1978). A multilevel approach is used to describe all phenomena and a multilevel description forms a critical element of our understanding of reality: "We call it multilevel because there is an observable hierarchy of mental functions" (Dąbrowski, 1972b, p. 39). This framework views levels of reality as objective entities that can be studied empirically, developing scientific, objective descriptions that allow us to differentiate and understand lower versus higher levels. Dąbrowski's application of multilevelness to psychology was based upon his observations that development involves changes in the qualitative character and expression of psychological functions and this allows us to see differences among the distinct levels of functions. Applying this multilevel approach to psychology, Dąbrowski was able to account for the range of human experience, from the lowest, most instinctual and primitive behaviors to the highest achievements of humankind.

Dąbrowski (1973) explained:

By multilevelness of reality we mean external and internal reality of various levels conceived by means of sensory perception, imagination, intellectual, intuitive or combined operations. Perception of the various levels of reality depends on the kind and level of receptors and transformers of an individual. Its objective discussion and description is grounded on empirical and discursive methods. (p. 5)

The traditional Western approach to development is based upon the idea that higher levels are characterized by increasing cognitive control of impulses, instincts, and emotions by seamless socialization. We learn to control our lower impulses (including our emotions) by incorporating social prescriptions and intellectual rationalizations (the "thou shalt" of Nietzsche and, later, Freud) in order to conform socially. This control and conformity represents the herd or tribal mentality and is a vital component of social order. It is informative to consider Freud's (1923/1984) model. Although it is somewhat cliché today, there is much insight in Freud's division of the id, ego, and superego. Freud (1923/1984) essentially described the id as the unconscious manifestation of our instincts, played out impulsively, with little insight and with little regard for the consequences. In response to social conditions, the ego develops to look at the realities of society, etiquette, and laws to decide how one ought to behave in a practical way. Although one might want to steal the candy from the jar, the ego would suggest this might be unwise upon noticing the storekeeper watching. Freud used the analogy that the ego is to the id as a rider is to a horse. The rider must "hold in check the superior strength of the horse" (Freud, 1923/1984, p. 364). If the horse has chosen a course, sometimes all the rider can do is "guide it where it wants to go"; similarly, "the ego is in the habit of transforming the id's will into action as if it were its own" (Freud, 1923/1984, p. 364).

McLeod (2016) provided a good summary describing how the superego incorporates the values, mores, and morals of a society as learned by parents and others.

As Freud (1923/1984) explained, using the father as a model, the superego enforces society's prohibitions and controls the id. Its task is also to pressure the ego to use moral codes over simple realistic and pragmatic choices. Ideally, the superego would inhibit stealing candy based on the principle that thievery is morally wrong. As McLeod (2016) pointed out, the superego has two methods to apply this pressure. First, if the individual strays from the path, the superego can use guilt to encourage the ego to comply in the future. Secondly, the superego develops an ideal picture of the self. Freud's (1923/1984) construct of ego-ideal represents an ideal self within one's social context—the ideal self needed to achieve successful career goals, to treat other people appropriately and, in general, to be a good member of society. Freud's construct of ego ideal is not based on one's understanding or appreciation of one's own character. In many cases with Freud's approach, one would have to modify oneself so as to fit within society's parameters, goals, aims, methods, and values. In describing the ego-ideal, Freud (1923/1984, p. 396) emphasized "the general character of harshness and cruelty exhibited by the ideal—it's dictatorial 'Thou shalt.'"

Dąbrowski suggested that the highest levels of individual development go beyond the external forces of socialization to involve individually determined characteristics and motives. At these highest possible levels, external control of behavior (socialization) fades, and behavior now stems from an inner locus of control that reflects uniquely personal values and motivations. These individual, internal motivations are created based upon one's core values—the personality ideal—and they reflect a conscious, multilevel experience of the reality function. With multilevelness, we see all the subtle shades of life—both high and low—and this contrast assists us in seeing and choosing the higher path over the lower. Conscious and volitional behavior in pursuit of higher alternatives replaces and transforms the robotic social and animal instincts inherent in the lower levels. In summary, the division between lower and higher levels parallels the distinction between the human as a herd animal or unthinking robot versus the authentic, autonomous, self-thinking and volitional human being.

Other authors have also suggested a multilevel approach to psychology; for example, William James (1890/1950) presented a multilevel perspective on the self:

> A tolerably unanimous opinion ranges the different selves of which a man may be "seized and possessed," and the consequent different orders of his self-regard, in a hierarchical scale, with the bodily Self at the bottom, the spiritual Self at the top and the extracorporeal material selves and the various social selves between. (p. 313)

Is not clear if Dąbrowski read James or not. Dąbrowski's ideas about multilevelness were likely influenced by the hierarchy presented by Pierre Janet (1859-1947), the prominent French neurologist and psychologist and one of Dąbrowski's teachers. Janet described five levels of reality and mental functions that could be used to measure mental health. Van der Hart and Friedman (1989) summarized these levels:

- the reality function [highest]
- disinterested activity (habitual, indifferent and automatic actions)
- functions of imagination (abstract reasoning, fantasy, daydreaming and representative memory)
- emotional reactions
- useless muscular movements [lowest] (p. 12).

Van der Hart and Friedman (1989) continued: "The first three levels were considered the superior functions, the last two levels inferior; each set requiring a lesser degree of involvement with reality in order to be performed" (p. 12). At Janet's highest level, Level 1, the reality function creates an integrated synthesis of all incoming data to yield a high level of perception and appreciation of reality as it exists in the here and now. To be functioning at this level is "to be in the moment." This highest level is also characterized by an abundance of energy that the individual can use to perceive and act on reality that Janet called psychological tension: "Psychological tension refers to the capacity to use one's psychic energy. The higher one's mental level, i.e., the more operations one can synthesize, the higher one's psychological tension" (van der Hart & Friedman, 1989, p. 12). Lower levels in the hierarchy are characterized by progressively lower and lower amounts of psychological tension and therefore lower levels are associated with inferior perception and poor integration of stimuli and functions. Individuals may consistently function at lower levels based on constitutional factors (genetics), or in Janet's model they may be suffering a temporary depression of psychic energy, a feature that both Janet and Dąbrowski referred to as psychasthenia— literally, a weakening of the psychic functions. In Janet's model, psychasthenia replaces a healthy reality connection (represented by the reality function) with symptoms such as anxieties and obsessions, each lower level being associated with a particular set of characteristic symptoms, forming a hierarchy of neurotic styles. In summary, Janet concluded that the perception of reality and psychological functions can be described as a hierarchy and that fundamental differences in perception of reality are a major feature differentiating lower from higher levels.

Charles Taylor provided another important multileveled analysis of the self (C. Taylor, 1989). His analysis considered what it is to be a person, first examining our understanding of our current moral, social, and spiritual situation; and then looking at the critical role played by a multilevel understanding of the good—including a discussion of what ought to be done and the objectivity of such judgments. C. Taylor (1989) said:

> Human life is irreducibly multileveled. The epiphanic and the ordinary but indispensable real can never be fully aligned and we are condemned to live on more than one level—or else suffer the impoverishment of repression. (p. 480)

Ben Rogers (2008) explained that the modern self as described by C. Taylor includes conflicting feelings and drives—some higher and some lower. The claim is made that individuals will develop a hierarchy of values, holding "some ethical values or ideals to be worthier and more important or more fundamental than others" (Abbey, 2004, p. 4). Although this is a multilevel approach, it is based upon the traditional model of reason controlling emotion. Part of C. Taylor's central thesis is that people seek reason and value by an internal examination and ordering of one's inner life—truth and virtue are reached by "getting our thoughts and emotions in order—by following logical procedures, listening to our conscience and subjecting our emotions to reason" (B. Rogers, 2008, para. 8). C. Taylor's main concern is therefore with the hermeneutical inquiry involved in self-interpretation, a critical component of one's identity, especially when one is called upon to re-examine what was previously accepted about oneself without question—the situation one finds oneself in during a disintegration. These self-interpretations are based upon the vertical—our hierarchy of values—as well as along the horizontal dimension of time (Abbey, 2004). With the passage of time, our self-interpretations become an ongoing narrative describing our life, open to the revision of our recollections and the projection of our imagined self into the future. Thus, C. Taylor anticipated the emphasis on interpreted narrative life stories that have become an important movement in contemporary psychology (McAdams, 2006).

C. Taylor's second central thesis is that the modern age is characterized by an emphasis on the ordinary life—work, family, play, sport and so forth. In this context, people can now attach greater value to self-expression and authenticity, a movement that now finds expression in every strata of society (B. Rogers, 2008). The everyday, ordinary life is affirmed by emphasizing our sense of respect and obligation for others, our understanding of what makes a life full, and by recognizing the importance of dignity. Everyday life today is also characterized by the idea that suffering must be avoided and reduced to a minimum. While a traditional focus of religion has been to give suffering meaning, today, in our secular society, we struggle with the role of suffering. As well, in reviewing C. Taylor, Mos (1994) observed:

> If relativism and subjectivism have obscured our sensitivity to the higher and better, our adherence to naturalistic explanations in the human sciences, even of individual freedom and reason, has banned all moral considerations in an

understanding of ourselves and our culture. (p. 449)

C. Taylor emphasized that in order to come to know oneself one must ask questions: questions about what is good, what is bad, and about who we have been and who we want to become. In considering the emphasis on individuality in today's consumer society, C. Taylor articulated the ironic concern that there is a risk that independence might become a "shallow affair" in which masses of individuals try to discover and express individuality in a stereotypic fashion (C. Taylor, 1989, p. 40). The remedy for this situation is for each person to carefully choose the parameters that will define his or her life and, in that way, make it unique and significant.

In summary, C. Taylor (1989) resonates with Dąbrowski:

My identity is defined by the commitments and identifications which provide the frame or horizon within which I can try to determine from case to case what is good, or valuable, or what ought to be done, or what I endorse or oppose. In other words, it is the horizon within which I am capable of taking a stand. (p. 27)

Dąbrowski approached his description of levels of development as a medical doctor and psychiatrist; neurology was always an integral part of his theoretical approach. As mentioned, Dąbrowski was a student of the prominent French psychologist and neurologist Pierre Janet, and also studied under neurologist and child psychologist Édouard Claparède (1873-1940). Dąbrowski also admired British neurologist Sir Charles Scott Sherrington (1857-1952). However, Dąbrowski was also influenced by another English neurologist, John Hughlings Jackson, and the hierarchical model of the nervous system he developed. In his influential 1884 Croonian lectures titled, "On the evolution and dissolution of the nervous system," Hughlings Jackson outlined an evolutionary, level-based model of the nervous system that described differences between lower and higher levels (Hughlings Jackson, 1884; see also Critchley & Critchley, 1998; J. Taylor, 1958). Dąbrowski outlined three major principles of Hughlings Jackson's that guided him:

- Evolution is the transition from the simplest [and most stable] toward the most complex [but least stable and most fragile] centers.

- Evolution is the transition from well-organized lower centers toward higher, less well-organized centers.
- Evolution is the transition from more automatic toward more voluntary functions. (Dąbrowski, 1970b, p. 103)

In addition, the operation of lower levels tends to be subordinate to the control of higher levels. Hughlings Jackson described evolution (development) as the movement from lower to higher levels and therefore toward more complexity, less organization and more deliberate voluntary actions. Dąbrowski (1972b) included these attributes in his definition of higher levels: "[B]y higher level of psychic development we mean a behavior which is more complex, more conscious and having greater freedom of choice, hence greater opportunity for self-determination" (p. 70). Thus, higher levels are characterized by increased functional autonomy and greater volitional control, reflecting recent evolutionary advancements. Lower levels are "holdovers" of early evolution and largely involve primitive survival instincts and other autonomic, habitual functions. The lowest levels essentially run automatically, maintaining our physiology and expressing our instincts with little (if any) conscious thought or volition involved. The lowest levels provide an instant, ready-made response set to respond immediately to situations that were once commonly encountered in life (e.g., LeDoux, 1996; Sokolov, 1963). In other words, the lower levels operate on a Stimulus-Response (SR) model, generally designed to help us flee or prepare to fight off danger. If higher levels do not develop, or if their inhibitory function somehow fails, then the lower levels are free to express their primitive nature unchecked, an idea similar to K. G. Bailey's (1987) theory of paleopsychological regression.

In summary, following Hughlings Jackson, Dąbrowski (1964b, 1972b) hypothesized that lower levels of development demonstrate simpler, more organized, more rigid, and more resilient psychological structures. Appearing earlier in evolution, the lower levels are more automatic (reflexive), better organized, and less vulnerable to damage or modification. Higher levels are associated with higher brain structures that appear more recently in our evolution, such as the neocortex. These structures are less automatic, allowing for more voluntary control, but they are also less well organized and thus more prone to disruption and reorganization (see also Kolb & Whishaw, 2014; Sapolsky, 2017).

Dąbrowski followed Hughlings Jackson's neurological orientation and described multilevelness in neurological terms as a "division of functions into different levels, for instance, the spinal, subcortical and cortical levels in the nervous system" (Dąbrowski, 1972b, p. 298). More reminiscent of Janet, Dąbrowski also gives a phenomenological description: "Individual perception of many levels of external and internal reality appears at a certain stage of development, here called multilevel disintegration" (Dąbrowski, 1972b, p. 298). Thus, in the multilevel experience of life—Janet's highest level—reality function provides a more complex and subtler reality than is experienced in unilevelness.[7] Dąbrowski emphasized that the individual is not totally a slave to his or her perceptions—recall Janet's emphasis on individual synthesis. Dąbrowski said people could develop their own synthesis of reality and thus consciously and volitionally move beyond the "is" of the given world. We can use our imagination to move towards a possible future. Multilevelness is a realization of the "possibility of the higher" (a phrase Dąbrowski frequently used) and of the contrasts and conflicts between the imagined higher and the actual lower in life.

As the process of hierarchization becomes stronger, the distinction between that which is more myself and that which is less myself becomes clearer. At the same time, the distinction between what is and what ought to be also becomes clearer. This creates an internal mental struggle between the lower and higher elements within one's self—a multilevel conflict—which is a hallmark for the potential of further psychological development.

By endorsing a multilevel approach, Dąbrowski developed a theory explaining how differences and levels in the nervous system are expressed as psychological phenomena. Alternatively, we can observe differences in psychological functions and now understand how they result from neural substrates on different levels.

Dąbrowski's five psychological levels underlie and explain the broader realms of human function. This approach allows a new flexibility in understanding the wide ranges seen in human behavior. Higher-level behavior is seen as moving beyond the largely unconscious, stimulus-response mode, to a model based on an individual's conscious, volitional autonomy. This also moves us into a deeper and more realistic philosophy of what it means to be an authentic human being, a philosophy emphasizing phenomenology and existentialism, which will be further discussed in Chapter Six.

2–2. MULTIDIMENSIONALITY

Dąbrowski combined the idea of multilevelness with a multidimensional analysis. Different dimensions can be described and their interactions analyzed based upon the level observed for each dimension under consideration. For example, intellectual function may be at a high level while emotional dimensions may function at a lower level.

A critical implication is that the features or characteristics of a given behavior or trait will be quite different on lower levels versus higher levels. Behaviors emerge from and represent traits, and it is essential "to identify the underlying physiological, psychological and social bases of traits" (Matthews, Deary, & Whiteman, 2009, p. 4). From the multilevel perspective, this means it is vital to recognize the level underlying a behavior/trait in question. Differences between the characteristics and expression of a given behavior or trait between levels may be more profound than differences between various particular traits. Dąbrowski (1996) gave the example that the differences between love and hate at the lowest level will be less than the differences between love at the lowest level compared to love at the highest level.

An important implication of this approach is that an individual will generally display different levels of development in different dimensions of psychological function. When this is the case, it becomes a complex issue to describe or assign a measurement to the overall developmental level of the individual.

Another important implication of multidimensionality is that ideal growth must eventually achieve a balance of development across the different dimensions. Although it is common for some dimensions to develop sooner than others, the lagging dimensions eventually must "catch up." If this does not occur, one-sided development is the result. In this situation, development is limited to one ability or to a narrow range of abilities. In the most common example, a person may be at a high level intellectually and at a low level emotionally. This is not a desirable situation because without the guidance of emotion, intelligence is used in the service of advancing an individual's primitive instincts or in advancing social agendas: "Grave affective retardation is usually associated with above average intelligence subordinated to primitive drives" (Dąbrowski, 1970b, p. 30).

2–3. LEVELS VERSUS STAGES

Dąbrowski (1976) differentiated "development through stages" versus "development through psychical levels." He said that development through stages concerns the development of many humans (also many animal species) and is determined biologically ("phylogenetically"). Individuals are born and pass through determined periods of development—for instance, puberty, adolescence, adulthood, old age, and death. Development through psychical levels is quite different and is only observed in "certain groups within the human society" (Dąbrowski, 1976, p. 134). This development is characterized by the progression through the five levels of the theory of positive disintegration. Disintegration, growth and reintegration on a higher level allow an individual to transcend the normal course of development through stages and thereby overcome his or her biological species development and move towards self-directed and self-conscious individual development.

Based on the above distinction, Dąbrowski was careful to emphasize that in his theory, he used the construct of development through levels and not stages. Stage theory dictates several unique features; e.g., people must start at the first stage; stages must be moved through sequentially; and no stage can be missed or jumped over. Also, once a stage is achieved, reverting to a previous stage is not permitted. A model using levels allows greater flexibility compared to a stage theory. In a level approach, not everyone has to begin at the first level; one can regress back to earlier levels; or levels can be skipped in development.

Dąbrowski, like Piaget, derived his levels from observational data. Thus, it is an inductive theory based upon a set of phenomena. In casual conversations, it is easy to talk about levels as if they were physical attributes of an individual; however, Marlene Rankel reminded us that "levels are not physical structures like train stations" (personal communication, ca. 2004). Several ideas are implied that we need to keep in mind:

- Levels do not represent milestones of development (they are not linked to developmental timelines).
- Levels are not necessarily attained one after the other. Different dimensions are likely to show different levels of development; therefore, the common picture will usually be one of development straddled over several levels.
- Levels and sub-levels within unilevel experience can be differentiated quantitatively and described on a continuum.
- The distinction between unilevel and multilevel experience involves a qualitative distinction describing a basic shift in one's reality function and perception of the world.
- Levels and sub-levels within multilevel experience can be differentiated quantitatively and described on a continuum.
- Multiple sub-levels may be differentiated within a level; for example, at the primary level.
- Dąbrowski was open to the idea that meaningful descriptions could eventually be developed of levels beyond his fifth level of secondary integration.

The division of psychological functions into discrete levels is largely a matter of judgment and definition. Dąbrowski would often emphasize that "there are no pure forms," and this must be considered when trying to describe phenomena such as levels, developmental potential (including overexcitability), and the dynamisms. It also bears keeping in mind that, although these descriptions are based on observations and are intended to describe psychological development as seen in the real world, they are metaphors and heuristic devices designed to help us imagine and better comprehend human psychology. Given our current understanding and measurement techniques, the tasks of interpretation and analysis risk being taken too literally.

Dąbrowski initially had limited interest in quantification; however, an empirical approach was requisite under the criteria of the Canada Council grants[8] that Dąbrowski used to pay the salaries and costs of the research team (Dąbrowski, 1972b, p. vi). Data collection and analysis began in 1969. The first numerical assignments to the five levels appeared in print in Dąbrowski (1972b).

2–4. DIAGNOSIS AND ASSESSMENT

In Dąbrowski's theory, diagnosis is not based on the identification of symptoms; rather, diagnosis is based upon an understanding and appreciation of the overall developmental situation and developmental potential of the individual. One's history, one's current situation, and one's potentials for development all must be taken into consideration in making a diagnosis. Symptoms and signs, both positive and negative, must be understood and analyzed within this overall context.

The purpose of diagnosis was primarily "to grasp all the positive factors, to introduce the patient to them and to make him a co-author of his diagnosis" (Dąbrowski, 1972b, p. 252). This point bears repeating: a diagnosis cannot be made primarily based on the symptoms displayed by an individual because the same symptom may represent two quite different phenomena in two different people. Symptoms must be understood based upon the positive or negative role they may play in the individual's life, and Dąbrowski (1964b) made the surprising point that it may take months or even years of observation and investigation for a psychiatrist to reach an opinion.[9] Likewise, the understanding or assessment of a specific trait yields little meaning unless considered within the context of the overall developmental diagnosis.

Dąbrowski (1972b) referred to his "multidimensional, multilevel descriptive-interpretive diagnosis." In referring to a "descriptive-interpretive" diagnosis, Dąbrowski was emphasizing the role played by observation, judgment, and interpretation. The clinician does not *give* a diagnosis to a client; the diagnosis is arrived at through discussion and consensus between the clinician and the client (Dąbrowski, 1972b). In addition, the descriptive-interpretive approach distinguished this type of diagnosis from that of a traditional clinical diagnosis, which is based upon categorizing an individual according to a classification scheme of disorders.

The basic thrust of the diagnosis is to determine if the client displays a unilevel or a multilevel disintegration, and this fundamental distinction will also determine the subsequent therapeutic approach taken. A diagnosis therefore also constituted an integral part of the overall therapy program—comprising essentially half of the psychotherapeutic process (Dąbrowski, 1967). In Dąbrowski's approach, the "client" largely conducts his or her own therapy program through self-education and autopsychotherapy. This reflected the philosophy that psychotherapy should not be focused on "treatment" of symptoms; instead Dąbrowski's emphasis was on a larger process of education, explanation, and encouraging self-discovery and self-awareness of the basic developmental process, both in general and as it related specifically to the client. Through understanding the developmental significance of symptoms, the client can benefit from their presence and, as development proceeds, the symptoms will naturally diminish.

Dąbrowski's primary focus was the application of hierarchization and multilevelness to reveal "the differentiated diagnosis of levels of emotional, instinctive and intellectual development" (Dąbrowski, 1972a, p. 59). Dąbrowski would use a combination of clinical judgment supplemented by conventional psychological testing. For example, the Wechsler Adult Intelligence Scale was used to assess intelligence. The Rorschach test was used to assess personality type based upon Herman Rorschach's (1884-1922) model of associating inner psychic transformation with the ambiequal type of personality: "The ambiequal type is usually associated with above-average intelligence, original thinking, affective stability and harmonious cooperation between intratensive and extratensive qualities" (Dąbrowski, 1973, p. 81).

Dąbrowski did not use conventional personality testing. As

mentioned above, he felt the one personality test that could be of benefit was the Rorschach. I had been exposed to the Minnesota Multiphasic Personality Inventory as a psychology student and asked Dąbrowski his opinion about the test; he replied, "Such tests are interesting but not very useful in understanding a person."

Dąbrowski also developed several diverse experimental tests. For example, he extended techniques emerging from depth psychology to develop a projective test using an array of photographs to measure an individual's likes and dislikes. As well, he developed an extensive neurological examination. Unfortunately, it is beyond the scope of the present work to provide a detailed examination of these techniques.

One of the more promising assessment approaches that Dąbrowski developed involved the analysis of verbal responses to reveal the presence of developmental dynamisms. Dąbrowski (1996) said:

> The expression of a function can be observed directly in behavior or it can be measured by appropriate tests, even if such tests still have to be constructed. This is the empirical aspect of multilevelness that consists in the collection of descriptive data. The theoretical aspect consists in uncovering the dynamisms involved in shaping the expression of behavior. . . . Thus, a dynamism as a theoretical abstraction is within easy grasp of what is observable and analyzable, at least in verbal behavior. A qualitative and quantitative analysis of responses representative of all the dynamisms of positive disintegration has been attempted. (p. 44)

Dąbrowski and Piechowski (1996) largely report such data.

In summary, Dąbrowski utilized an intuitive rather than an empirical approach to assessment. A diagnosis was based on a comprehensive review of symptoms and signs in the context of the overall history, current situation, and potential for development of an individual. Symptoms were understood in the context of an individual's life.

2–5. DĄBROWSKI'S FIVE LEVELS OF HUMAN FUNCTIONING

Just as Plato outlined a theory of levels of reality, Dąbrowski described several levels of psychological development and function. Dąbrowski's differentiation of human development into levels was based upon his perception of reality as being multileveled, with lower, intermediate, and higher levels of reality: "This refers not only to thinking, feeling, imagining and human behavior; but includes all kinds of mental functions, groups of functions or specific higher functions" (Dąbrowski, 1973, p. 4). Dąbrowski (1996) defined the construct of level as the operation of a characteristic constellation of developmental factors creating an identifiable and distinct developmental structure: "Going from the lowest to the highest level one sees a broadening and deepening in the way a human individual approaches the aspects of life," ranging from "the complete egocentrism of the primitive level to the full alterocentrism of the highest level" (Dąbrowski, 1970b, p. 98).

Dąbrowski (1973) linked the differentiation of reality with the psychological characteristics of the viewer: "By multilevelness of reality we mean external and internal reality of various levels conceived by means of sensory perception, imagination, intellectual, intuitive or" (p. 5) a combination thereof. Further, he claimed that because different observers can consistently describe differences between levels, they should be considered objective phenomena (Dąbrowski, 1970b). Dąbrowski (1973) developed the construct of "multilevel empiricism" to reflect the idea that knowledge derived from experience constitutes an empirical understanding of the world: "Multilevel empiricism is a consequence of the fundamental fact of the multilevelness of mental structures and activities of man" (Dąbrowski, 1973, p. 9). This model avoided the statistical normative approach which traditionally describes and characterizes large groups of individuals in recognition of the fact that special methods are required to study rare phenomenon occurring in a small number of individuals; for instance, the few individuals reaching advanced individual development.

Multilevel perception is based on more than just sensory inputs. It includes all of the psychological functions available to humans—

thinking, feeling, imagination, instincts, empathy, intuition and so forth. Therefore, Dąbrowski suggested that his level structure could be used to describe a wide range of properties associated with development: "typological characteristics; instincts; intelligence; social, moral, religious and aesthetic emotions; inner psychic milieu; volition; creativity; and mental disturbances" (Dąbrowski, 1970b, p. 99). The various levels of function observed in everyday behavior and characteristics reflect distinct structures and levels of the nervous system as elaborated by Hughlings Jackson.

Reflecting Dąbrowski's fundamental idea that development occurs through crises, each of the three levels of disintegration is associated with a corresponding type of crisis or disturbance and a characteristic set of symptoms. Dąbrowski described these symptoms as a hierarchy of interneurotic and intraneurotic levels of mental function. For instance, when illustrating interneurotic levels, different types of psychoneuroses will be seen on different levels. Within a given psychoneurosis, higher and lower levels (intraneurotic differences) can also often be described. Dąbrowski introduced considerable subtlety and complexity in the way he analyzed psychological features.

Dąbrowski distinguished five levels of mental development within three major divisions:

- 1. An initial integration (Level I).
- 2. Three types of disintegration (Levels II, III, and IV).
- 3. A second integration (Level V).

The names Dąbrowski chose are descriptive of the idea of each level:

- 1. Primary integration (I)
- 2. Unilevel disintegration (II)
- 3. Multilevel disintegration: Spontaneous (III)
- 4. Multilevel disintegration: Organized or Directed (IV)
- 5. Secondary integration (V)

Dąbrowski made it clear that values were a central component in the hierarchy of levels: "To each level of mental development there is a corresponding level of value experience. Mental development of man and the development of a hierarchy of values are, in fact, two names for the same process. One cannot separate the two" (Dąbrowski, 1970b, p. 98). Each level was described on the basis of emotional and instinctive functions corresponding to a level of value experience. Dąbrowski also made it clear that this initial outline of levels is an approximation, open to modification and future refinements.

Table 1 (following) presents a synopsis of the levels of development.

Table 1. Summary of the Major Features of Each Level

Dąbrowski Level	Key Descriptor	Dominant Factor	Locus of Control	Typical Conflicts	Values	Personality	Suicide
Secondary Integration. [V]	Personality. Inner Harmony.	Third.	Strongly internal.	External. (Social injustice)	Self-determined hierarchy of values. Unique, authentic.	Full unique self-created personality ideal.	Transcend. Heroic: save another. Social protest.
Directed Multilevel Disintegration. [IV]	Higher psychoneurotic processes.	Emerging third.	Emerging internal.	Internal. (Weakening)	Personalized values emerge.	Personality ideal forms.	Partial— "kill" lower self.
Spontaneous Multilevel Disintegration. [III]	Lower psychoneurotic processes.	Third appears: Conflicts with Second	Weakly internal.	Internal. Strong vertical. Complex.	Hierarchization of personalized values begins.	Self-identity emerges.	Life betrayal. Intense inner conflicts.

Table 1. Summary of the Major Features of Each Level (continued)

Dąbrowski Level	Key Descriptor	Dominant Factor	Locus of Control	Typical Conflicts	Values	Personality	Suicide
Unilevel Disintegration. [II]	Neuroses. Chaos. Extreme stress.	Second. (In crises)	In flux.	Internal. Horizontal.	Status quo under scrutiny.	Ambiguity. (Don't fit anywhere)	Intense or prolonged stress.
Primary Integration [I]	Borderline Average Person ~ Asocial ~ Psychopath	Second First	Strongly external. (Social mores) Strongly internal. (Ego)	External. (Social goals blocked) External. (Ego goals blocked)	Values reflect social mores, rules and conventions. Values reflect self-interest.	Individuality. (No personality per se)	Escape. Shame. Revenge. Impulsive. Cowardice. Anger.

2–5–1. Level I: Primary (or primitive) integration, integrated unilevelness

Dąbrowski used the terms psychopath, psychopathy, primitive and primary synonymously in describing Level I (Dąbrowski, 1964b, pp. 73-75). He differentiated sociopathy from psychopathy; sociopathy is the failure to achieve one's full development due to the influence of social or environmental factors. Psychopathy is the failure to achieve full development due to biological and genetic causes (e.g., Blair, 2001; Hare, 1995/1999, pp. 23-24; Harpur, Hare, & Hakstian, 1989; Hosking et al., 2017; Lykken, 1995; Millon, Simonsen, & Birket-Smith, 1998). Thus, Dąbrowski's use of the term psychopath is appropriate given his definition of advanced development (achieving a unique and autonomous personality) and his observation that the average person lacks sufficient developmental potential (a set of genetic features) necessary to achieve this ideal.[10]

Level I is characterized by automatic impulses and rigid structures. In the average person, behavior is controlled by a combination of primitive instincts and drives and by the external forces of socialization. Behavior occurs reflexively and automatically in response to stimuli, with little consciousness or awareness; thus, there is no opportunity for reflection or real self-control. Behavioral responses occur in stereotypic fashion, emanating from social conditioning. Both thinking and emotions are experienced through this social filter with an emphasis upon roles, expectations, and socially correct responses. Although high levels of intelligence may be seen, Dąbrowski (1996) emphasized that in primary integration, intelligence is used in the service of lower instincts and to achieve social goals. The primary characteristic of Level I is an adjustment to the social milieu—an adjustment lacking any significant individual review or deep reflection. As Dąbrowski (1996) described,

> The characteristic of cognitive and emotional structures and functions of primary integration is that they are automatic, impulsive, and rigid. Behavior is controlled by primitive drives and by externality. Intelligence neither controls nor transforms basic drives; it serves the ends determined by primitive drives. There is no inner conflict while external

conflicts are the rule. The overall picture is of little differentiation, primitive drive structure, and predominant externality. (p. 18)

Level I is characterized by an inner harmony—although many conflicts may exist between the individual and his or her external environment. Here there are no internal conflicts present; people at this level

> are not capable of having internal conflicts, although they often have conflicts with their external environment. They are unaware of any qualities of life beyond those necessary for immediate gratification of their primitive impulses and they act solely on behalf of their impulses (Dąbrowski, 1964b, p. 4).

The theory describes three factors that influence behavior. The *first factor* encompasses the heredity ("constitutional endowment") influences on an individual. The *second factor* are external influences, primarily one's social environment. The *third factor* is an internal drive to achieve autonomy.

At Level I, people display either prominent first factor and/or second factor. The majority of people show a mixture of the influence of both factors: certain primitive drives may coincide with social expectations and are expressed through socially sanctioned behaviors. The drive for recognition and status may be expressed through success in the "dog-eat-dog" corporate world, leading to socially respected and sanctioned individual wealth and power.

A continuum of degrees of integration characterizes Level I: "Among normal primitively integrated people, different degrees of cohesion of psychic structure can be distinguished" (Dąbrowski, 1964b, p. 66). Within the continuum, Dąbrowski (1964b) highlighted two basic groups: the psychopath and the socialized person (see Figure 1). The antisocial psychopath represents a small subset of Level I (about 5% of the population) primarily characterized by relatively unimpeded first factor (heredity) drives and impulses. These individuals "see what they want and take it" without regard for the law, social sanctions or consequences. Individuals in this small subset tend to be extremely rigid and display little potential for development. The socialized group includes the "average person," primarily characterized by the dominance of the second factor (the influence of environment). Social conditioning inhibits primitive instincts, leading to socially conforming and law-abiding behavior. Conscience is largely socially determined and exceptions of behavior are socially rationalized. To illustrate, during the Vietnam War, in 1968, Lt. William Calley was prosecuted for the My Lai massacre (William Calley, 2017). His behavioral rationale was that he was simply doing his duty by following orders. Justifications can also be socially sanctioned; for instance, "all's fair in love and war" or in the "unpleasant but necessary" bloodletting that is often required to maintain one's "business edge." Dąbrowski distinguished the two major subgroups of Level I by degree and related the potential to develop to the degree of integration present (Dąbrowski, 1964b):

> The state of primary integration is a state contrary to mental health. A high degree of primary integration is present in the average person; a very high degree of primary integration is present in the psychopath. The more cohesive the structure of primary integration, the less the possibility of development; the greater the strength of automatic functioning, stereotypy and habitual activity, the lower the level of mental health. The psychopath is only slightly, if at all, capable of development; he is deaf and blind to stimuli except those pertaining to his impulse-ridden structure, to which intelligence is subordinated. The absence of the development of personality means the absence of mental health. (pp. 121-122)

Research has supported the idea that the "severity" of psychopathy is a continuum. Studies have demonstrated that non-criminal and criminal psychopaths differ by degree and do not constitute qualitatively distinct populations and that the two groups share similar physiological and neuropsychological characteristics (Mahmut, Homewood, & Stevenson, 2008).

As mentioned, second factor—socialization—inhibits and controls the basal animal and biological instincts (first factor) in the "average" person. This group, most of Level I, is categorized at the primitive level because their social conformity is based upon a blind or rote following and does not reflect consciously, individually chosen moral positions. Dąbrowski's observation was that the influence of socialization also robs the individual of the opportunity to express genuine autonomy and to develop a unique personality. Dąbrowski (1970b) suggested that the average person simply incorporates the value structure and social roles and expectations of his or her culture; the development of an autonomous value structure and of an autonomous personality is largely dissuaded by social factors. In Dąbrowski's terminology, there is no opportunity for third factor (autonomy) to emerge. The emphasis on group conformity increases the inertia associated with primary integration and thus makes breaking free difficult even for those individuals who possess significant potential to develop. Socialization as a process can make it difficult to achieve advanced individual development.

Dąbrowski painted a bleak view of Level I, saying that the majority of the population can be categorized here. These individuals lack substantial potential to develop and do not develop an individual personality; therefore, in Dąbrowski's opinion, these individuals are not mentally healthy. This claim is unusual, and it is helpful to review its justification in more detail. First, as discussed above, is Dąbrowski's specific usage of the term psychopath. As well, his usage of the terms primary and primitive are appropriate descriptive terms when seen in contrast to his definition of ideal personality development.

Second, it is helpful to consider selected contemporary works on psychopathy—works that use conventional definitions—that examine the prevalence and success of psychopaths. In a well-known and controversial essay, in 1957, Norman Mailer[11] noted that:

> If it be remembered that not every psychopath is an extreme case, and that the condition of psychopathy is present in a host of people including many politicians, professional soldiers, newspaper columnists, entertainers, artists, jazz musicians, call-girls, promiscuous homosexuals and half the executives of Hollywood, television, and advertising, it can be seen that there are aspects of psychopathy which already exert considerable cultural influence. (p. 282)

More recently, Lykken (1995) noted, "some psychopaths, [however], are at least superficially socialized, some have learned the rules and do generally obey them" (p. 22).

Several recent constructs of psychopathy are also relevant. The "successful psychopath" is based upon the idea that psychopathy confers advantages that, in some contexts, and in some occupations, lead to life and career success (e.g., Gao & Raine, 2010; Glenn & Raine, 2014; Hanson & Baker, 2017; Kantor, 2006; Macur, 2014). Also relevant are "subclinical psychopathy" (e.g., Akhtar, Ahmetoglu, & Chamorro-Premuzic, 2013; Fennimore & Sementelli, 2016; LeBreton, Binning, & Adorno, 2006) and the "prosocial psychopath" (e.g., Galang, 2010; Galang, Castelo, Santos, Perlas, & Angeles, 2016; B. A. White, 2014). Psychopaths in politics are considered by Ashcroft (2016) and by Lilienfeld et al. (2012).

In an aptly titled work, *Snakes in Suits*, Babiak and Hare (2006) explore the construct of corporate psychopathy. Other works also consider the prevalence, toxicity, and success of these so-called "white-collar" psychopaths (e.g., Babiak, Neumann, & Hare, 2010; Boddy, 2011, 2014; Hanson & Baker, 2017; Lykken, 1995; Walker & Jackson, 2016). Finally, more general works on psychopathy provide context to Dąbrowski's usage of psychopathy (e.g., Adams, 2016; Cleckley, 1988; Coid, Freestone, & Ullrich, 2012; Dutton, 2012; Fallon, 2013; Raine, 2018).

I will also provide several direct quotations to elaborate.

- Dąbrowski observed that "the average person" (about 65% of the population) is at Level I: "Individuals with some degree of primitive integration comprise the majority of society" (Dąbrowski, 1964b, p. 4) (see also Dąbrowski, 1964b, pp. 4-10 and pp. 121-122).

- The number of people who complete the full course of development and attain the level of secondary integration is limited. A vast majority of people either do not break down their primitive integration at all, or after a relatively short period of disintegration, usually experienced at the time of adolescence and early youth, end in a reintegration at the former level or in partial integration of some of the functions at slightly higher levels, without a transformation of the whole mental structure. (Dąbrowski, 1970b, p. 4)

- "In the primitive integration pattern, there is little possibility of transformation to another type" (Dąbrowski, 1964b, p. 71).
- In the context of the theory of positive disintegration, psychopathy also represents a primitive instinctual structure. Intelligence is subjugated to this structure and plays a purely instrumental role. A psychopath is one whose personality structure is strongly integrated at a low level. (Dąbrowski, 1972b, p. 154)
- "This character pattern is a stabilized, primitive level of integration in which development of personality does not take place. Its occurrence seems strongly influenced by constitutional factors" (Dąbrowski, 1964b, pp. 65-66).
- "The state of primary integration is a state contrary to mental health" (Dąbrowski, 1964b, p. 121).

Not everyone will pass through Level I. Dąbrowski (1967) believed that a few rare individuals may exhibit such strong development that they never become integrated at the first level and can pass directly into higher levels:

It should also be kept in mind that there are people, though rarely met, whose initial integration belongs to the higher level, whose rich structure, constantly improved by life's experiences and reflections, does not undergo the process of disintegration, but harmoniously and without greater shock develops into a full personality. (p. 58)

In summary, primary integration is characterized by the strong influence of socialization. Typically, there is little internal conflict and limited consciousness; awareness, especially of the self and the autonomous forces of development (third factor), is minimal. Behavior tends to be stereotypic and reflexive, with little self-reflection. There is generally an absence of developmental potential and disintegration; when disintegrations actually occur, they tend to be minor, short-lived, and resolved through a reintegration at the primary level. Figure 1, below, presents the sublevels of Level I, the first and second factors, and a scale of the relative rigidity of socialization. At the lowest level, adherence to socialization is perfunctory and self-serving. The Figure is based on Mika (2015).

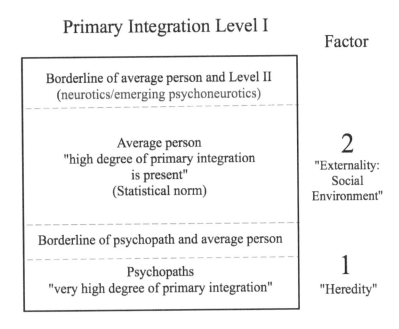

Primary Integration Level I

Factor

> Borderline of average person and Level II
> (neurotics/emerging psychoneurotics)
>
> Average person
> "high degree of primary integration
> is present"
> (Statistical norm)
>
> Borderline of psychopath and average person
>
> Psychopaths
> "very high degree of primary integration"

2
"Externality:
Social
Environment"

1
"Heredity"

Figure 1. Primary Integration Level I

2–5–2. Level II: Unilevel disintegration

The definition of Level II is reflected in its name: Unilevel Disintegration. The prominent features of this level are initial, brief, and often intense crises. The security and automatism of day-to-day adjustment breaks down, creating an opportunity for the individual to examine his or her life, to become aware and, ideally, to take one's life and one's development into one's own hands. This idea encapsulates the most fundamental principle of development in Dąbrowski's theory—development cannot occur during times of adjustment: "The individual who is always adjusted is one who does not develop himself" (Dąbrowski, 1970b, p. 58).

Dąbrowski's (1996) description of unilevel disintegration is helpful:

> It consists of disintegrative processes occurring as if on a single structural level. There is disintegration but no differentiation of levels of emotional or intellectual control. Unilevel disintegration begins with the loosening of the cohesive and rigid structure of primary integration. There is hesitation, doubt, ambivalence, increased sensitivity to internal stimuli, fluctuations of mood, excitations and depressions, vague feelings of disquietude, various forms of mental and psychosomatic disharmony. There is ambitendency of action, either changing from one direction to another, or being unable to decide which course to take and letting the decision fall to chance, or a whim of like or dislike. Thinking has a circular character of argument for argument's sake. Externality is still quite strong. Nuclei of hierarchization may gradually appear, weakly differentiating events in the external milieu and in the internal milieu but still there is continual vacillation between 'pros' and 'cons' with no clear direction out of the vicious circle. Internal conflicts are unilevel and often superficial. When they are severe and engage deeper emotional structures the individual often sees himself caught in a "no exit" situation. Severe mental disorders are associated with unilevel developmental structure. (p. 18)

It takes a fairly major disruption of the adjustment and homeostasis of primary integration in order to precipitate an experience of unilevel disintegration. As seen in the quotation above, Dąbrowski felt that the "storm and stress" associated with adolescence and puberty or major life transitions such as retirement or menopause could precipitate periods of unilevel disintegration. In addition, stressful external events, especially when compounded by strong overexcitability, could precipitate the type of crisis leading to Level II experiences.

Dąbrowski (1996) was clear that this initial disintegration could represent a severe shock and threat to the individual and he associated the possibility of "severe mental disorders" with Level II. The individual experiencing unilevel crises usually experiences great ambivalence—one choice seems as good as another. This ambivalence leads to what Dąbrowski called ambitendencies: the individual experiences many conflicting tendencies at the same time and no one course of action takes preference over another. The individual is often immobilized by the inability to decisively choose a course of action, and he or she is often overwhelmed by feelings of ambiguity. Frustration and despair are also common emotions at Level II; the individual often turns to "seek immediate palliatives like alcohol, drugs, or suicide" (Dąbrowski, 1972b, p. 306)[12].

Two critical transitional aspects are associated with Level II: first, it represents the transition from integration to disintegration; second, the transformation from Level II to Level III is the critical shift from unilevel to multilevel experience. If an individual is to move on to the higher levels in Dąbrowski's theory, this critical shift to multilevelness must occur. If a person does not have the developmental potential to fully move ahead into a multilevel view, he or she commonly falls back from the crises of Level II to reintegrate at Level I.

Level II is a transitional period. Dąbrowski said an individual entering Level II must fall back, move ahead, or end in suicide or psychosis: "Prolongation of unilevel disintegration often leads to reintegration on a lower level, to suicidal tendencies, or to psychosis" (Dąbrowski, 1964b, p. 7). Dąbrowski (1970b) emphasized this point a second time, making it one of the 72 hypotheses he suggested for further study. Here, Dąbrowski (1970b, p. 135) suggested that unless a reintegration back into Level I occurred or there was further transcendence into Level III, an individual risked falling into "a trap of a rapidly growing mental tension," creating a drama "without exit" and likely eventually culminating in suicide or negative disintegration (mental illness).

In summary, unilevel disintegration is characterized by conflicts with a horizontal focus—conflicts between impulses, features, and emotional states on the same level. These conflicts are expressed through strong ambivalence and ambitendency—the individual is equally pulled, first one way and then the other; however, there is little practical difference between the available alternatives. There is limited consciousness or self-consciousness involved in decision making at this level. These conflicts are not developmental per se, because they do not provide "a way up" and they involve little insight or transformation. Unilevel disintegrations are transitory and usually end in a reintegration back at the initial level; without reintegration, prolonged periods of unilevel disintegration may create crises "without exit" (Dąbrowski, 1970b, p. 135), leading to suicidal tendencies or psychosis.

2–5–3. Level III: Spontaneous multilevel disintegration

The fundamental feature qualitatively distinguishing Level III from Level I and Level II is the beginning of multilevel experience—an extensive vertical differentiation of mental life (Dąbrowski, 1996). The ambiguity of Level II is replaced by a growing sense of an emerging vertical struggle between "what is" versus "what ought to be." The contrasts between the lower realities and the higher possibilities create many new internal conflicts. As the individual comes to grips with these internal conflicts, there is a growing sense of self-control over one's behavior.

Level III marks the appearance of three critical new features:

- A "new" focus on one's inner life characterized by multilevel processes of introspection, self-examination and self-evaluation (Piechowski, 2008).
- The process of multilevel disintegration, a feature Dąbrowski believed was indispensable for development.
- The inner psychic milieu—the combined emergence and operation of creative and transforming dynamisms that come to control and direct one's development.

The multilevel disintegration at this level reflects Dąbrowski's fundamental belief that: "What is new, higher, richer, must in a large measure grow from the loosening and disruption of what is old, simple, poorer, integrated and nondynamic" (Dąbrowski, 1964b, p. 122).

Dąbrowski (1964b, p. 123) described the features associated with multilevel disintegration:

- A disruption of the integrated and rigid internal environment,

thereby allowing modifications.
- The rise of a sense of subject-object.
- The emergence of an awareness of higher and lower levels in one's values.
- The development of an attitude of prospection and retrospection.
- The consequent elevation of the disposing and directing center to a higher level.
- The emergence of the third factor.
- The development of a personality ideal.

In addition to these factors, Dąbrowski (1996) described additional developmental forces he called dynamisms that characterize this level:

They reflect the nature of multilevel conflicts crucial to the progress of development: positive maladjustment, astonishment with oneself, feelings of shame and guilt, disquietude with oneself, feeling of inferiority toward oneself and dissatisfaction with oneself, positive maladjustment. (p. 19)

In addition, the developmental instinct emerges as a powerful force helping to direct and move development in an upward direction.

As Dąbrowski (1996) observed, the developmental transformations occurring here affect the whole personality structure. The key shift in the developmental process occurs in the transition from Level II to Level III. This transition is an awkward and complicated notion. For one thing, Dąbrowski clearly saw it as a process that could either occur all at once or incrementally. Thus, development may involve many partial disintegrations and reintegrations as the self slowly changes, or things can change in a more dramatic, sudden, and global fashion.

This transition is a difficult time, demanding a significant amount of energy. The developmental process sweeps one along, and as it does the person and their view of life change. It is a time of great uncertainty and ambiguity: "Where am I going?" "What should I do?" "I thought I understood life; now I don't understand anything." The inner self (inner psychic milieu) struggles to find its new voice in the old and rigid status quo environment. New views lead to new values and, often, to a new sense of injustice. The birth of the multilevel experience of life creates a powerful new phenomenon, a new experience—the vertical conflicts that become so vital in directing growth. As the higher is seen and endorsed, the lower must give way—must be inhibited, overcome, or transformed and transcended.

2–5–4. Level IV: Organized or directed multilevel disintegration

With further development, conflicts lose their spontaneous character as the person assumes more and more control of his or her disintegrations and development. The individual begins to direct and consciously shape his or her crises and so begins to direct his or her own development.

At one point, Dąbrowski (1976) used the phrase "organized, systematized multilevel disintegration" to refer to this level and to emphasize the idea that the individual is now introducing his or her own system of development. This marks another vital aspect of advanced growth—the conscious and volitional involvement of the individual in controlling and directing his or her own development. Subsequently, Dąbrowski used the term, "directed multilevel disintegration." This self-control and self-directed development is the hallmark of Level IV disintegration. This level marks the solidification of autonomy and a sense of an individual hierarchy of aims, goals, and values. The answers and solutions to life's problems fully and finally shift from external sources to a strong sense of self-responsibility to find internal solutions, particularly through efforts to educate oneself (self-education) and to rise above one's problems (autopsychotherapy). The general instincts of self-development become focused on creativity and, ultimately, on self-perfection. The personality ideal becomes clearer and more tangible.

Dąbrowski (1996) summarized the prominent features at this level:

The developmental factors (dynamisms) characteristic for organized multilevel disintegration are: subject-object in oneself, third factor (conscious discrimination and choice), inner psychic transformation, self-awareness, self-control, education-of-oneself and autopsychotherapy. Self-perfection plays a highly significant role. (p. 19)

2–5–5. Level V: Secondary integration—integrated multilevelness

Secondary integration marks the emergence of a new cohesive organization and the emergence of the personality. There is a harmonization. The conflicts and disintegrative struggles between "is" and "ought" are now relegated to memory. The full operation of the advanced features of development (for instance, of the hierarchy of values, of the inner psychic milieu, of the disposing and directing center and so forth) mark an end to internal conflict.

There is an inner harmony as one's behavior emerges from one's values, reflecting one's personality ideal. Behavior now reflects an integrated cooperation and symbiosis between cognitive and emotional aspects. One's conflicts and disagreements with the lower level "as is" world are expressed compassionately in doing what one can to help solve problems and through genuinely pro-social, altruistic behavior. This is not an end state but an ongoing striving to put one's principles into day-to-day action. As Dąbrowski (1996) said: "The developmental dynamisms characteristic of secondary integration are: responsibility, autonomy, authentism and personality ideal. Those who achieve the level of secondary integration epitomize universal compassion and self-sacrifice." (p. 20)

2–6. CHAPTER SUMMARY

Dąbrowski described a multilevel reality that included a description of empirically distinct and meaningful levels of internal and external reality and psychological development. These higher and lower levels of perception and development arise from levels in the structure of the nervous system. Many people will live in a primary integrated harmony, characterized by socialized conformity. Individuals possessing sufficient developmental potential may begin to experience conflicts and disintegrations. These conflicts may eventually take on a vertical character marking multilevelness—a significant step forward in development. Advanced development is characterized by the emergence and operation of a complex series of interacting developmental factors and dynamisms that ultimately come under the conscious control of the individual. Eventually disintegration fades and development culminates in establishing a secondary harmonious integration. This secondary integration differs markedly from the first, primarily in that experience and life are now experienced as a multilevel phenomenon. The individual's behavior is now controlled internally through a synthesis of emotion and cognition that reflects his or her own unique hierarchy of values, aims, and goals reflecting his or her personality ideal.

3

DEVELOPMENTAL POTENTIAL

As mentioned in Chapter One, Dąbrowski emphasized that his approach to development was, in part, non-ontogenetic. To recap, most developmental theories are ontogenetic—development is a function of accumulating experience (or age) and proceeds in a stage-to-stage fashion. In non-ontogenetic development, new features may appear without precursors and some developmental features may not automatically or naturally occur in every individual. This has two major implications. First, in this framework, not everyone can achieve advanced development because not everyone has sufficient developmental potential. Second, as Dąbrowski described it, developmental potential is a constellation of features and forces that amalgamate and work synergistically to contribute to positive disintegration and to coordinate higher-level development. The central features of developmental potential include psychic overexcitability, the three factors, special abilities and talents, dynamisms and psychoneuroses. Not everyone with developmental potential will display all of these developmental features, and there will be differences in the strength of these features between individuals. As well, the interaction of these features will differ in each individual. Thus, for those who have sufficient developmental potential, not all will display the same features or sequence of steps on the pathway to advanced personal development.

3–1. THE THREE FACTORS OF DEVELOPMENT

Developmental potential is a relative measurement of the interaction and activity of each of three factors: *heredity*—innate, genetic influences; *externality*—the influence of the external, family and social environment; and a third, *internal autonomous* factor of self-directed development (Dąbrowski, 1970b, 1996).

Dąbrowski (1970b) said,

> The first factor is in most part the genetic endowment that an individual inherits from his parents plus all lasting effects of pregnancy, birth defects, nutrition, drugs, etc. The second factor represents the influences of the external environment, mainly family and social milieu. The third factor represents the autonomous forces of self-directed development. In this sense, the term "third factor" is used to denote the totality of the autonomous forces. In a stricter sense of a dynamism, the third factor is the agent of conscious choice in development. The third factor assumes gradually an essential part in human destiny and becomes the dominant dynamism of multilevel disintegration. (pp. 72-73)

The first factor plays a critical role in setting parameters and potentials for future development. Dąbrowski believed that the basis of individual essence and the factors that determine an individual's traits and development have their basis in his or her genetic endowment: "Our personality is shaped throughout our lives; our inborn characteristics constitute the basis determining our potential for inner growth" (Dąbrowski, 1967, p. iv). As we will see in more detail below, although Dąbrowski believed that people could influence their lives through the choices they make, writing under his pseudonym,[13] he said: "no experiences, no shocks, no breakdowns will trigger growth if the embryo of what is to develop is not there" (Cienin, 1972, p. 38). In addition to being positive or negative, Dąbrowski (1970b) recognized that these hereditary elements could also be more specific or more general.

Dąbrowski described an interaction between the first and second factors that we would today understand as the interaction between genetics and environment in the determination of phenotype. Dąbrowski suggested that the environment often played a secondary role depending upon the strength of the initial genetic factors present. As he used to say: "The best genetics will find a way to overcome the worst environment, the worst genetics can't be helped by the best environment" (K. Dąbrowski, personal communication, October, 1977) We see this anecdotally every day—"bad" kids sometimes come from good homes and good kids sometimes overcome the worst environments. Dąbrowski (1970b) described three major interactions between genetics and the environment:

- If the developmental potential is distinctly positive or negative, the influence of the environment is less important.
- If the developmental potential does not exhibit any distinct quality, the influence of the environment is important and it may go in either direction.
- If the developmental potential is weak or does not exhibit any distinct quality, the influence of the environment is important and may prove decisive, positively or negatively. (p. 34)

In Dąbrowski's theory, the "best genetics" are affected the least by the worst environment; the best environment has only a modest positive impact over the "worst genetics." Environment has a significant impact in determining the outcome of development when genetic factors are equivocal.

Dąbrowski's view of the genetics of development potential is confirmed by modern research. Toga and Thompson (2005) concluded:

Nature is not democratic. Individuals' IQs vary, but the data presented in this review and elsewhere do not lead us to conclude that our intelligence is dictated solely by genes. Instead genetic interactions with the environment suggest that enriched environments will help everyone achieve their potential, but not to equality. Our potential seems largely predetermined. (p. 17)

Initial developmental challenges often pit the first two factors against each other—"Do I follow my instincts (first factor) or do I follow my teachings (second factor)?" The emergence of the third factor introduces a new and significantly different element into this formula: "Or do I follow my personality ideal (third factor)?" Dąbrowski said that in the common course of maturation a "premature" integration of mental structures occurs based on "the desire to gain a position, to become distinguished, to possess property and to establish a family" and that "the more the integration of the mental structure grows, the more the influence of the third agent weakens" (Dąbrowski, 1964b, p. 57). Dąbrowski lamented the fact that many people accept essentially all social rules, values, and roles so casually. The average person becomes "mature" too quickly, and he suggested that advanced, authentic development requires a protracted maturation. People with strong developmental potential:

> must have much more time for a deep, creative development and that is why you will be growing for a long time. This is a common phenomenon among creative people. Simply, they have such a great developmental potential, "they have the stuff to develop" and that is why it takes them longer to give it full expression. (Dąbrowski, 1972b, p. 272)

The developmental solution to crises is to become more authentic—we have to transform what is in us that is less human, our lower instincts. In addition, one has to develop an autonomous personality by learning to choose for oneself and not simply follow socialized protocols. A developmental answer to the question posed above might be "listen to your heart, transform your biological instincts into positive features (for instance, motivation) and carefully think about and evaluate ready-made, rote, socially derived answers."

Dąbrowski (1972b) made it clear that the third factor focused upon the individual's active role in shaping his or her personality and in selecting an environment corresponding to one's character. Thus, the third factor involves a process of "conscious choice (valuation) by which one affirms or rejects certain qualities in oneself and in one's environment" (Dąbrowski, 1972b, p. 306). As Dąbrowski (1996) explained, this process of choice also allows the individual to differentiate and select higher positive elements from negative lower elements. This creates the vertical aspect so critical to multilevelness—"at the roots of the third factor are the ability to distinguish between lower and higher mental strata" (Dąbrowski, 1973, p. 77). As Dąbrowski (1964b) explained, the individual can now inhibit, reject, and transform the lower demands of instinct and socialization while selecting, affirming, and accepting the positive aspects from both the internal and external environments:

> Along with inborn properties and the influence of environment, it is the "third factor" that determines the direction, degree and distance of man's development. This dynamic evaluates and approves or disapproves of tendencies of the interior environment and of the influences of the external environment. (p. 53)

Two meanings are associated with the third factor: 1) a specific context defining third factor as a dynamism and 2) a broader meaning that incorporates all autonomous factors of development under the umbrella of third factor. As a dynamism, third factor provides a mechanism of conscious choice leading to either affirmation or negation of alternatives in both the internal and external environments. This mechanism implies self-examination and motivation to improve the self: "The first two factors allow only for *external motivation*, while the third is a factor of *internal motivation* in behavior and development" (Dąbrowski, 1996, p. 15). Dąbrowski (1996) said in a general sense:

> The third set of factors represents those autonomous processes which a person brings into his development, such as inner conflict, self-awareness, choice and decision in relation to personal growth, conscious inner psychic transformation, subject-object in oneself. When the autonomous factors emerge, self-determination becomes possible, but not before. (p. 14)

Third factor ultimately allows an individual to transcend the second factor and, at least to a degree, the initial parameters imposed on him or her by the first factor, "and by the maturational stages of the life cycle" (Dąbrowski, 1996, p. 14).

In describing the third factor, Dąbrowski (1973) realized he was creating a paradoxical construct: the elements of the third factor must initially be determined by and stem from hereditary (first factor) and be influenced by environment (second factor). However, Dąbrowski (1970b) was clear that the third factor is ultimately an emergent factor generated by the individual:

> We can only suppose that the autonomous factors derive from hereditary developmental potential and from positive environmental conditions; they are shaped by influences from both. However, the autonomous forces do not derive exclusively from heredity and environment, but are also determined by the conscious development of the individual himself. They appear at various developmental periods; they can be described and differentiated. (p. 34)

With advanced development, the third factor becomes independent in relation to the first and second factors and Dąbrowski (1964b) made it clear that the third factor emerges to play a dominant role in determining personality development:

> The appearance and growth of the third agent is to some degree dependent on the inherited abilities and on environmental experiences, but as it develops it achieves an independence from these factors and through conscious differentiation and self-definition takes its own position in determining the course of development of personality. (p. 54)

Again, we see Dąbrowski (1973) associating the origin and operation of the third factor with advanced growth itself:

> The genesis of the third factor should be associated with the very development with which it is combined in the self-consciousness of the individual in the process of becoming more myself i.e., it is combined with the vertical differentiation of mental functions. (p. 78)

In summary, Dąbrowski presented three factors of development. The first two factors are commonly associated with primary integration and concern the struggle of socialization to control and inhibit the free expression of our lower instincts. In the average "good citizen," the second factor dominates and mediates the first factor. A third internal and autonomous factor is associated with advanced growth. The third factor becomes an emergent force, surpassing its genetic roots and social influences to become a critical motivating force in an individual's development. The third factor operates in a coordinated and orchestrated fashion along with other developmental features, including developmental and creative instincts, dynamisms, and developmental potential. As these constructs are explored, a view of Dąbrowski's coordinated approach to development will coalesce.

3–2. THE ROLE OF INSTINCTS

Instincts play a critical role in Dąbrowski's theory; however, he formulated three important postulates concerning how instincts operate.

First, in a traditional approach, Dąbrowski (1973) described a group of basic, primitive, genetically based instincts that are common to both lower species and to man.

Second, in keeping with his non-ontogenetic approach, Dąbrowski described several human instincts not seen in lower species, including the developmental instinct, the instinct of self-development, creative instincts, and the instinct of self-perfection. These instincts have profound effects in contributing to the course and magnitude of development. Human instincts are characterized by the following attributes:

- They are a genuine force which is differentiated in the course of development from other instinctive forces.
- Their tension is equal to or higher than the tension of the basic, primitive instincts.
- They constitute a compact, strong and distinctly structured force.
- They appear and grow, not only in phylogenesis, but also in ontogenesis. (Dąbrowski, 1973, p. 11)

Finally, based on his non-ontogenetic initiative, Dąbrowski postulated that not all individuals will display the same instincts;

some individuals display developmental instincts, and some may not. Also, using his multilevel approach, Dąbrowski differentiated higher and lower instincts and, in addition, higher and lower levels within one instinct.

All development is associated with the strength and action of the developmental instinct. Dąbrowski (1970b) said:

> The developmental instinct [is an] instinct of a most general and basic nature, a "mother instinct" in relation to all other instincts; the source (in nucleus) of all developmental forces of an individual. It finds its expression particularly in such dynamisms as dissatisfaction with oneself, feelings of inferiority towards oneself, the third factor, inner psychic transformation, disposing and directing center at a higher level, autonomy and authentism, personality ideal. It acts differently at different stages of development, pushing the individual towards higher and higher developmental levels. It operates with variable intensity in most human individuals; among those with the ability for accelerated development it takes the form of education-of-oneself and autopsychotherapy. (p. 164)

In his studies of exemplars, Dąbrowski observed cases where an individual came to inhibit and transform lower instincts by exerting conscious control over "forces" that arise in the service of human development. The idea that development needs to involve the self-control of one's natural instincts dates back in Dąbrowski to at least 1937: "Exercises in submitting the natural instincts to the authority of the intellect and moral principles of a philosophy of life in order to reach a high degree of self-control and inner harmony is by all means desirable" (Dąbrowski, 1937, p. 100). I quote Dąbrowski (1964b) again because his words convey the exact meaning we need to understand:

> Throughout the course of life of those who mature to a rich and creative personality there is a transformation of the primitive instincts and impulses with which they entered life. The instinct of self-preservation is changed. Its direct expression disintegrates and it is sublimated into the behavior

of a human being with moral values. The sexual instinct is sublimated into lasting and exclusive emotional ties. The instinct of aggression continues in the area of conflicts of moral, social and intellectual values, changing them and sublimating itself. (p. 2)

Dąbrowski went on to describe what he perceived as a recent advance in human evolution involving the appearance of a general developmental instinct. The developmental instinct, while not universal, is a strong and irrepressible force of development. This instinct plays a critical role in the development of personality (Dąbrowski, 1964b):

Stimulated by this instinct the personality progresses to a higher level of development—the cultural human being—but only through disintegration of narrow biological aims. Such disintegration demonstrates that the forces of the developmental instinct are stronger than the forces of primitive impulses. The developmental instinct acts against the automatic, limited and primitive expressions of the life cycle. (p. 2)

Dąbrowski (1964b, p. 2) linked the developmental instinct to disintegration and ascribed the fundamental basis of growth to it, saying that "by destroying the existing structure of personality," the developmental instinct "allows the possibility of a reconstruction at a higher level." Dąbrowski's definition of developmental instinct showed its position relative to other instincts as an "instinct of a most general and basic nature, a 'mother instinct' in relation to all other instincts; the source (in nucleus) of all developmental forces of an individual" (Dąbrowski, 1970b, p. 164).

Dąbrowski differentiated two phases of the developmental instinct. The first phase reflects biological factors that determine its expression and is comprised of sub-instincts like self-preservation, fighting, sexual drive, herd instincts and so forth. In the second phase, the developmental instinct manifests itself through a loosening and disintegration of the individual's initial sense of him or herself ("the internal milieu") and by challenging the individual's adaptations to the environment. As one realizes how much of oneself is externally based and as one becomes more aware of one's internal psychological milieu, disappointments and dissatisfactions arise, creating the disease necessary to trigger a review of the status quo and to motivate change. This awareness is the first step in constructing and shaping one's personality. Subsequently, further development is directed by the unique expression of the developmental instinct as it becomes individualized to the unique aspects of one's character. This personality-building phase sees the emergence of the third factor, wherein an individual takes over conscious control and direction of his or her development, moving beyond the biological forces and beyond adaptations and reactions to the external environment. In this process, a picture of one's personality ideal forms and cognitive functions begin to be directed, and work toward, the realization of this ideal. Moments of new unification (partial secondary integrations) begin to appear, representing higher-level reintegrations of the individual's personality. This upward movement reflects the operation of several dynamisms and instincts that flow from the developmental instinct and that are characteristic of the higher levels of human development.

As the developmental instinct expresses itself, several "new instincts" subsequently and sequentially emerge: the instincts of self-development, of self-improvement, of creativity and, ultimately, of self-perfection. As just mentioned, concomitant with the operation of these instincts is the contribution of the third factor. Once again, we see an integrated and multilevel analysis differentiating lower animal-like instincts from higher, conscious, autonomous, and authentically human instincts associated with development. This hierarchization of instincts also contributes to Dąbrowski's description of the levels of development, the hierarchy of dynamisms, and the hierarchy of values. In development, the individual is able to exert control over his or her lower instincts in order to achieve idealized aims and goals or to express higher values. Dąbrowski (1964b) cited the example of Gandhi's hunger strike as proof of one's ability to control the instincts of self-preservation and hunger. Dąbrowski (1967) summarized his position in this idealistic quote:

The greater our experience in life, the greater our sensitivity; the more intensive and thorough our elaboration of experiences, the clearer our ideal of personality; and the more we are apt to sacrifice, to subordinate our instinctive needs in favor of personality, the stronger is our disposition to the attitude of courage and heroism. (p. 19)

To cite another example: At the level of secondary integration, the instinct of self-preservation is transformed and becomes a functional ambassador of one's personality, gradually merging with self-perfection to create a feeling of empathy and communion with other people and with all living creatures (Dąbrowski, 1970b). In contrast to the developmental picture just described, the basic primitive instincts in primary integration (the first phase of the developmental instinct) struggle to express themselves against the externally imposed control of the second factor, creating a self-centered, pleasure seeking and primitive orientation to life, ruled by drives, instincts, and stimulus-response reactions.

3–3. DEVELOPMENTAL POTENTIAL

The definition of developmental potential offered by Dąbrowski emphasized its genetic character and the fact that it sets parameters on development. Dąbrowski (1972b) described developmental potential as the "constitutional endowment that determines the character and the extent of mental growth possible for an individual" (p. 293).

Developmental potential is a relative measurement of the interaction and activity of each of the three factors. For instance, Dąbrowski (1996) said an individual's developmental potential may be limited to first factor or, more commonly, may display first and second factor influences:

In that case we are dealing with individuals who throughout their life remain in the grip of social opinion and their own psychological typology (e.g., social climbers, fame seekers, those who say "I was born that way" or "I am the product of my past" and do not conceive of changing). (pp. 14-15)

Dąbrowski (1996) continued that, ideally, an individual would initially display an interaction among all three factors of development:

The developmental potential may have its full complement of all three sets of factors. In that case the individual consciously struggles to overcome his social indoctrination and constitutional typology (e.g., a strongly introverted person works to reduce his tendency to withdraw by seeking contacts with others in a more frequent and satisfying fashion). Such a person becomes aware of his own development and his own autonomous hierarchy of values. He becomes more and more inner-directed. (p. 15)

From the initial mix of the three factors, the third factor emerges to become the dominant and critical developmental force in guiding and organizing the inner psychic milieu.

Dąbrowski (1996) recognized that the description of developmental potential based upon the contribution of the three factors "does not allow one to measure it independently of the context of development" (p.15). Thus, he identified the need to describe additional specific and measurable factors of developmental potential. Illustrating the latter, Dąbrowski suggested that "developmental potential can be assessed on the basis of the following components: psychic overexcitability, special abilities and talents and autonomous factors (notably the third factor)" (Dąbrowski, 1972b, p. 293). Dąbrowski (1996) noted: "The five forms of overexcitability are the constitutional traits which make it possible to assess the strength of the developmental potential independently of the context of development" (p. 16).

Dąbrowski (1972b) also linked developmental potential with the presence of psychoneuroses, an early and necessary early step in development:

It is the task of therapy to convince the patient of the developmental potential that is contained in his psychoneurotic processes. Obviously, to achieve that one has to show him this clearly and precisely on the concrete creative and "pathological" dynamisms that are active in his case. (p. viii)

Thus, the presence of psychoneurotic dynamisms can be taken as another measurable sign of developmental potential.

Dąbrowski (1996) made it clear that developmental potential is a necessary, but not sufficient, component of advanced development. Other conditions also must be met for development to proceed. Dąbrowski made the following observations about developmental potential:

- The degree of developmental potential varies among people and strong developmental potential is the exception, not the norm.
- Developmental potential may be positive or negative; may be general or specific; and may be strong, equivocal or weak.
- Strong developmental potential causes an individual to rebel "against the common determining factors in his external environment" (Dąbrowski, 1970b, p. 32).
  o If the potential is positive, one develops an individually chosen set of values reflecting how one can best be oneself and best work to elevate one's society.
  o If negative, the individual rejects social prohibitions and allows base instincts to run amok, injuring those who are unfortunate enough to be caught in his or her path.
- Strong developmental potential (either positive or negative) is expressed regardless of the environment. Mild developmental potential may not be expressed unless the environment is optimal. If the potential is "not universal and of weak tension," the "environmental influence is to a very great degree responsible for the path which will be taken" (Dąbrowski, 1972b, p. 12).
- Although Dąbrowski identified the third factor as a means to assess developmental potential, no test or measure of this factor has yet been developed, and none of the subsequent research on overexcitability has included the third factor as a component.

3–3–1. Overexcitability

In 1899 Clouston provided one of the first references to overexcitability in a description of "the conditions of neurotic children." These conditions were described as "pathogenetic states of deranged reactiveness of the neurons of the higher regions of the brain" (Clouston, 1899, p. 481). Clouston believed these conditions were primarily hereditary and essentially developmental.

The descriptions provided by Clouston (1899) resemble Dąbrowski's own:

> The first of those morbid states to which I would direct attention is a simple hyper-excitability; an undue brain reactiveness to mental and emotional stimuli. This may come on at any age, from three years to puberty. The child becomes ceaselessly active, but ever changing in its activity. It is restless and so absolutely under the domination of the idea which has raised the excitement that the power of attending to anything else is for the time being gone. (p. 483)

Clouston (1899) noted children sometimes become over-sensitized to external stimuli: "any loud noise will startle them and 'upset' them badly or will put them into a condition of trembling and terror. Any unusual or terrible sight will cause sleeplessness, tendency to nightmare and a condition bordering on hallucination." (p. 483)

Clouston (1899) was also articulate in his description of imaginational overexcitability, saying that "the intensity and actuality of their imaginations are greater than is consistent with sound working brain" and, at times, these children become "slaves of their over-excited imagination" (p. 484). Clouston (1899) continued:

> Children become for a time so over-imaginative that they cannot distinguish between their objective experiences and their subjective images and where, without stimuli from without, mental or bodily, they conjure up fancies so vivid that they mistake them for realities and talk about them accordingly. (p. 484)

Clouston (1899) recommended the use of "bromide of potassium [potassium bromide] with a minute quantity of arsenic every day" (p. 486) and said, "the bromides must be given fearlessly in large doses" (p. 489) and for long periods as a "treatment" for such cases.

William James (1907) noted that "scientific psychology" had completely ignored the notion of energy within individuals. In this essay, James observed that an individual's energy could vary widely;

some days one feels energetic; some days one feels lethargic; and he concluded that the average person utilized little of the energy potentially available to him or herself. James (1907) also described a barrier or dam holding back one's energy reserves that can sometimes be breached—for instance, in the case of an individual who is exhausted but who reaches down to tap his or her energy reserves and thus finds a "second wind." "The excitements that carry us over the usually effective dam are most often the classic emotional ones, love, anger, crowd-contagion, or despair. Life's vicissitudes bring them in abundance" (James, 1907, p. 6).

James (1907) described the average person's limited consciousness:

> Most of us feel as if we lived habitually with a sort of cloud weighing on us, below our highest notch of clearness in discernment, sureness in reasoning, or firmness in deciding. Compared with what we ought to be, we are only half-awake. Our fires are damped, our drafts are checked. We are making use of only a small part of our possible mental and physical resources. (p. 3)

In *The Varieties of Religious Experience*, James presented a connection between genius and neurosis and concluded that the combination of a "neurotic temperament" along with a superior quality of intellect would make it more probable that an individual would leave a mark and affect his or her age (James, 1902/1929, p. 26). James also connected the notion of excess energy ("ardor and excitability of character") with the neurotic temperament and went on to emphasize the "extraordinary emotional susceptibility" displayed by such a person (James, 1902/1929, p. 24). James (1902/1929, p. 256) also emphasized that differences in excitement are a major component of individual differences: "where the character, as something distinguished from the intellect, is concerned, the causes of human diversity lie chiefly in our *differing susceptibilities of emotional excitement* and in the *different impulses and inhibitions* which these bring in their train."

James described impulses pushing us one way (toward "yes") with dissonant obstructions and inhibitions resisting and saying "no"—this struggle forms the basis of one's moral attitude. Within an individual, James viewed emotional excitability as part of an "energetic character" being "exceedingly important" in overcoming one's lower inhibitions. James also suggested that differences among people could also be explained in a similar way: "When a person has an inborn genius for certain emotions, his life differs strangely from that of ordinary people, for none of their usual deterrents check him" (James, 1902/1929, p. 259). In such individuals, the typical struggle between impulses and inhibitions is not seen; rather, they are free of "inner friction and nervous waste" and consequently they are able to boldly pursue their ideals without inhibition (James, 1902/1929, p. 260). James (1902/1929) concluded:

> The difference between willing and merely wishing, between having ideals that are creative and ideals that are but pinings and regrets, thus depends solely either on the amount of steam-pressure chronically driving the character in the ideal direction, or on the amount of ideal excitement transiently acquired. (pp. 260-261)

In a footnote, James emphasized the importance of the higher excitabilities: "The great thing which the higher excitabilities give is *courage*; and the addition or subtraction of a certain amount of this quality makes a different man, a different life" (James, 1902/1929, p. 260).

In carefully reviewing James's (1899) work, we also find another passage that seems to describe various types of increased excitability ("eagerness") quite similar to the schema that Dąbrowski arrived at:

> Wherever a process of life communicates an eagerness to him who lives it, there the life becomes genuinely significant. Sometimes the eagerness is more knit up with the motor activities, sometimes with the perceptions, sometimes with the imagination, sometimes with reflective thought. But, wherever it is found, there is the zest, the tingle, the excitement of reality; and there is "importance" in the only real and positive sense in which importance ever anywhere can be. (pp. 9-10)

Dąbrowski may have been exposed to the work of James during

the year he spent visiting Harvard University in 1933, although Dąbrowski makes no reference to James.

The construct of overexcitability was evident in Dąbrowski's writing from the beginning. The basic forms of "hyperexcitability," "psychic overexcitability," and "overexcitability" (synonymous terms) were described in his 1937 monograph (Dąbrowski, 1937). The five specific forms of overexcitability were first articulated in English in Dąbrowski (1964b): "Loosening of structure occurs particularly during the period of puberty and in states of nervousness, such as emotional, psychomotor, sensory, imaginative and intellectual overexcitability" (p. 6). Dąbrowski (1972b) clearly placed overexcitability in a neurological context, explaining:

> Each form of overexcitability points to a higher than average sensitivity of its receptors. As a result, a person endowed with different forms of overexcitability reacts with surprise, puzzlement to many things, he collides with things, persons and events, which in turn brings him astonishment and disquietude. One could say that one who manifests a given form of overexcitability and especially one who manifests several forms of overexcitability, sees reality in a different, stronger and more multisided manner. Reality for such an individual ceases to be indifferent but affects him deeply and leaves long-lasting impressions. Enhanced excitability is thus a means for more frequent interactions and a wider range of experiencing. (p. 7)

In this definition, Dąbrowski mentioned higher-than-average sensitivity of the nerves (receptors). Additionally, Dąbrowski (1972b) also emphasized a higher-than-average responsiveness of the nerves to stimuli. Dąbrowski also explained why he used the term overexcitability: "The prefix over attached to 'excitability' serves to indicate that the reactions of excitation are over and above average in intensity, duration and frequency" (Dąbrowski, 1996, p. 7).

In summary, two critical neurological aspects define overexcitability: a lowered threshold to stimuli making one more sensitive and, second, heightened responses to stimuli compared to the average person.

Dąbrowski also mentioned that individuals will usually display a characteristic response type—one of the five forms of overexcitability will generally be dominant: "For instance, a person with prevailing emotional overexcitability will always consider the emotional tone and emotional implications of intellectual questions, i.e. what do they mean for people's feelings and experiences" (Dąbrowski, 1996, p. 7). An individual will "channel" his or her overexcitability into the form most appropriate for him or herself. For example, a person with dominant imaginational overexcitability will tend to

> close themselves in the world of imagination, they isolate themselves in the outdoors or in their room, they read, they think or meditate, they go to see plays or films in order to see things other than those they tire of because of familiarity and lack of freshness. (Dąbrowski, 1972b, p. 66)

Dąbrowski (1972b) also suggested that overexcitability "widens and enhances the field of consciousness" (p. 66), an important aspect because development in general is accompanied by increasing degrees of consciousness, both of the self and of one's environment.

Dąbrowski talked about overexcitability in yet another context, describing it as "a term introduced to denote a variety of types of nervousness," and he used the terms overexcitability and nervousness synonymously (Dąbrowski, 1996, p. 7). In his glossary, Dąbrowski (1972b) defined nervousness as enhanced psychic overexcitability and listed the five types.

The following descriptions of overexcitability are direct quotations from Dąbrowski (1996, p. 72), and each is followed by another description in square brackets from Dąbrowski (1972b, p. 7).

> *Sensual overexcitability* is a function of a heightened experiencing of sensory pleasure. It manifests itself as need for comfort, luxury, aesthetics, fashions, superficial relations with others, frequent changes of lovers, etc. As with the psychomotor form it also may, but, need not be, a manifestation of a transfer of emotional tension to sensual forms of expression of which the most common examples are overeating and excessive sexual stimulation. In children, sensual overexcitability manifests itself as a need for cuddling,

kissing, clinging to mother's body, early heightened interest in sexual matters, showing off and need to be with others all the time. [An individual who is excessively sensitive sensually possesses a more or less superficial sensitivity to beauty, is suggestible, is more exposed to the difficulties of life.]

Psychomotor overexcitability is a function of an excess of energy and manifests itself, for example, in rapid talk, restlessness, violent games, sports, pressure for action, or delinquent behavior. It may either be a "pure" manifestation of the excess of energy, or it may result from the transfer of emotional tension to psychomotor forms of expression, such as those mentioned above. [An individual who is psychomotorically overexcitable is restless, curious, cannot sit still in one place, wanders around, has an insatiable need of change and of "wandering into space."]

Imaginational overexcitability in its "pure" form manifests itself through association of images and impressions, inventiveness, use of image and metaphor in verbal expression, strong and sharp visualization. In its "impure" form emotional tension is transferred to dreams, nightmares, mixing of truth and fiction, fears of the unknown, etc. Imaginational overexcitability leads to an intense living in the world of fantasy, predilection for fairy and magic tales, poetic creations or invention of fantastic stories. [An individual who is overexcitable in respect to imagination is sensitive toward "imaginational realities," is usually creative, has vivid fantasy and is often full of ideas and plans. He displays abilities in poetry, art or music. He has his "kingdom of dreams and fantasy."]

Intellectual overexcitability in contrast to the first three does not distinctly manifest the transfer of emotional tension to intellectual activity under specific forms. This does not mean that intellectual and emotional processes of high intensity do not occur together. They do, but they do not appear to take on such distinct forms. Intellectual overexcitability is manifested as a drive to ask probing questions, avidity for knowledge, theoretical thinking, reverence for logic, preoccupation with theoretical problems, etc. [An individual intellectually overexcitable shows strong interests early in inner and in external life, has strong nuclei of analysis and synthesis. Early in life he is capable of asking questions and demanding logical answers.]

Emotional overexcitability is a function of experiencing emotional relationships. The relationships can manifest themselves as strong attachment to persons, living things or places. From the developmental point of view presented here, intensity of feelings and display of emotions alone are not developmentally significant unless the experiential aspect of relationship is present. [An individual who is emotionally overexcitable is sensitive, takes everything to heart, is syntonic and even more often empathic, though not necessarily in a highly developed manner. He has a need of exclusive and lasting relationships, of help and protection, of understanding suffering.]

It is the nature and expression of the mix of many developmental features that initially determines developmental potential and, ultimately, its expression. In terms of overexcitability, Dąbrowski (1972b) talked about "the big three," referring to the fact that three forms appear to be more important than the other two: "Some forms of overexcitability constitute a richer developmental potential than others. Emotional (affective), imaginational and intellectual overexcitability are the richer forms. If they appear together they give rich possibilities of development and creativity" (p. 7).

In another passage, Dąbrowski (1996) said:

Developmental potential is strongest if all, or almost all forms of overexcitability are present. The three forms, intellectual, imaginational and emotional, are essential if a high level of development is to be reached. The highest level of development is possible only if the emotional form is the strongest, or at least no less strong than the other forms. Great strength of the psychomotor and the sensual forms limits development to the lowest levels only. (p. 16)

Overexcitability has several profound impacts on a person. One effect is quite visceral: overexcitability heightens the impact of experiences on the autonomic nervous system, expressed in such symptoms as trembling of the hands, headaches, unpleasant feelings of tension, and flushing of the skin (Dąbrowski, 1970a). Overexcitability may also represent an experiential challenge, creating overwhelming feelings, especially for a younger person. As one becomes more aware of the overall impact of overexcitability, and especially of its developmental aspects, one commonly comes to manage these challenges in stride.

Dąbrowski called overexcitability a "tragic gift." One of Dąbrowski's students, Peter Jensen (2009), explained that Dąbrowski:

called them gifts because, for example in the case of emotional overexcitability, these people really feel the world. They are in touch with all the joy and the suffering; they experience at an emotional level all that they and others are going through. He called them tragic because the world was not yet ready for people who felt at such a deep level. (p. 12)

Dąbrowski (1996) said that when an overexcitable person experiences "higher highs" and "lower lows" it helps bring into consciousness a multilevel view of life:

Enhanced excitability, especially in its higher forms, allows for a broader, richer, multilevel and multidimensional perception of reality. The reality of the external and of the inner world is conceived in all its multiple aspects. High overexcitability contributes to establishing multilevelness, however in advanced development, both become components in a complex environment of developmental factors. (p. 74)

Dąbrowski (1970a) differentiated and highlighted the two roles played by overexcitability:

It is, on one hand, a basis for excitement, inner and external conflicts, tension, sadness, depression, anxiety and so on and—on the other hand—a basis for [a] universal and more complicated view of reality but in a different light: vital, full of contrasts and non-automatic. (pp. 2-3)

Finally, and perhaps most significantly, Dąbrowski (1970b) made overexcitability an integral part of disintegration, both by definition and by clinical observation:

First, psychic hyperexcitability, whether general or more differentiated (emotional, psychomotor or, intellectual) provokes conflicts, disappointments, suffering in family life, in school, in professional life; in short, it leads to conflicts with the external environment. Hyperexcitability also provokes inner conflicts as well as the means by which these conflicts can be overcome. Second, hyperexcitability precipitates psychoneurotic processes and third, conflicts and psychoneurotic processes become the dominant factor in accelerated development. (p. 38)

Overexcitability increases an individual's sensitivity to both the external environment and to his or her internal psychic environment, thus creating disappointments, unpleasant emotional reactions, and conflicts (Dąbrowski 1970a).

Overexcitability also creates the basis and opportunities for new, higher, and more complicated solutions to conflicts and crises. Dąbrowski (1973) emphasized the importance of overexcitability to development: "It is mainly mental hyperexcitability through which the search for something new, something different, more complex and more authentic can be accomplished. All this is associated with the loosening and disintegration of primitive homeostasis" (p. 15).

As a person moves forward through development, the character and expression of the different forms of overexcitability change and "undergo extensive differentiation" (Dąbrowski, 1996, p. 16). "The characteristics of a low level of development as being primitive, of little consciousness (reflection) and control, ahierarchical, egocentric, selfish and non-creative, apply also to the manifestations of overexcitability" (Dąbrowski, 1996, p. 74). At lower levels, the five forms tend to be disjointed and may occur in isolation; for example, psychomotor and intellectual overexcitability may occur with little imaginational or emotional overexcitability. If strong psychomotor and sensual forms exist in isolation, development is limited to the lowest levels. At higher levels, the expression of the five forms of overexcitability becomes more integrated and coordinated, and all five work together. As well, at higher levels, the fundamental nature and expression of the overexcitabilities changes. When influenced by emotional, imaginational, and intellectual overexcitability, the character and expression of the sensual and psychomotor forms "are transformed and serve, among other things, to energize individuals" (Mendaglio & Tillier, 2015, p. 222). Dąbrowski (1996, pp. 75-78) presented brief descriptions of each overexcitability at each of the five levels.

To illustrate, I will provide examples of three overexcitabilities, detailing Level I through Level IV (he did not give Level V examples), quoted directly from Dąbrowski (1996, pp. 75-78).

Psychomotor Overexcitability

Level I

> Violent irritability and uncontrollable temper with easy return
> to equilibrium, general restlessness, impulsive actions, need
> for frequent changes of jobs and places, primitive wanderlust
> (impulse to be constantly on the go), juvenile delinquency
> (frequent running away from home, frequent attempts to
> escape from detention, stealing cars, getting into fights, etc.).

Level II

> Ambivalences and ambitendencies bring about, from time to
> time, a suspension of the drivenness of activity and replace it
> instead by somewhat more controlled activity.

Level III

> Psychomotor overexcitability comes into closer linkage with
> higher forms of overexcitability (emotional, imaginational and
> intellectual) and begins to be transformed and modified by
> them. Within the drivenness of psychomotor overexcitability
> appear inhibitions, multilevel conflicts, energetic search for
> channels "upward." Psychomotricity plays thus a role in the
> formation of a new DDC at a higher level because of the
> person's decisiveness.

Level IV

> Psychomotor overexcitability provides the dynamics and
> energy for carrying out a developmental program of action. In
> Patanjali's *Yoga Sutras* we find a statement: "Success in yoga
> comes quickly to those who are intensely energetic" (aphorism
> 21, Prabhavananda and Isherwood, 1953). At this level,
> psychomotor overexcitability is totally subordinated to higher
> forms of overexcitability and provides theta with "executive"
> power.

Imaginational Overexcitability

Level I

Imagination is in the service of sensualism and impulsiveness. It is manifested in confabulation, facile mendacity, identification with such externally defined roles as, for instance, the office of the president or "I am the boss." It is also manifested in acting out such roles with theatrical gestures to enhance the effect. Mesmerism of rally and revival speakers belongs here as well.

Level II

Productive and seemingly fertile creativity, primitive suggestibility (magic, witchcraft, spiritism), success in acting on stage but not as the highest and universal art. Unselective taste for fantasy and adventure stories. Occasionally intense visions of the future, egocentric fantasy (self-delusion) and anxiety states. Frequent dreams and daydreaming, interest in dream symbolism, especially sexual.

Level III

Imaginational overexcitability becomes more closely associated with emotional and intellectual forms. There is differentiation of the "lower" from the "higher" in imagination and creativity. Dreams and symbolic contents are distinctly multilevel. Dreams and visions of the ideal. Creative instinct makes contact with the instinct of self-perfection.

Level IV

The multilevel characteristics of imaginational overexcitability described for Level III become intensified at this level. They serve as tools of conscious development of personality; they become more fully engaged in the realization of transcendental needs.

Emotional Overexcitability

Level I

Aggressiveness, irritability, lack of inhibition, lack of control, envy, unreflective, periods of isolation or an incessant need for tenderness and attention, which can be observed, for instance, in mentally retarded children.

Level II

Fluctuations, sometimes extreme, between inhibition and excitation, approach and avoidance, high tension and relaxation or depression, syntony and asyntony, feelings of inferiority and superiority. These are different forms of ambivalence and ambitendency.

Level III

Interiorization of conflicts, differentiation of a hierarchy of feelings, growth of exclusivity of feelings and indissoluble relationships of friendship and love. Emotional overexcitability appears in a broader union with intellectual and imaginational overexcitability in the process of working out and organizing one's own emotional development. The dynamisms of spontaneous multilevel disintegration are primarily the product of emotional overexcitability.

Level IV

Emotional overexcitability in association with other forms becomes the dominant dimension of development. It gives rise to states of elevated consciousness and profound empathy, depth and exclusivity of relationships of love and friendship. There is a sense of transcending and resolving of one's personal experiences in a more universal context.

Recent works have criticized the construct of overexcitability as largely the same construct as openness to experience, part of the five-factor model (Vuyk, Kerr, & Krieshok, 2016; Vuyk, Krieshok, & Kerr, 2016). "Openness facets and OEs appear to represent the same construct, and thus the giftedness field would benefit from discussing the construct as the personality trait of openness to experience" (Vuyk, Krieshok, & Kerr, 2016, p. 205).[14] Vuyk and her colleagues take the position that overexcitabilities in the field of gifted education have been applied as atheoretical—standalone descriptive traits, often assumed to be normally distributed in the population—and that overexcitability research has been conducted in isolation of Dąbrowski's broader theory. As has been noted before (Mendaglio & Tillier, 2006, p. 83), *at least* research on overexcitability should be expanded to look at the other basic components of development potential (especially the third factor). I concur with the fundamental observations of Vuyk and her colleagues in concluding that the existing research on overexcitabilities leaves much to be desired. In particular, this research views the overexcitabilities as unitary constructs and does not consider the different expressions of each overexcitability on each different level of development. This would seem *prima facie* to invalidate these studies.

In an interesting article, Karpinski, Kinase Kolb, Tetreault, and Borowski (2017) made the case that intellectual overexcitability (hyper brain) is connected to a general overexcitability of the body (hyper body) and that intellectual overexcitability is associated with a number of severe disorders, including: mood and anxiety disorders, ADHD/ADD, autism spectrum disorders, food and other allergies, and asthma and autoimmune disorders. The authors presented a theoretical model of the impact of intellectual overexcitability on both psychological disorders and physiological diseases—an impact that results in a significantly greater prevalence of several significant disorders.

3–3–2. Sensory Processing Sensitivity

Elaine Aron has presented a construct generally referred to as sensory processing sensitivity (SPS) (e.g., Acevedo et al., 2014; Aron, 1996, 2002, 2006, 2010, 2012; Aron & Aron, 1997; Aron, Aron, &

Jagiellowicz, 2012; Boterberg & Warreyn, 2016; Homberg, Schubert, Asan, & Aron, 2016; Miu, Bîlc, Bunea, & Szentágotai-Tătar, 2017). Research has found that individuals fall into "3 distinct groups with different levels of Environmental Sensitivity—low (approx. 25–35%), medium (approx. 41–47%), and high (20–35%)" (Pluess et al., 2017, p. 1). The latter group comprises what Aron has called the highly sensitive person (HSP). Aron, Aron, & Jagiellowicz (2012) presented SPS as a genetically determined trait—motivated by higher emotional reactivity, SPS triggers deeper levels of processing of sensory information and deeper cognitive processing of stimuli.

Aron's work on the HSP has become very popular and the construct she has described certainly appears to overlap with Dąbrowski's observations of overexcitability. On the other hand, the way these two authors view the impact of being sensitive is quite different. Aron views sensitivity almost like a doctor would treat an allergy—one must act to minimize overstimulation. Aron (1996) advocated that if stimuli are overwhelming, one should modify the environment to protect oneself, for example, by changing jobs if necessary. In another example, those bothered by noise should wear noise cancelling headphones. Aron (1996) advocated striving for homeostasis—to find and maintain one's optimal level of arousal. Dąbrowski advocated that overexcitability plays a vital role in personality growth that often leads to feelings of intense dis-ease; the motivation needed to break homeostasis and to develop.

Other approaches to environmental sensitivity are found in the literature on psychiatry. For example, in 1995, Kendler et al. (1995) studied the differential effects of stressful life events in the induction of depression. A summary of this research was provided in Kendler and Prescott (2006). It appears that the genetic risk for depression is expressed in two ways: genetics influences the overall liability to depression (independent of the environment), and genetics controls an individual's sensitivity to the depressogenic effects of the environment (variance in susceptibility to stressful life events). The authors call this the genetic control of sensitivity to the environment (stress sensitivity) (Kendler & Prescott, 2006). In other words, "the importance of environmental influences can vary dramatically as a function of genetic factors" (Dick et al., 2015, p. 3). This environmental sensitivity has been linked to depression, a broad range of stress-linked pathology, and personality traits (Caspi, Hariri, Holmes, Uher, & Moffitt, 2010).

Another line of research suggests that a variation in a gene involved in serotonin transport is implicated in environmental sensitivity (Caspi et al., 2010). Specifically, people who carry the short version of the 5-HTTLPR allele are thought to be more sensitive to emotional cues and stimuli in the environment than people with the long allele version (Conway, Slavich & Hammen, 2014; see also Palma-Gudiel & Fañanás, 2017).

Fox and Beevers (2016) explored the molecular genetics and environmental context (G × E interactions) that "might underlie individual variation in sensitivity to the environment" (p. 1). Their model suggests "that biased cognitive processing of emotional information may be one critical pathway through which differential susceptibility influences psychological wellbeing" (Fox & Beevers, 2016, p. 1; see also Halldorsdottir & Binder, 2017).

A review of this research area supported the social/differential susceptibility approach, described above, and made recommendations to improve research methodology (Leighton, Botto, Silva, Jiménez, & Luyten, 2017).

3–3–3. Other aspects of developmental potential

Special abilities and talents, another aspect of developmental potential, also play a major role in development as one takes what one does well and incorporates it into one's development. Examples include intellectual ability, musical ability, artistic ability, kinesthetic aptitudes, and other specialized traits and abilities. Conventional measurements of these abilities and traits are used in assessing an individual. It's important to keep in mind that in advanced development an individual will ideally display an integration and balance between special abilities and talents and his or her overall personality growth, including multilevel and emotional development.

In some cases, an individual ability or talent may be particularly strong in isolation—lacking overall personality development. Dąbrowski called this situation "one-sided development." Dąbrowski (1996) gave the example of a female musician who:

spends a lot of energy perfecting her music and feels highly responsible for the quality of her skill, even to the point of feeling that others should not end up taking blame for her imperfections. But we do not observe her spending much energy in perfecting herself as a person. (p. 164)

In these cases, talents may be used in the service of lower individual interests—for example, in trying to achieve status or fame, or in the service of social goals. A scientist working for the military may be an illustration. Essentially these are expressions of "ability without morality." This is why high intelligence alone cannot be used as an index of developmental potential and why Dąbrowski (1970b) was concerned with the high likelihood for damage done by individuals with high intelligence but low emotional development:

We find this negative type of development in its less successful form in individuals inhabiting prisons, in its more forceful, one-sidedly perfected form among political and military national leaders, labour union bosses, etc. In this last case, grave affective retardation is usually associated with above average intelligence subordinated to primitive drives. Leaders of criminal gangs belong to this group. Two eminent psychopaths Adolf Hitler and Joseph Stalin displayed this kind of mental structure characterized by lack of empathy, emotional coldness, unlimited ruthlessness and craving for power. (p. 30)

At lower levels, people tend to do what they do well at (behavior is determined and driven by genetic ability in a given area). For instance, tall children often play basketball (but they may not really have a passion for it). With balanced development, the focus of special abilities and talents shifts: one directs (subjugates) the expression of one's talents in the service of one's higher goals, personality ideal, and values (the tall child may quit the basketball team and join the chess club because that is his or her real passion).

3–4. CHAPTER SUMMARY

Development is based upon a complex interaction of many

different genetic elements including instincts, specific abilities, and talents, plus various uniquely developmental features. Dąbrowski used the phrase "developmental potential" to refer to a constellation of features he observed in exemplars of advanced personality development. Developmental potential is not a universal attribute—Dąbrowski only observed it in a minority of cases. Advanced development invariably involves clear signs of strong developmental potential. Perhaps the central feature in this formulation is a developmental instinct, expressed largely through an autonomous, conscious, and internal factor of development (the third factor). Dąbrowski also described overexcitability as a necessary precondition of development. Overexcitability involves a heightened sensitivity and over-reactivity to stimuli that contribute to generating crises and to establishing a multilevel view of reality. As we will see in the subsequent two chapters, strong developmental instinct and developmental potential lead to the loosening and disintegration of the initial psychological structures which, in turn, provide opportunities for the advanced features of development to become active in creating and shaping one's personality.

4

THE DEVELOPMENTAL PROCESS
AND PSYCHONEUROSES

4–1. APPROACHES TO INTEGRATION

Dąbrowski carefully differentiated states of integration and disintegration as a central element of the theory. Dąbrowski (1967) acknowledged significant influences, saying: "The terms integration and disintegration were used by Descartes and later by Spencer, Hughlings Jackson, then by Sherrington, Pavlov and others" (p. 58). In fact, Dąbrowski culminated and synthesized the ideas of several theorists who discussed integration and levels within the nervous system.

Herbert Spencer (1820-1903) described a cycle where a first phase dominated by integration—what we call growth—is followed by a middle phase which includes alternating excesses of both integration and disintegration, leading to a final phase characterized by disintegration and ultimately death (Spencer, 1900). The notions of integration and disintegration were broadly applied to all existence, including biology, geology, astronomy, sociology, and psychology. Accordingly, Spencer linked the ideas of integration and disintegration with the dominant scientific paradigm of the day, matter and motion: dissolution is "the absorption of motion and disintegration of matter; we shall everywhere mean by Evolution, a process which is always an integration of matter and dissipation of motion" (Spencer, 1900, p. 261).

Spencer used the term integration to describe the process of growth, and he also associated a shift from "incoherent homogeneity" to a "coherent heterogeneity" with growth and evolution, having observed that higher animals display a well-integrated nervous system not found in lower types. As Fullinwider (1983) explained:

> Herbert Spencer had been describing a central nervous system featuring integrative levels, the lower levels corresponding to more primitive functions. Man, with his higher levels, was said to be able to cognize, thus manifesting a much more refined adjustment to his world than the fight-flight functioning of animal. It was Spencer's model that Hughlings Jackson adopted to account for the behavior of the brain-damaged and mentally ill. He urged a "level theory" in which "integration," "re-integration," and "re-reintegration" take place at several anatomical levels. (p. 152)

Hughlings Jackson (1884) made it clear that each level of the nervous system is a functional level represented by its own operational integration. The hierarchy of levels observed represents a phylogenetic model of successive, newer levels of integration and function. At its highest level, consciousness, as defined by speech, supersedes lower levels, allowing their activities to go on unconsciously in the background.

One of the implications of Hughlings Jackson's (1884) theory is that each level of the nervous system is more or less self-contained and displays internal integration. In addition, higher order integration occurs when higher levels exercise integrative and control functions over lower levels. There is an overall vertical "meta-integration" in the healthy nervous system—a coordinated system of subareas, each playing their role and contributing to the gestalt of the whole, a view reflected in modern neuropsychology (e.g., Kolb & Whishaw, 2014, 2015). This meta-integration is similar to Maturana and Varela's (1987) idea of second order unity.

Sir Charles Sherrington's 1906 volume, *The Integrative Action of the Nervous System,* brought the construct of integration to the neurological lexicon (Sherrington, 1906/1948). In addition, several authors contributed to introducing the integration construct to personality. Morton Prince (1854-1929), an American neurologist, wrote in 1929:

> If traits are mental processes why can we not change them at will and so change our personalities—change our sentiments, our prejudices, our ideals, our attitudes and feelings, as we can change our thoughts from one topic to another, or change our clothes? . . . To my mind the most satisfying theory, to which I am forced by long continued observation and studies, is that of "Integration of Dispositions." According to this theory traits depend upon the organization of inherited and acquired psychophysiological dispositions. That is to say, they are the functioning of organized integrates of such dispositions. (p. 429)

It is worthwhile to consider Prince's (1929) analysis of personality in detail:

> Accordingly, we may say, as a final analysis of traits: Personality is the sum total of all the biological innate dispositions of the individual and of all the acquired dispositions and tendencies—acquired by experience. And it is limited to these.
>
> The former would embrace the emotions, feelings, appetites and other tendencies manifested in instinctive reactions to the environment; the latter the memories, ideas, sentiments and other complexes of intellectual dispositions acquired and organized within the personality by the experiences of life.
>
> The integration into one functioning organism or whole of all these innate and acquired dispositions, with their mechanisms and inherent forces by which they come into play, is personality. (p. 431)

Prince (1929) described the dynamic potentiality of traits within the personality structure as emotional or instinctive mechanisms that create energy. Prince described three important corollaries of his approach:

1. That human behavior and personality will not be determined by a single vital principle such as libido, *"but rather* [by] *the motivating energy derived from and inherent in the different inherited (instinctive) dispositions and the many multiform, integrated and organised systems of acquired dispositions created by the experiences of life."* (p. 432)

2. *"A second corollary is that personality is a synthetic product . . . of which the properties are determined by the number, combinations and configurations of selected elements."* (p. 432)

3. *"A third corollary is that any personality theoretically can be modified or reconstructed or transformed into another synthetic product with traits corresponding to the new synthesis."* (p. 432)

In conclusion, Prince (1929) believed that "personality can be changed by modifying, reconstructing its traits and organizing new ones by the creative force of new experience" (p. 432).

Another important milestone was a lengthy discussion of personality integration in a popular 1938 textbook by Louis Thorpe, *Psychological Foundations of Personality.* Following Sherrington, Thorpe said integration "stands for a wholeness in personality which gives direction to the coordination of parts" (Thorpe, 1938, p. 434). Thorpe's (1938) perspective is important for us to understand; the integrated personality is:

characterized by unity of action in which the responses of parts or aspects have meaning only in terms of their relation to the action of the whole; all work together under the direction of a central self and in harmony with the plans and purposes of the individual concerned. (p. 434)

Thorpe advocated adjustment to one's social milieu, concluding that the combination of "rational analysis" and volition—a push or a drive that acts to buttress one's thoughts—leads toward integration.

Dąbrowski (1972b) defined integration as "an organization of instinctive, emotional and intellectual functions into a coordinated structure" (p. 296). He described two types; primitive (or primary) integration (Level I) and secondary integration (Level V). In Dąbrowski's view, the common route of maturation (development through stages) leads to a "premature integration" of mental structures reflecting a "desire to gain a position, to become distinguished, to possess property and to establish a family" (Dąbrowski, 1964b, p. 54). Dąbrowski was clear that the stronger this initial integration, the less the individual can influence his or her development. Dąbrowski (1964b) said that "the more the integration of the mental structure grows, the more the influence of the third agent weakens" (p. 54). However, as mentioned above, some individuals may break free of the forces governing normal ontogenetic development. A key early feature of this shift in development entails a loosening and disintegration of the primitive instincts. This disintegration also rocks the unity of the individual's personality structure, creating opportunity for change—the reconstruction of a new integration on a higher level.

Various other works have examined integration in personality (e.g., Fajkowska & DeYoung, 2015; Hearn & Seeman, 1971; Royce, 1983; Seeman, 1959, 1966, 1983, 1989; Seeman, Barry, & Ellinwood, 1963; Widiger, 2016).

4–2. APPROACHES TO DISINTEGRATION

Tracing the idea of disintegration also takes us back to Herbert Spencer. As Rizzo (1999) pointed out, Spencer's view of the cosmos was one of mechanical processes of evolution and dissolution. Spencer said, "evolution involves 'loss of motion and consequent integration' while dissolution is the 'gain of motion and consequent disintegration' that follows evolution" (Rizzo, 1999, p. 122). Just as Spencer described evolution as creating more complex and more integrated structures, dissolution reduces complexity and integration. Spencer went on to describe an oscillation between forces predisposing evolution and forces creating dissolution.

Given Spencer's influence on Hughlings Jackson, it comes as no surprise that evolution and dissolution were equally prominent in Hughlings Jackson's work. Hughlings Jackson (J. Taylor, 1958, vol.

II) explained:

> The higher nervous arrangements evolved out of the lower to
> keep down those lower, just as a government evolved out of a
> nation as well as directs that nation. If this be the process of
> evolution, then the reverse process of dissolution is not only "a
> taking off" of the higher but is at the very same time a "letting
> go" of the lower. (p. 58)

William James (1902/1929) also outlined the process of
disintegration:

> Now in all of us, however constituted, but to a degree the
> greater in proportion as we are intense and sensitive and
> subject to diversified temptations and to the greatest possible
> degree if we are decidedly psychopathic, does the normal
> evolution of character chiefly consist in the straightening out
> and unifying of the inner self. The higher and the lower
> feelings, the useful and the erring impulses, begin by being a
> comparative chaos within us—they must end by forming a
> stable system of functions in right subordination. Unhappiness
> is apt to characterize the period of order making and struggle.
> If the individual be of tender conscience and religiously
> quickened, the unhappiness will take the form of moral
> remorse and compunction, of feeling inwardly vile and wrong
> and of standing in false relations to the author of one's being
> and appointer of one's spiritual fate. This is the religious
> melancholy and "conviction of sin" that have played so large a
> part in the history of Protestant Christianity. The man's
> interior is a battleground for what he feels to be two deadly
> hostile selves, one actual, the other ideal. (pp. 167-168)

The above quotation encapsulates several Dąbrowski notions:

- The propensity of the character to evolve is associated with
  increased intensity and sensitivity.
- This evolution is accomplished by modifications ("a
  straightening out") and subsequent reintegration of the self
  ("unifying of the inner self").

- Multilevel conflicts arise when higher versus lower feelings are contemplated.
- This period of unhappiness and chaos (disintegration) is resolved after changes and a reordering of the self.
- James (1902/1929, p. 168) pointed out that one's inner experience (inner psychic milieu) is a "battleground" between the actual self ("the is") versus the ideal self ("the ought to be").
- James used the phrase "psychopathic temperament" and "psychopathic degeneration" in *The Varieties of Religious Experience*; however, he used the terms in describing what is essentially a neurotic constitution—in our terminology, a sensitive individual prone to anxiety and self-doubt. For example, in describing the Christian writer and preacher, John Bunyan (1628-1688), James said he "was a typical case of the psychopathic temperament, sensitive of conscience to a diseased degree, beset by doubts, fears and insistent ideas and a victim of verbal automatisms, both motor and sensory" (James, 1902/1929, p. 154).

Another important author who discussed integration and disintegration was Frederick Thorne (1909-1978). Thorne (1976) presented "a new approach to psychopathology based on a psychology of integration as applied to psychological states" (p. 751). Thorne reasoned that because all behavior occurs in psychological states, psychopathology must refer to disorders of integration—disintegration is found in all mental disorders and lack of integration is associated with failure to adapt. There are many interesting parallels between Thorne's approach and Dąbrowski's. For example, Thorne's integrative psychopathology begins with the assumption that complex integrated states are achieved through hierarchical organizing factors and that "psychic development depends on the organization of progressively higher levels of integration, in the absence of which the person is mentally retarded" (Thorne, 1976, p. 751). In listing the various types of integrative disorders, Thorne described disintegrations that may be acute, chronic, global or partial, and that are characterized by a disruption of the function of inner processes. Further, Thorne suggested: "The goal is for each person to transcend his own previous levels of integration and even possibly to establish new world records of specific achievements," and, "The highest integration levels make possible increasingly complex levels of self-control, i.e., the person becomes more and more the cause of his own effects" (p. 754). Thorne (1976) described the process of development:

> In the developmental process, growth proceeds in stages and patterns of increasing integrative complexity. The person normally transcends lower levels of integration in a process that even may eventuate in striving to transcend the highest previous human accomplishment, i.e., to achieve new world records for qualitative or quantitative peak experiences. Literally, "the sky is the limit," and no one knows what he can accomplish unless he struggles to achieve progressively higher levels of controlled performance.
>
> The young person often is satisfied with lower levels of accomplishment (which in themselves may represent excellent achievement), but still be unaware of higher levels of peak experience simply because he has not yet lived long enough to know what they involve or to have achieved the experience that makes them possible. (p. 758)

Thorne's perception was that the average person is in a state of limited integration and is essentially "half awake." In describing the current situation as he saw it, Thorne (1976) painted a grim picture:

> From the scientific psychobiologic viewpoint, every living thing starts out as an experiment of nature; only a few relatively perfect specimens ever occur. Man has an average mental age of 14 years, is subject to all kinds of developmental trauma, is conditioned more or less haphazardly by imperfect educational systems and rarely achieves maximal self-actualization of resources. Any realistic evaluation of the nature of Man must result in a characterization of immaturity, imbalance, inadequacy, ineffectuality, nonproductivity and lack of achievement as demonstrated by the huge hordes of also-rans who never

achieve distinction. (p. 760)

Dąbrowski (1972b) used the term disintegration to mean a "loosening, disorganization or dissolution of mental structures and functions" (p. 293). Dąbrowski (1964b) elaborated a continuum of disintegration: "The term disintegration is used to refer to a broad range of processes, from emotional disharmony to the complete fragmentation of the personality structure, all of which are usually regarded as negative" (p. 5). Dąbrowski (1967) was clear that disintegration involves fundamental changes for an individual:

> When a man oversteps the normal, common life cycle there begin to act such new tendencies and aims and such attractive values, that, without them, he sees no more meaning in his own existence. He must leave his present level, lift himself to a new, higher one and, on the other hand, must, as we have said before, retain his unity, retain the continuity of his psychophysical life, his self-awareness and identity. (p. 49)

Dąbrowski (1967) continued: "The development of personality, therefore, takes place in most cases through disintegration of man's present, initial, primarily integrated structure and, through a period of disintegration, reaches a secondary integration" (p. 49).

4–3. DĄBROWSKI'S TYPES AND DEGREES OF DISINTEGRATION

Dąbrowski differentiated disintegration into distinct types and degrees: positive and negative disintegration; unilevel disintegration (Level II); two types of multilevel disintegration: spontaneous multilevel disintegration (Level III) and organized multilevel disintegration (Level IV); partial disintegration; and finally, global disintegration.

Dąbrowski described the subtypes of disintegration as follows:

- *Unilevel*: involves "conflicts between drives and emotional states of a similar developmental level and of the same intensity" (Dąbrowski, 1970b, p. 165).
- *Multilevel*: "conflicts between higher and lower levels of

instinctive, emotional or intellectual functions" (Dąbrowski, 1970b, p. 165).

- *Negative disintegration*: also called involutional disintegration. "Characterized by the presence and operation of dissolving dynamisms and by the lack of developmental dynamisms. It occurs almost solely at the stage of unilevel disintegration" (Dąbrowski, 1970b, p. 165). May result in serious, chronic mental illness.
- *Positive disintegration*: "effects a weakening and dissolution of lower level structures and functions, gradual generation and growth of higher levels of mental functions and culminates in personality integration" (Dąbrowski, 1970b, pp. 165-166).
- *Spontaneous*: an initial form of multilevel disintegration. A relative preponderance of spontaneous developmental forces.
- *Organized or self-directed*: the second, higher form of multilevel disintegration. A period of conscious organization and direction in the application of the processes of disintegration.
- *Global disintegration*: involves all mental functions. Can result from one major disintegration or from many partial disintegrations: "It transforms the whole mental structure and thus paves the way for a new global integration at the level of personality" (Dąbrowski, 1970b, p. 166).
- *Partial disintegration*: Dąbrowski (1972b) said:

> Disintegration within one or a few related dynamisms. It may lead either to reintegration at a previous level, to reintegration at a lower level (primitive integration), to partial integration at a higher level, or to global disintegration. Partial disintegrations followed by partial integrations at a higher level characterize the developmental pattern of people with average developmental potential. In contrast, global disintegration and global secondary integration (if any) are the privilege of people with rich endowment for accelerated development. (p. 300)

- *Partial multilevel disintegration*: occurs within one or a few interconnected dynamisms. It can either regress back to a lower primitive disintegration, advance into a global disintegration, or lead to a partial integration at a higher level than previously existed. As Dąbrowski (1970b) explained:

> Partial multilevel disintegration is a result of limited hereditary endowment and psychic experiences limited to a narrow sphere. These cause a loosening or disintegration of narrow, primitive structures. The partial secondary integration at a higher level, which usually follows, is a result of inner psychic transformation within a limited area. An accumulation of a great number of partial integrations at a higher level may culminate in a global disintegration and later formation of personality. Partial disintegrations culminating in partial integrations at higher levels are the usual endpoint of mental development of people with average sensitivity and average endowment. (p. 166)

4–4. POSITIVE DISINTEGRATION

There is no question that the idea of positive disintegration was formed early in Dąbrowski's life. We clearly see it in his first major English work in 1937 (Dąbrowski, 1937):

> Frequently, independent of disease, or after having gone through a psychotic episode, great mental suffering because of conflicts, or a crisis, stabilization of the personality at a higher level occurs (Beers, Dostoyevsky). States of struggle of conflicting complexes, suppression and torture of one complex by another often produce outbursts of energy from a strong tension in the form of creative activity (Dostoyevsky, Schopenhauer, Nietzsche, Weininger, Zeromski and others). (pp. 99-100)

The origins of Dąbrowski's framework likely began in response to Hughlings Jackson and his disciple, Jan Mazurkiewicz (1871-1947).

Mazurkiewicz, a prominent Polish psychiatrist, was Dąbrowski's medical professor and was a major influence. Hughlings Jackson and Mazurkiewicz described dissolution as the opposing force of evolution. Hughlings Jackson (1884) stated that the highest levels with the most complexity will display the least organization and will therefore be less stable, more fragile, and prone to breakdown. This approach was influential in the early understanding of mental illness. In Hughlings Jackson's widely accepted view, mental illnesses involved "dissolution" of higher levels that normally exert control over lower, simpler, and more automatic structures. If the dissolution of higher levels becomes too great, the inhibitory effects of the higher levels fail and allow the lower levels to function unchecked. For Hughlings Jackson, initial neurotic symptoms were a sign of this dissolution process and the first step in a cascade towards major mental illness and total mental "involution."

Dąbrowski (1970b) rejected the Hughlings Jackson/Mazurkiewicz position and countered with the observation that in many cases, the breakdown of higher-level integrations appeared to play a key role in one's evolution; these disintegrations are *required* developmental features, needed to transform and reorganize one's internal psychological makeup. Dąbrowski (1970b) said:

> In the process of multidimensional disintegration, the individual goes beyond his biopsychological developmental cycle, his animalistic nature, his biological determination and slowly achieves psychological and moral self-determination. The human individual, under these conditions ceases to direct himself exclusively by his innate dynamisms and by environmental influences but develops autonomous dynamisms such as "subject-object" in oneself, the third factor, or personality ideal. (p. 60)

Dąbrowski called this process positive disintegration to stress its developmental direction and to differentiate it from the traditionally negative views of disintegration as described by Hughlings Jackson and that went on to influence conventional views of mental illness.

From the beginning, Dąbrowski recognized the role of pain and suffering in personality development. For instance, in his monograph on self-mutilation Dąbrowski said: "The endurance of pain, discomforts and fear were indispensable qualifications of a leader or of a high personality" (Dąbrowski, 1937, p. 34). In this early work, Dąbrowski was beginning to lay the foundations for his approach to personality based upon the experience of suffering. He suggested that suffering which leads to guilt causes introspection, self-sufficiency and introversion—attributes that Dąbrowski (1937) considered the "mark of personality." Finally, Dąbrowski (1937) viewed suffering as an indispensable bridge to reach intense spiritual experiences and, eventually, the transition to a spiritual life.

Continuing throughout his work, Dąbrowski emphasized the vital role of suffering and crisis in human life and made it clear that it is this suffering that defines our humanity: "We are human inasmuch as we experience disharmony and dissatisfaction, inherent in the process of disintegration" (Dąbrowski, 1970b, p. 122). Dąbrowski's (1973) description of the magnitude of the disintegrative process is often shocking to many people:

> Every authentic creative process consists of "loosening," "splitting" or "smashing" the former reality. Every mental conflict is associated with disruption and pain; every step forward in the direction of authentic existence is combined with shocks, sorrows, suffering and distress. (p. 14)

This quotation also includes another important construct in Dąbrowski's model—that one's experience of reality (the reality function) changes and is transformed during the developmental process.

Dąbrowski (1964b) observed that periods of developmental crises are characterized by symptoms of positive disintegration and that there is a close and clear relationship between personality development and the process of disintegration. Development pits the emerging personality against the negative elements of both the internal and external milieus, creating day-to-day conflicts and stress. In addition, severe external stressors, such as a car accident or death of a loved one, also may be linked to symptoms of positive disintegration; such symptoms may be evidence of both distress and growth. Major crises usually involve a great deal of emotion and often lead to deep reflection about life and about one's self: "Crises are periods of increased insight into oneself, creativity and personality development" (Dąbrowski, 1964b, p. 18).

Dąbrowski linked the effect of stress with the level of developmental potential of the individual. Severe stress in the absence of developmental potential cannot generate developmental transformations: "The chances of developmental crises and their positive or negative outcomes depend on the character of the developmental potential, on the character of social influence and on the activity (if present) of the third factor" (Dąbrowski, 1972b, p. 245).

Dąbrowski also observed that the lives of people who display advanced development invariably exhibit significant periods of disintegration, characterized by strong conflicts, crises, and suffering. Examples I offer include, William James (1842-1910), Carl Jung (1875-1961), Clifford Beers (1876-1943), Charlie Parker (1920-1955), Ingmar Bergman (1918-2007), William Blake (1757-1827), Agatha Christie (1890-1976), Winston Churchill (1874-1965), Joseph Conrad (1857-1924), T. S. Eliot (1888-1965), Ernest Hemingway (1899-1961), Henry James (1843-1916), Kurt Vonnegut Jr. (1922-2007), Jackson Pollock (1912-1956), Sylvia Plath (1932-1963), Vincent van Gogh (1853-1890), and Soren Kierkegaard (1813-1855).

Dąbrowski (1970b) made it clear that disintegration is an integral and fundamental part of development:

> The consequence of these observations was a hypothesis that in normal individuals every manifestation of development is, to a greater or lesser degree, related to disintegration and that in very creative individuals, development is strongly correlated with inner disharmony, nervousness and some forms of neurosis. (p. 20)

In contrast to traditional approaches where higher levels transcend and include the features and qualities of lower-levels (e.g., Wilber, 1996), positive disintegration is a process of transition whereby lower functions are replaced by higher ones. Through positive disintegration, "normal man" undergoes a restructuring of mental functions, evolving into a highly developed individual: "In the course of evolution from higher animals to man and from the normal man to the universally and highly developed man, we observe processes of disintegration of lower functions and an integration of higher functions" (Dąbrowski, 1972b, p. 62). In Dąbrowski's (1964b) theory, disintegration allows an opportunity for developmental forces to reorganize the initial structures, culminating in a higher-level reconstruction:

> Disintegration of the primitive structures destroys the psychic unity of the individual. As he loses the cohesion that is necessary for feeling a sense of meaning and purpose in life, he is motivated to develop himself. The developmental instinct, then, following disintegration of the existing structure of personality, contributes to reconstruction at a higher level. (p. 3)

As disintegration and growth continue, the features of development become linked to volition—the individual comes to exert conscious control over his or her development. A high level of self-awareness of internal conflicts allows volitional control and, in turn, allows for the conscious restructuring and transformation of internal psychic structures. Another critical element of advanced development was Dąbrowski's (1964b) observation that this developmental reorganization is not primarily cognitive or intellectual. Instead, it involves a basic breakdown and reconstruction of the emotional structures, facilitating deep empathy and connections with other people.

The developmental process that James described was also similar to Dąbrowski's—the "intense and sensitive" individual experiences multilevel conflicts. He or she must volitionally differentiate his or her various possible selves, actively choose among the selves, deny many, and actively choose one higher self under which to subordinate one's lower selves. James wrote: "So the seeker of his truest, strongest, deepest self must review the list carefully and pick out the one on which to stake his salvation" (James, 1890/1950, p. 310).

As described above, the theory of positive disintegration delineates three phases of disintegration—unilevel disintegration and two types of multilevel disintegration. Unilevel disintegration involves horizontal conflicts leading to strong ambivalence and ambitendency. There is little consciousness or self-awareness at this level. Horizontal conflicts are not developmental and unilevel disintegrations are transitory, usually ending in a reintegration back at the initial level.

For Dąbrowski, the crux of development is heralded by a qualitatively new type of conflict, a vertical or multilevel conflict between higher and lower levels of functions. The discovery of higher levels in the external environment and the subsequent discovery and self-examination of higher levels in one's own psychological milieu create the forces necessary for multilevel positive disintegration. "As soon as the process of hierarchization becomes more pronounced, the differences between that which is closer to 'more myself' and that which is more distant ('less myself'), between 'what is' and 'what ought to be,' becomes clearly distinguishable" (Dąbrowski, 1970b, p. 22). The "vertical solution" to internal conflicts is to choose higher over lower alternatives, thus moving upward and signaling the hallmark of development: "One also has to keep in mind that a developmental solution to a crisis means not a reintegration [at the same or lower level] but an integration at a higher level of functioning" (Dąbrowski, 1972b, p. 245).

4–5. NEUROSES AND PSYCHONEUROSES

4–5–1. Historical overview

It is helpful to have a context of the history of the terms neurosis and psychoneurosis. William Cullen (1710-1790), an influential Scottish doctor, was the first to use the term neurosis in 1769, to describe "disordered motions or sensations of the nervous system" (Knoff, 1970, p. 80). Cullen's belief was that healthy function was based upon the operation of a "vital principle" reflected by normal "nervous energy" and the movement of nervous ("etheric") fluid that, in its excited state, coordinated bodily functions and transmitted sensation throughout the body (Forget, 2003). Abnormal movement of this fluid was the root of all disease. For Cullen, neurosis referred to any symptom or disorder characterized by abnormal nervous or mental dysfunction and located in the nervous system (Neve, 2004).

Accordingly, mental disorders had a corresponding physical location in the nervous system and were thus neurological (physical) in origin.

Neve (2004) described the subsequent influences of Franz Anton Mesmer (1734-1815), known for his research on animal magnetism, the prominent French neurologist Jean-Martin Charcot (1825-1893) and fellow French neurologist Hippolyte Bernheim (1840-1919):

> Neurosis began to mean a fairly mild mental state in which there was no loss of contact with reality but rather various forms of defensive exaggeration present. Acute anxiety, obsession, compulsion, phobias—these were now neuroses, with all connections to the Cullenite organic causes jettisoned. (p. 1170)

Knoff (1970) noted that Philippe Pinel (1745-1826) accepted the nervous component of neuroses but also believed they had a moral component as well. This implied that these disorders were at least in part caused by psychological factors and therefore psychological treatments or "moral treatments" could be used in cases of neurosis. Pinel's approach set the stage for Sigmund Freud.

4–5–1–1. Sigmund Freud's views on neuroses

Freud's influence was significant, and his approach again changed how neuroses were viewed. Dąbrowski (1972b) gave an excellent overview of Freud's position:

> The cause of various unconscious processes is the contradictory action of two opposite desires (or purposes), one of which is apparent and the other hidden and unconscious. The subconscious and the unconscious processes are expressed in dreams often in symbolic form, acceptable to the censor or "guard" who watches, as it were, on the borderlines of consciousness. This censor, according to Freud, is a function of the "ego" (*Ich*), or our personal consciousness, developed by the instinct of self-preservation. Corresponding to the conscious "ego" is the dark and primitive aspect of our personality, the "id" (*Es*). In the subconscious there is also the "superego" (*hber-Ich*). "Superego" is the subconscious representative of our relations with our parents, it represents

the internalization of parental prohibitions, expressing the need for penance and punishment; it is the source of religious and social sentiments. . . . Neuroses, according to Freud, result from the conflicts between the "ego" and the "id". The "ego" depends on reality and in trying to adjust to reality, represses part of the "id": the "ego" is then transferred from the pleasure principle to the reality principle. The action of the pleasure principle is thereby thwarted. This results in an improper development. (pp. 226-227)

In other words, the individual unconsciously struggles to repress certain elements of the id. These thoughts, conflicts, desires, memories and so forth, often focus on unacceptable sexual desires, or memories of intense, inappropriate (for example, murderous) feelings toward a parent or other loved one. If these ideas were to become conscious, they would be quite threatening and upsetting to the person, so the ego must unconsciously try to repress them and block their expression. Anxiety arises when these types of thoughts are only partially repressed or when they threaten to resurface back into one's consciousness. As anxiety mounts, neurotic symptoms will occur either to directly express the anxiety or to act as a defense against it. Freud (1920) stated:

We believe that civilization was forged by the driving force of vital necessity, at the cost of instinct-satisfaction, and that the process is to a large extent constantly repeated anew, since each individual who newly enters the human community repeats the sacrifices of his instinct-satisfaction for the sake of the common good. Among the instinctive forces thus utilized, the sexual impulses play a significant role. They are thereby sublimated, i.e., they are diverted from their sexual goals and directed to ends socially higher and no longer sexual. But this result is unstable. The sexual instincts are poorly tamed. Each individual who wishes to ally himself with the achievements of civilization is exposed to the danger of having his sexual instincts rebel against this sublimation. Society can conceive of no more serious menace to its civilization than would arise through the satisfying of the sexual instincts by their redirection toward their original goals. (p. 8)

In another quote, Freud (1920) said:

I frequently noticed that a man who contented himself with incomplete sexual gratification, with manual anonism [masturbation], for instance, would suffer from a true neurosis (p. 335) . . . These neuroses [are] disturbances in sexual metabolism. It may be that more sexual toxins are produced than the individual can dispose of, or that inner, even psychic conditions, stand in the way of the proper elaboration of these substances. (p. 337)

Freud's "true neuroses" included neurasthenia, anxiety neurosis, and hypochondria—physical neuroses, much as Cullen had described them. In these cases, the cause and the symptom appear at the same time and no psychic trauma is apparent. For Freud, actual neuroses are organically (physically) generated by sexual etiology. As explained in the quotation above, anxiety neuroses occur due to the accumulation of somatic excitation which either goes undischarged or is incompletely satisfied by masturbation (because it results in only a partial relief) (Knoff, 1970). Freud suggested that all energy was derived from the libido, and as we can clearly see, he was afraid of the consequences of an individual allowing his or her energy free expression. Rather, he believed that a healthy individual should sublimate his or her libido into many controlled activities and subroutines that gave some pleasure, while preventing the expression of their "true, darker desires." These latter desires must be prevented because they would involve acts abhorrent to a civilization (incest, rape, murder, stealing and so forth). A "civilized libido" gives its owner the energy to succeed and accomplish great things in society, whereas the unrepressed libido runs amok and ruins one's life.

4–5–1–2. Abraham Maslow's views on neuroses

Another relevant author to consider on the topic of neuroses is Abraham Maslow. Unfortunately, Maslow's thoughts on neuroses are presented in a disjointed and somewhat contradictory manner. In an article originally published in 1967 and reprinted in Maslow (1971/1976), it was proposed that practically all people have an active impulse or will to grow and move toward actualizing one's potential;

however, few people (one in a hundred, or one in two hundred, adults)[15] achieve this goal (Maslow, 1968, p. 163, p. 204). The question was asked, "What blocks it?" Maslow's answer was that on one hand, part of our human nature is a "will to health" encouraging the individual to develop and creating "pressure to self-actualization" (Maslow, 1968, p. 193). In describing the will to health, Maslow said it was "the urge to grow, the pressure to self-actualization, the quest for one's identity" (Maslow, 1962, p. 180). Individual differences are seen in this will to health, and therefore some people display stronger growth motivation relative to others. On the other hand, there are strong forces of regression in ungratified deficiency-needs and it takes significant willpower and courage to leave the relative safety and defensive posture of the status quo in order to take chances and grow (Maslow, 1968). Maslow (1966) emphasized the dichotomy between growth versus fear, saying that "fear must be overcome again and again" (p. 22).

Even when deficiency needs are satisfied and growth is chosen, this is no guarantee that self-actualization will be achieved. The result of failure is a general illness of the personality, created by any "falling short of growth, or of self-actualization, or of full-humanness" and caused primarily by the frustration of one's basic needs, the B-values, individual potentials, and the individual's tendency to grow in his or her own style and at his or her own pace (Maslow, 1968, pp. 193-194).

B-values are "being values," important universal values that define one's being. Self-actualized people tend to incorporate more B-values than those at lower levels. Examples include truth, goodness, wholeness, perfection, uniqueness, justice, simplicity, playfulness, self-sufficiency, etc.

Maslow described a continuum ranging from failure to growth—from diminution to a full growth that he referred to as full humanness: "Maslow seems to interpret the psychoneuroses as representing a weakness in the capacity of a person for the healthy realization of self, as a diminution in humanness" (Dąbrowski, 1972b, pp. 247-248). Maslow (1970) said, "it is now seen clearly that most psychopathology results from the denial or the frustration or the twisting of man's essential nature" (p. 269) and he asked, "What is psychopathological? Anything that disturbs or frustrates or twists the course of self-actualization" (Maslow, 1970, p. 270).

Given the contrast with full humanness, Maslow suggested the term "human diminution" better captured failures of growth and was preferable to the term neurosis "which is anyway a totally obsolete word" (Maslow, 1971/1976, p. 29). Maslow (1971/1976) went on:

> Strictly speaking, neurosis means an illness of the nerves, a relic we can very well do without today. In addition, using the label "psychological illness" puts neurosis into the same universe of discourse as ulcers, lesions, bacterial invasions, broken bones, or tumors. But by now, we have learned very well that it is better to consider neurosis as rather related to spiritual disorders, to loss of meaning, to doubts about the goals of life, to grief and anger over a lost love, to seeing life in a different way, to loss of courage or of hope, to despair over the future, to dislike for oneself, to recognition that one's life is being wasted, or that there is no possibility of joy or love, etc. (p. 30)

In an excellent review of Maslow, Colin Wilson[16] (1972) noted Maslow's view that neuroses represented a kind of stabilization of the impulses to grow, and this stasis removed one's motivation to pursue higher growth opportunities, resulting in a negative passivity that causes both depression and neuroses. Thus, a neurosis represents an essentially passive state—noise without action—that is essentially self-destructive largely due to frustrated life energies turned inward (Wilson, 1972, p. 173). For Maslow, neuroses represent a failure of personal growth—a "blockage of the channels of self-actualisation" (Wilson, 1972, p. 198).

Maslow (1970) also described the neurotic as being "psychologically retarded," failing to overcome his or her childhood perceptions and acting as if he or she is afraid of receiving a spanking: "Such a person behaves as if a great catastrophe were almost always impending, i.e., he is usually responding as if to an emergency" (Maslow, 1970, p. 42).

Maslow (1970, p. 142) also endorsed the Freudian view of neuroses as coping mechanisms. According to this view, neurotic behaviors are primarily functional or provide coping mechanisms and do an actual job for the person such that he or she is better off for having the symptom. Maslow (1970) observed that the necessary role played by these symptoms, analogous to a foundation holding up a house, made therapy "dangerous for truly neurotic symptoms" (p. 142).

In another passage, Maslow (1968, p. 205) described a neurosis as a defense against one's inner core, or an evasion of it, as well as a distorted expression of it. One expresses one's neurotic needs, emotions, attitudes, definitions, etc., at the expense of expressing one's true inner core or real self. These neurotic expressions reduce the capacity of an individual to be him or herself, thus producing a "diminished human being."

In discussing perceptions of reality, Maslow (1970) said that "the neurotic is not emotionally sick—he is cognitively wrong!" (p. 153). In another major discussion of Maslow, Goble (1970) explained that neuroses and psychoses represent a stunting of growth and are "cognitive diseases" contaminating one's perceptions, learning, remembering, attention and thinking (Goble, 1970, p. 74). A person diminishes psychological health by allowing desires to distort perceptions of the world. It is only the truly mature (self-actualizing) individual who can see him- or herself and reality as they truly exist and not as he or she wishes them to be. Goble (1970) further elaborated Maslow's position:

> Neuroses may also be recognized as the inability to choose wisely: that is, to choose in conformance with one's true psychological needs. People may be divided into good and bad choosers, just as chickens may be. Some people who are poor perceivers can believe in falsehoods year after year even though truth continually stares them in the face. (p. 74)

Maslow's position implied that neuroses are self-created: "People who fail to develop their talents, who live dull, uninteresting lives, who never develop workable methods of relating to other people, subconsciously know that they have wronged themselves for it. From this, 'neurosis' develops" (Goble, 1970, p. 74). To emphasize the point, Maslow found "intelligent people leading 'stupid lives' which led to boredom, loss of zest, self-disapproval and even physical deterioration" (Goble, 1970, p. 76).

Adding confusion in Maslow's interpretation of neuroses was his suggestion that personality required challenge to facilitate growth. Discipline, deprivation, frustration, pain, and tragedy help an individual to discover his or her inner nature and, when successfully overcome, contribute to a sense of achievement, self-esteem, and self-confidence. The untested person has doubts that he or she could overcome such obstacles (Maslow, 1968). Maslow (1971/1976) elaborated:

Conflict itself is, of course, a sign of relative health as you would know if you ever met really apathetic people, really hopeless people, people who have given up hoping, striving and coping. Neurosis is by contrast a very hopeful kind of thing. It means that a man who is frightened, who doesn't trust himself, who has a low self-image, etc., still reaches out for the human heritage and for the basic gratifications to which every human being has the right simply by virtue of being human. You might say it's a kind of timid and ineffectual striving toward self-actualization, toward full humanness. (p. 33)

Neuroses as a positive feature were again implied in a passage from Maslow (1968) when he said:

All his [the neurotic's] conflicts and splits turn out to have a kind of sense or wisdom. Even the constructs of sickness and of health may fuse and blur when we see the symptom as a pressure toward health, or see the neurosis as the healthiest possible solution at the moment to the problems of the individual. (p. 92)

Moss (2001) makes an insightful remark summarizing Maslow's approach to neuroses:

Maslow envisioned humanistic psychology as a psychology of the whole person, based on the study of healthy, fully functioning, creative individuals. He criticized the psychologists of his time for spending too much time studying mentally ill and maladjusted humans and for seeking to explain higher levels of human experience by means of neurotic mechanisms. (p. 15)

In summary, Maslow presented several different viewpoints and interpretations of neuroses. Frustratingly, he did not present a coherent approach and his references to a positive view of neuroses were vague. Perhaps his most dominant view was that neuroses were the result of an individual's failure to satisfy his or her needs and to achieve self-actualization, and that lack of will and fear hold most people back from making day-to-day decisions to grow; they choose instead to remain in a secure and defense-oriented stasis—a crippling passivity leading to depression and neurosis. Although Maslow indicated that growth required successfully overcoming challenge, his overall view of neuroses was negative, perceiving them as blockages to growth. Thus, Maslow did not agree with Dąbrowski's view that these mental conditions and their symptoms help define what makes us human or that they were a prerequisite for, or even a form of, growth.

4–5–1–3. Psychoneurosis

The term psychoneurosis was introduced by Thomas Smith Clouston (1840-1915), a pioneer in the psychiatric study of adolescence, in his 1883 book, *Clinical Lectures on Mental Diseases*. *The Oxford English Dictionary* defined psychoneurosis as "mental disease, especially without organic lesion or recognized mental weakening" (Weiner & Simpson, 1991, p. 2347).

Freud described three psychoneuroses: conversion hysteria, anxiety hysteria (phobia), and obsessional neurosis (Rycroft, 1968/1995, p. 145). These conditions result from psychic (psychological) excitation, primarily caused by sexual conflicts occurring in childhood and often the result of psychological trauma. Unlike the neuroses, where symptoms and causes appear at the same time, the psychological conflicts causing psychoneuroses were thought to occur prior to the appearance of symptoms, usually many years before.

Historically, usage was disjointed, and neurosis and

psychoneurosis were often used synonymously (Townsend & Martin, 1983). Psychoneurosis (psychoneurotic disorder) was originally used in the *Diagnostic and Statistical Manual of Mental Disorders* (1st ed., American Psychiatric Association, 1954, p. 44). The *Diagnostic and Statistical Manual of Mental Disorders* (2nd ed., American Psychiatric Association, 1968) dropped psychoneurosis but described several types of neurosis, as did the *Diagnostic and Statistical Manual of Mental Disorders* (3rd ed., American Psychiatric Association, 1980). Neurosis did not appear after DSM-III. The *International Classification of Diseases and Related Health Problems* (ICD-10 version: 2016) still uses the term "psychoneurotic personality disorder."

4–5–2.   Dąbrowski's   perspective   on   neuroses   and psychoneuroses

Dąbrowski rejected traditional perspectives on the roles played by neuroses and psychoneuroses. He developed a multilevel, hierarchical description of mental symptoms that reflected his belief that such symptoms are often associated with development. It must be kept in mind that at the lower levels, little development is seen; therefore, the presence of symptoms lacks the developmental connotations and implications compared to symptoms appearing at higher levels where significant developmental potential exists. For example, at the level of primary integration individuals may experience feelings of anxiety and depression. These emotional states are invariably the result of interactions and conflicts with the external environment and lack the developmental implications they have at higher levels.

For example, an individual may feel anxiety over an upcoming test, or may be depressed over losing a job. At the level of primary integration, the individual attempting to seek solutions in the environment, for instance, by studying harder or by getting a new job, generally copes with these experiences. The individual's integration may not be penetrated—his or her integrated sense of self is not brought into question.

One of the hallmarks of developmental crises is that developmental potential intensifies those crises, making them break through the individual's integration and thus leading to deep and inescapable questions focused upon the self: "Why can't I be smarter, stronger? What's the matter with me?" This increased focus upon the self may lead to increased self-awareness, self-doubts and, often, feelings of anxiety and dissatisfaction focused on the self. These feelings create the dis-ease necessary to motivate further self-development. While external crises may produce intense feelings, they do not generally involve much internal conflict in the absence of developmental potential and there is little impetus for individual development or growth in resolving such situations.

Traditional psychiatry viewed neurotic and psychoneurotic symptoms as pathological obstacles to growth. Dąbrowski said this view was "responsible for inhibition, isolation, non-creative feeling of inferiority and lack of a creative and rich development" (Dąbrowski, 1972b, p. 12). This lack of acceptance created the "loneliness of psychoneurotics," as was eloquently described in Dąbrowski's poem, "Be Greeted Psychoneurotics!"[17] (Dąbrowski, 1972b, p. xvi).

The idea that psychoneuroses could play a positive role was a major source of disagreement between Dąbrowski and his peers and is arguably one reason why the psychiatric and psychological community was reluctant to embrace the theory of positive disintegration. We have seen Hughlings Jackson's influential position that a neurosis was the beginning of a complete mental breakdown. Dąbrowski (1972b) disagreed with this position and said that "if anything, psychoneuroses prevent the development of mental breakdown" (pp. 220-221). In a more contemporary example, Maslow and Dąbrowski disagreed over the role of psychoneuroses, an issue we will discuss further in Chapter Eight. Maslow saw psychoneuroses as blockages or "holes" that needed to be "patched" before development could proceed. Most contemporary theorists continue to reject the idea that symptoms may play a positive developmental role.

As we have seen, Freud was a major influence in creating the contemporary understanding of the nature and role of neurosis. Dąbrowski was quite critical of the lack of lower versus higher differentiation (multilevelness) in Freud's approach, as well as Freud's lack of appreciation for any major ongoing psychological development. Specifically, Dąbrowski (1972b) rejected Freud's approach to neurosis, saying it was "permeated with pansexualism, having a dominance of the 'libido' principle without properly appreciating psychoneurotic processes in personality development and without noticing the role of 'developmental drive'" (p. 229).

One of Dąbrowski's major contributions was in making a paradigm shift in the perception of symptoms and their role in development. "The theory of positive disintegration places a new orientation on the interpretation of nervousness, anxiety, neurosis, hysteria, psychasthenia, depression, mania, paranoia and schizophrenia" (Dąbrowski, 1964b, p. 14). In describing the process of development, Dąbrowski (1972b) made the roles of neuroses and psychoneuroses explicit:

> Nervousness, neuroses and especially psychoneuroses, bring the nervous system to a state of greater sensitivity. They make a person more susceptible to positive change. The higher psychic structures gradually gain control over the lower ones. The lower psychic structures undergo a refinement in this process of inner psychic transformation. This transformation is the fruition of the developmental potential that makes these states possible and makes possible further development. (p. 160)

Dąbrowski's glossary entry for neurosis reads: "psychophysiological or psychosomatic disorders characterized by a dominance of somatic processes. There are no detectable organic defects, although the functions may be severely affected" (Dąbrowski, 1972b, p. 299). Dąbrowski (1972b) said, "we shall apply the term 'neurosis' or 'somatic neurosis' only in those cases where physiological components (organs or systems of organs) are involved" (p. 40). Dąbrowski went on to note that the defects involved in the neuroses are psychosomatic, with no structural abnormality in underlying nerves.

In defining psychoneuroses, Dąbrowski (1970c) said: "psychoneuroses are structures, syndromes and processes of disharmony and conflicts within the inner psychic milieu and with the external environment" (p. 2). The expression of a particular psychoneurosis depends on several factors including the individual's dominant overexcitability and his or her developmental level.

Dąbrowski (1973) also linked psychoneuroses directly with development, referring to them as "those processes, syndromes and functions which express inner and external conflicts and positive maladjustment of an individual in the process of accelerated development" (p. 151). Psychoneuroses cause sadness and stress that can be quite intense, leading to feelings of resignation and suicidal tendencies. The individual may be overwhelmed by "the antinomies" within him or herself and in the external environment, or by his or her inability to make a decision or by feelings of strangeness (Dąbrowski, 1970a). An individual with developmental potential will react by emotionally hardening himself or herself against these difficulties and by becoming familiar with them, first as enemies to be defeated but later as friends bringing new opportunities for creativity, new and rich experiences, and a strong sense of individual development (Dąbrowski, 1970a). Initially becoming aware of these tensions and forces "as enemies" creates a prophylactic aspect to psychoneuroses—this awareness helps to protect the individual and prevent him or her from disturbances that could lead to more serious mental illness such as psychosis (Dąbrowski, 1970a). In addition, psychoneuroses create an awareness of a richer and broader experience of reality and thus reassure the individual by demonstrating that there exist other higher realities and solutions to pursue.

Dąbrowski (1972a, 1972b) differentiated and detailed a hierarchy of neuroses and psychoneuroses based upon a number of factors, such as the degree of self-awareness present, the degree of self-control expressed and the level of empathy present. The neuroses are considered lower and psychoneuroses higher; see Table 2 for a summary. Lower forms are characterized by biological functions, psychophysiological reactions, and limited awareness. Lower forms do not display the involvement of higher mental functions. Dąbrowski (1972b) noted that "psychoneurosis is a psychical or more mental form of functional disorder, while neurosis is a more nervous or somatic form" (p. 41). Psychoneuroses can be further differentiated into a series of higher functions not observed in the neuroses.

Dąbrowski (1972b) further associated psychoneurosis with "highly conscious internal struggles whose tensions and frustrations are not anymore translated into somatic [neurotic] disorders" (p. 303). Higher forms are associated with mental functions such as anxiety and depression, greater levels of intensity, awareness of inner conflict and alterocentric components. The somatic aspects of these conditions have dissipated. The higher levels of psychoneuroses are characterized by the philosophical attitude they represent, for instance, by attitudes encouraging self-control, self-development, and by identification and concern for others. Solutions are sought in the search for the new and unknown, in the reality or possibility of higher levels, and through creativity. With further development, psychoneuroses dissipate, leaving their constructions behind. For example, obsessions of heroism, self-sacrifice and responsibility become transformed into a personal philosophy expressing attitudes reflecting these traits. In turn, one's actions come to be in harmony with these traits and goals as reflected by one's personality ideal as expressed in secondary integration.

Dąbrowski's hierarchy of neuroses and psychoneuroses can be summarized briefly (from lowest to highest):

- Neurotic disorders dominated by somatic processes, affecting internal organs; for example, heart palpitations, "butterflies" in the stomach (the hockey player who throws up before every game), and muscular tics.
- Neurotic disorders of systems and functions; for example, circulatory issues (the public speaker who occasionally faints), digestive, urogenital.
- Overexcitability as a neurosis: nervousness/overexcitability is an introductory neurosis appearing at the early stages of accelerated and universal development. Relatively undifferentiated. Overexcitability causes an individual to be sensitized to both the internal and external environment and to discover different kinds and levels of reality. Mental tension increases and suggests a readiness for development.

Table 2. Dąbrowski's hierarchy of neuroses and psychoneuroses

Nervousness / Neurosis (primarily somatic)

- Neurotic disorders of organs
- Neurotic disorders of systems and functions
- Overexcitability as an introductory neurosis
- Neurasthenia
- Neurotic depression

Psychoneuroses (primarily psychic / psychological)

- Anxiety psychoneurosis
- Obsessional psychoneurosis
- Compulsions
- Psychasthenia
- Psychoneurotic depression
- Psychoneuroses

- Neurasthenia: A lower psychoneurosis exhibiting the basic mechanisms of disintegration. Asthenia literally means a weakness; hence neurasthenia is a weakness of the nerves. Displays as a cyclic pattern of excitation and inhibition; for example, in periods of creativity followed by fatigue. Neurasthenia is a lower form of psychasthenia.
- Neurotic depression: Mild breaks with the environment; for example, an individual mulling over his or her past and present mistakes. Mild maladjustment to the actual situation but only weak adjustment to what ought to be.
- Anxiety psychoneurosis: Mild and general anxiety, not well articulated, phobias may be present; for example, the fear of being robbed. At low levels, consciousness is limited and few existential aspects are present. At their highest levels, anxiety

psychoneuroses are associated with self-control of lower level fears, expansion of awareness and growth of an existential attitude, concern and empathy for others, and growth of personality. At this level, anxieties over one's personal issues are inhibited in favor of experiencing anxieties related to a feeling of responsibility and concern for others, especially those who suffer injustice or who are in difficulty—this is the birth of courage and heroism. Anxiety moves from objects toward anxiety over the unknown, anxiety over becoming anxious, and existential anxiety. Existential anxiety may be experienced as a general feeling of overwhelming "fear and trembling." Anxiety or even agony may be experienced over general world matters (the environment, wars, cruelty to others and so forth). There is awareness that these states of anxiety provide the foundation for growth.

- Obsessional psychoneurosis: Concentration upon the "most important things." For example, an individual may wash his or her hands repeatedly in protest of the "impurity of the world." At higher and more conscious levels, obsessions may represent moving away from lower levels of reality through disintegration in search of the "unknowable." For example, obsessions related to self-sacrifice, self-perfection, creativity, responsibility, love, heroism, and suffering may be observed. At the highest levels, obsessions concerning protesting injustice and perfecting the world may be seen.

- Compulsions: As with obsessions, a differentiation of the levels of compulsiveness is necessary to differentiate lower pathological forms from higher developmental forms. Compulsions may be seen manifested in self-sacrifice or suicidal decisions motivated by high moral aims.

- Psychasthenia: The weakening of mental functions. For example, an individual may become unable to handle the daily affairs concerned with ordinary life. A higher type of psychoneurosis associated with advanced development and with a clearly active disposing and directing center. Characterized by mental processes; for example, by phobias, obsessions, anxiety, and existential depressions. At high levels, examples may include altruistic feelings, concerns about morality and values, and existential and transcendental preoccupations.

- Psychoneurotic depression: Characterized by strong levels of tension produced by sensitivity and by a strong fear of being psychologically hurt, producing withdrawal, isolation, and inferiority feelings. When occurring with strong developmental potential, these depressions are usually of internal origin expressing feelings of dissatisfaction with oneself, feelings of guilt, or feelings of inferiority. Depression often arises when a contrast becomes conscious between one's "higher levels" versus one's "lower levels." One sees these lower levels negatively and feels weakness, misery, humiliation, and worthlessness. Seeing the sorrows experienced by others creates an accompanying feeling of being caught in a pointless reality. There is the beginning of conscious organization and control over one's depression. Maladjustment is accompanied by the need for adjustment to what ought to be, an active seeking of freedom from lower levels of reality and access to the higher. Autopsychotherapy becomes possible.

Dąbrowski's observations led him to conclude the following general points:

- Psychoneuroses are "connected with the tension arising from strong developmental conflicts" (Dąbrowski, 1973, p. 149).
- Psychoneuroses "contain elements of man's authentic humanization" (Dąbrowski, 1973, p. 152).
- "In psychoneuroses the highest neuropsychic centers are active and provide a decisive source of psychotherapeutic and developmental energies" (Dąbrowski, 1972b, p. 160).
- "'Psychoneurotic experiences,' by disturbing the lower levels of values, help an individual to gradually enter higher levels of values; i.e., the level of higher emotions. These emotions, becoming conscious and ever more strongly experienced, begin to direct our behavior and bring it to a higher level" (Dąbrowski, 1972b, p. 3).

- "The psychoneurotic problem is one of the lack of adjustment manifesting protest against actual reality and the need for adjustment to a hierarchy of higher values—to adjust to that which 'ought to be'" (Dąbrowski, 1972b, p. 3).
- "Psychoneurotics, rather than being treated as ill, should be considered as individuals most prone to a positive and even accelerated psychic development" (Dąbrowski, 1972b, p. 4).
- "Nervousness and psychoneuroses are structural conditions of sensitivity within and towards one's own inner psychic milieu wherein positive development through unilevel and multilevel disintegration finds especially favorable ground" (Dąbrowski, 1972b, p. 159).

The hierarchy presented above contains two terms that Dąbrowski frequently used and that are unfamiliar to most readers: *neurasthenia* and *psychasthenia*. Asthenia means a loss or lack of strength, weakness or debility. Dąbrowski (1972b) defined neurasthenia as a "type of psychoneurosis characterized by cycles of excitation followed by excessive fatigue, even exhaustion. Lower level of psychasthenia, frequently associated with obsessions and phobias" (p. 299). George Miller Beard (1839-1883), an American neurologist and pioneer in the use of electricity as a therapy in medicine, introduced the term neurasthenia in 1869. As used by Freud, neurasthenia was caused by masturbation leading to excessive dissipation of somatic excitation and exhaustion. Freud used the term to describe a fundamental disorder in mental functioning. The term has now largely been abandoned.

Pierre Janet introduced psychasthenia in 1903 (van der Hart & Friedman, 1989). Dąbrowski (1972b) defined psychasthenia as:

a type of psychoneurosis characterized by lowered bio-psychic tonus, especially in regard to primitive functions and adjustment to actual reality. Psychasthenia is characterized by feelings of inadequacy, obsessions, anxieties (especially existential), depressions. (p. 303)

Although the term is no longer in general usage, it has been retained in one important application in current psychology—psychasthenia was the basis of one of the scales for the Minnesota Multiphasic Personality Inventory (MMPI), a common personality test.[18]

Dąbrowski (1970c) went into considerable detail to describe the specific psychoneuroses associated with each type of overexcitability and at the various levels of development. To give a flavor of this complex analysis, I will elaborate the psychoneuroses characteristic of emotional overexcitability (Dąbrowski, 1970c, pp. 7-8):

- The higher the psychoneurotic level, the broader and deeper the range of emotional experiences an individual will display; conversely, the broader and deeper the emotions a person experiences, the higher the level of psychoneurotic functions he or she will display.

- At the lowest level are hypochondria and neurasthenia, featuring ambivalences, ambitendencies, egocentric despondency and fear. Emotional tensions are restricted to a narrow focus and display temperamental and psychosomatic character.

- At the level of spontaneous multilevel disintegration, we find psychasthenia. Positive obsessive tendencies are common; for example, a great love that disregards all conventions and ignores the restrictions of reality. Here we see creative systematization—penetrating attempts to move into a higher-level reality, to learn about it and to introduce its dominant principles into one's life. Multilevel vertical conflicts are common, as are states of anxiety, depression and high tension. Psychoneurosis of failure is encountered and usually dealt with in a creative way, often through suffering and transformation.

- On the level of organized multilevel disintegration, we find psychasthenia with a focus on existential philosophy, transcendental creative ideas and "a developed creative systematization." Empathy, self-control and "the awareness of taking advantage of psychoneurotic dynamisms in order to build one's own personality and that of others" (Dąbrowski, 1970c, p. 8).

We see again the holistic and systemic nature of Dąbrowski's approach—psychoneuroses do not simply appear as symptoms; they are the outcome of living with strong developmental potential, in particular of strong overexcitability, which commonly creates a series of experiences involving anxiety, depression, and crises. Together, these features may provoke a psychoneurosis and positive disintegration. In turn, Dąbrowski (1972b) explained the loosening of integration along with a psychoneurosis allows the individual to exercise volitional control over his or her development:

> Psychoneuroses—especially those of a higher level—provide an opportunity to "take one's life in one's own hands." They are expressive of a drive for psychic autonomy, especially moral autonomy, through transformation of a more or less primitively integrated structure. This is a process in which the individual himself becomes an active agent in his disintegration, and even breakdown. Thus, the person finds a "cure" for himself, not in the sense of a rehabilitation but rather in the sense of reaching a higher level than the one at which he was prior to disintegration. (p. 4)

The critical importance of psychoneuroses was emphasized by Dąbrowski in the title of his 1972 book, *Psychoneurosis is Not an Illness*. It is not an illness; it is a critical and necessary element for personality growth: "It is our opinion based on extensive experience that there is never, or almost never, a case of accelerated development and even more so of eminent development, without a psychoneurotic constitution" (Dąbrowski, 1972b, p. 6). Dąbrowski (1972b) did not appear to have much doubt when he said:

> The presence of neurotic or psychoneurotic positive developmental potential guarantees creative development through higher forms of psychoneurotic processes such as internal conflicts, hierarchization, development of autonomous and authentic dynamisms, towards a high level of personality and secondary integration. (p. 12)[19]

Thus far we have seen the developmental role and impact of psychoneuroses, but there is one more critical construct that Dąbrowski introduced: A given psychoneurosis may exert its developmental impact and then dissipate, or at the highest levels, a psychoneurosis may be transformed with its basic elements, becoming part of the forming personality. Dąbrowski (1972b) said:

> Psychoneurosis is a disorder of function, which like the neurosis, is reversible, i.e. it can be "cured" or even transformed into a developmentally higher form of psychological functioning. This higher form is no longer a psychoneurosis but a new personality structure in which the psychoneurotic history remains recorded. (p. 40)

The reader unfamiliar with Dąbrowski's use of psychiatric descriptive terminology is likely to be quickly overwhelmed by the literal lexicon presented. The timing and location of Dąbrowski's psychiatric training is also obvious when looking at this obscure list of turn-of-the-century European terms—terms that appear in Dąbrowski's writings, presented in Table 3.

Table 3. Dąbrowski's Descriptive Terminology

Altruistic fears	Anxiety neuroses
Anxiety psychoneurosis	Anxious, anxiety
Asthenic	Asthenic-schizothymic type
Borderline schizophrenia	Catatonic schizophrenia
Characteropathic (psychopathic) hysteria	Compulsive neuroses
Contact introversion	Conversion hysteria
Cyclothymic, cyclothymes	Depressive psychoneurosis
Dual personality	Dysplastic type
Egocentric, egocentrism	Existential hysteria
Existential psychoneurosis	Failure psychoneurosis
Hebephrenia	Hebephrenic schizophrenia
Hypochondria	Hysteria
Hysteric characteropathy	Infantile neurosis

Infantile types	Introvert-extravert
Introvertization	Intuitive type
Manic-depressive psychosis	Mental retardation
Migratory neuroses	Mixed depression/anxiety neurosis
Nervousness/overexcitability neurosis	Neurasthenia, neurasthenic
Neuroses of specific organs	Neurotic depression
Obsessional psychoneuroses	Obsessive neuroses
Obsessive psychoneurosis	Organ neuroses
Paranoia	Paranoid schizophrenia
Perversion neurosis	Phobias
Primitive criminal behavior	Psychasthenia
Psychoneurotic anxiety	Psychoneurotic depression
Psychoneurotic infantilism	Psychoneurotic obsessional
Psychopathy	Psychosis
Psychosomatic disorders	Schizoid
Schizoneurosis	Schizophrenia simplex
Schizophrenic	Schizothymes
Schizothymic constitution	Schizothymic
Schizothymocyclic	Sexual psychoneurosis
Simple schizophrenia	Somatic neuroses
Somnambulistic conditions	Nervousness (psychic sensitivity)
System (psychosomatic) neuroses	Tetanoid types

In reviewing this list, it is easy to see why Dąbrowski's theory, with its heavy emphasis on psychiatry, challenging new constructs, clinical diagnosis, and outdated clinical terminology, was not readily embraced by the American mental health community in the 1960s and 70s. This was a shame, as the theory clearly offers, at the very least, a substantive counterpoint to better-known approaches (as we have seen, for example, with Freud and Maslow). The theory's emphasis on emotion would have been a refreshing contribution to the cognitive paradigm, then taking over academic psychology, and the idea of a potential developmental role for crises would have laid an early foundation for the study of post traumatic disorders and growth. As well it promises potentially beneficial therapeutic practices for supporting individuals in crisis through its emphasis on growth versus disorder.

Including a positive role for anxiety and psychoneurosis adds a major degree of complexity to Dąbrowski's theory, making it a clinical theory of growth. The core psychoneuroses feature depressive and anxiety symptoms. At their peak, these psychoneuroses express existential concerns and help the person work out his or her understanding of the meaning of life in general and of his or her life in particular.

4–6. CHAPTER SUMMARY

This chapter presented Dąbrowski's unique and controversial view of the role played by "so-called symptoms" in development. Psychoneuroses were linked to development by Dąbrowski's observations of eminent personalities and a review of their life histories. Dąbrowski came to the conclusion that the process of development is inextricably bound with the expression of symptoms of anxiety and depression. Accordingly, Dąbrowski defined psychoneuroses in a developmental context and described a complicated hierarchy of symptoms that parallel the developmental levels comprising the theory of positive disintegration. This classification can also be seen in Dąbrowski's description of the different types of disintegration.

In Chapter Three, the foundation of developmental factors was presented, including instincts, dynamisms, and developmental potential. Developmental potential, especially overexcitability, contributes to an experience of life that predisposes conflict, crisis, anxiety and depression—in short, the neuroses and psychoneuroses discussed in this chapter. These positive symptoms create the tension and disruption of the normal integration of psychological structures and motivate an individual to seek new and different answers. The process leads to disintegration and creates an opportunity for the individual to actively participate in his or her development by constructing new realities, new values, new ideals and, for the first time, a unique personality. This process of construction involves many psychological features and structures that will be described in Chapter Five.

5

KEY PSYCHOLOGICAL STRUCTURES OF DEVELOPMENT

We could use the analogy of a symphony orchestra in describing the process of development. Dąbrowski described a large orchestra—a broad constellation of developmental factors including the five overexcitabilities, three factors of development, some 20 dynamisms, special abilities and talents, and four critical instincts. How do these diverse factors come together and work as a unit in promoting development? To answer this question, Dąbrowski (1996, p. 25) concluded that a meta-organizing developmental factor, a conductor of sorts, appears to be "a logical necessity"—and he suggested that the developmental instinct plays this critical role in coordinating and organizing development.

Dąbrowski described many different developmental features and structures, all operating together in a coordinated fashion. It can be daunting at first to grasp what Dąbrowski is describing because each structure must be described and understood on its own merits. But no one structure stands alone and ultimately all must be seen and understood as they function together as an integrated whole.

5–1. DYNAMISMS

While overexcitability and the third factor are the main driving forces of development, they are expressed in day-to-day behavior through "dynamisms." Dynamisms can be a difficult construct to grasp, in part because Dąbrowski was inclusive in his thinking; he described some 20 dynamisms covering a wide variety of developmental features. Dąbrowski defined a dynamism as a "biological or mental force controlling behavior and its development. Instincts, drives and intellectual processes combined[20] with emotions are dynamisms" (Dąbrowski, 1972b, p. 294). Dąbrowski (1996) also made it clear that dynamisms are an active component in shaping development: "There are many factors involved in development. Our concern here is with the intrapsychic factors which shape development and the expression of behavior. The intrapsychic factors of positive disintegration are called dynamisms" (p. 13).

The ultimate dynamisms are the instinct of life and in particular the developmental instinct—because it is the most pervasive and basic developmental drive. As we will see, Dąbrowski also described many other features and structures as dynamisms that play a distinct role in personality development.

Dąbrowski (1967) also used the terms instinct and dynamism somewhat interchangeably and said that within instincts there are transforming dynamisms. "In the instincts themselves, therefore, there exist transforming dynamisms, for which the conflictive experiences and participation of gnostic mechanisms[21] are fundamental factors determining the development of a man" (Dąbrowski, 1967, p. 51).

Dąbrowski described a hierarchy of dynamisms. At different levels, different dynamisms are operational. For illustration, at the lowest level there are primitive instinctual dynamisms strongly influenced by the biological life cycle, most predominantly seen in the instinct for survival and often expressed through the need to compete and win at all costs, thus elevating one's sense of self-importance and primitive well-being. As development proceeds, new dynamisms appear and become prominent; they become more and more developmental in their character. The hierarchy of dynamisms corresponds to the basic levels in the theory; for example, in addition to primitive dynamisms, different dynamisms will reflect unilevel, spontaneous multilevel, organized multilevel, and finally secondarily integrated forms.

The dynamisms can also be categorized as disintegrative or as integrative. "Disintegrating dynamisms destroy the more primitive ways of thinking that are linked to satisfying both instinctive drives and social needs. Emotional pain created by persistent inner conflict leads either to negative or positive disintegration" (Mendaglio 2017, p. 11). Examples of dynamisms contributing to disintegration include anxiety over one's self, dissatisfaction with oneself, feelings of shame and guilt, and the feeling of inferiority to oneself. Organizing dynamisms include subject-object in oneself and the dynamism of third factor. Secondary integration dynamisms include the disposing and directing center on a high level and the personality ideal.

5–1–1. Unilevel dynamisms

Lower level dynamisms associated with unilevel disintegration:

5–1–1–1. Ambivalence

Conflicting and opposing attitudes, such as feelings of inferiority and superiority or feelings of love and hate characterize this dynamism. These conflicting or mixed feelings are felt to be of equal value (unilevel), and there is no hierarchization present. These conflicting feelings can produce great frustration and the feeling that one is trapped by the situation and by one's inability to choose.

5–1–1–2. Ambitendency

Ambi- as a prefix means both. Ambitendencies are simultaneous tendencies to act in opposing or contrary directions. For example, two contrary drives may struggle with each other for dominance, neither able to assert itself. Dąbrowski (1972b) gave the example that greed and the desire to accumulate money may compete with the desire to spend money to acquire goods and enjoy oneself, or, for instance, suicidal tendencies may conflict with the drive for self-preservation. As with ambivalences, ambitendencies do not display any differentiation as to higher and lower; they are unilevel. Competing tendencies are on the same level and therefore their struggle is experienced as seemingly endless.

5–1–2. Spontaneous multilevel dynamisms

At this level, dynamisms are characterized by spontaneity and a lack of organization. These dynamisms are seen in the first phases of multilevel disintegration.

5–1–2–1. Astonishment with oneself and one's environment

A sudden feeling of surprise and excitement usually associated with an unexpected accomplishment and often of a cognitive nature. For example, a person is surprised when he or she solves a difficult problem that he or she had believed was unsolvable. Astonishment combined with curiosity creates the urge to seek further knowledge of the world in general and in some cases, astonishment and curiosity can be used to generate self-knowledge. Astonishment with oneself must be differentiated from astonishment or surprise with events occurring in the external environment or by the actions of others. These "external" surprises are less developmental as they are not directly focused upon the self.

5–1–2–2. Disquietude with oneself

A dynamism characterized by a general feeling of uneasiness or mild anxiety with oneself. This is an early dynamism expressing an individual's cognitive and developmental drives and marking the beginning of multilevel disintegration.

5–1–2–3. Dissatisfaction with oneself

This dynamism involves the early expression of subject-object in oneself and is an expression in opposition to one's own structure. It suggests an initial differentiation between what is lower and what is higher within one's self. Lower dissatisfactions tend to focus upon the feeling that there is something wrong with others or with the environment or world in general. Dissatisfaction with oneself could be described as a feeling that "there is something wrong" and the growing sense that it is something "within you."

5–1–2–4. Feelings of inferiority toward oneself

Most psychological approaches to inferiority refer to inferiority in relation to others or in relation to the social environment. For example, Dąbrowski (1967) mentioned Alfred Adler (1870-1937) and his suggestion that a feeling of inferiority in relation to the environment may be dealt with by social attitudes and compensations such as through self-criticism. Dąbrowski used the construct to refer to a feeling of inferiority in relation to one's own inner environment. Dąbrowski (1967) said: "It seems that general mental development and also development of moral personality, would not be possible without participation of the feeling of inferiority and particularly without this feeling in relation to oneself" (p. 99).

Dąbrowski (1967) went on to describe the feeling of inferiority in relation to oneself as a sign of the process of disintegration. Within the individual, these feelings involve a comparison of lower elements with higher, and a comparison of one's internal experience in relation to one's personality ideal. At times an individual may progress and then "slide back" to a lower developmental level. If this happens, the individual will feel dissatisfaction and feelings of inferiority with him- or herself, often associated with a Kierkegaardian "fear and trembling" (Dąbrowski, 1967). The feeling of inferiority towards oneself is a reflection of an intense internal moral and cultural development not observed in feelings of inferiority in relation to others or to the environment. The feeling of inferiority towards oneself works closely with the process of self-education and the consciousness of one's personality ideal. As feelings of inferiority are felt, a conscious redirection of activity "upward" can take place involving a number of dynamisms, including the third factor along with the disposing and directing center. Dąbrowski observed that inferiority towards oneself is common in the great majority of creative individuals.

5–1–2–5. Feelings of shame and guilt

Initial primary integrations are often associated with feelings of self-assurance and a confidence expressed as arrogance. Feelings of guilt, shame, and responsibility characterize the early stages of multilevel disintegration. Shame is initially associated with a loss of confidence, especially in relation to the external environment. Strong anxiety causes the individual to want to flee from the situation. As the individual begins to perceive the reasons for his or her actions, a sense of self-consciousness begins to develop, and shame shifts to an internal focus. Guilt is an internalization of shame that expresses remorse over past events, primarily focused upon one's moral failures—either real or imaginary (Dąbrowski, 1970b, p. 68). Guilt derives from disappointments involving the contrast between one's thoughts and actions versus the standards suggested by one's developing hierarchy of values and personality ideal. The feeling of personal failure can produce strong tension, even "fear and trembling." These feelings fuel positive disintegration.

5–1–2–6. Positive maladjustment

An important developmental feature characterized by a strong inner protest against any situation that fails to correspond to an individual's hierarchy of values and aims.

5–1–2–7. Creativity

In advanced development, creativity emerges in conditions of emotional crisis and conflicts, both internal and external. Creativity grows from an appreciation of the contradictions between the "is" of the external world versus the "ought" of the inner world. Creativity can be generally thought of as a conscious, highly aware attempt to build a new reality. Creativity is an important outlet for the anxiety and tension produced by the internal conflicts associated with disintegration, and as such, creative dynamisms are an important prophylactic for mental illness. With advancing self-development and awareness, the creative instinct is transformed into the instinct of self-perfection.

5–1–3. Organized multilevel dynamisms

At the highest levels, dynamisms organize, shape, and assimilate positive disintegration, moving toward reintegration(s) on the secondary level.

5–1–3–1. The third factor

In Dąbrowski's schema, three factors contribute to and determine the ultimate developmental outcome of an individual. As mentioned above, these factors are, respectively, heredity, environment, and the third factor. In the theory, the construct of the third factor plays a number of different and critical roles, acting in conjunction with subject-oject, self-education, self-control, and autopsychotherapy in promoting intrapsychic transformation. "It plays a decisive role in the transition from a biologically and socially determined development to the specifically human self-determination" (Dąbrowski, 1973, p. 80).

Initially, Dąbrowski presented the third factor as a genetic, ontogenetic component of developmental potential. Later it becomes a non-ontogenetic, emergent force of development. This creates some confusion over the role of the third factor. This confusion perhaps mirrors the changes in the nature and role of the third factor which, as it emerges in development, transcends its genetic roots and becomes an independent force as development advances. Ultimately, the third factor acts as a rudder guiding a person in implementing his or her personality ideal—the authentic self—by making value choices that select what is "more me" and reject what is "less me."

5–1–3–1–1. Origins of the third factor. Dąbrowski was well aware of the contradiction in initially presenting the third factor as an ontogenetic component of development that, *in* some *cases*, emerges into an advanced developmental force—thus becoming non-ontogenetic. "It is not easy to strictly define the origin of the third factor, because, in the last analysis, it must stem either from the hereditary endowment or from the environment" (Dąbrowski, 1973, p. 78).

Dąbrowski elaborated that "The dynamism of the third factor arises from cross-influences of the first two factors, but represents a new ability, irreducible to its sources" (Dąbrowski, 1970b, p. 25), and further, "the autonomous forces do not derive exclusively from heredity and environment, but are also determined by the conscious development of the individual himself" (Dąbrowski, 1970b, p. 34).

5–1–3–1–2. Definition. The construct of the third factor is both frustratingly complicated and vague at the same time. It is defined in a general sense as the totality of autonomous forces participating in self-directed and self-chosen development. These forces include "self-objectivity, self-criticism, self-control, and [the] objective evaluation of the social environment" (Dąbrowski, 1964b, p. 54).

In a stricter sense, it is a dynamism or force of conscious choice. Once brought to fruition, third factor becomes the dominant dynamism of organized multilevel disintegration coordinating all inner psychic transformation.

Dąbrowski (1970b) explained that:

Its selective role consists in accepting and fostering or rejecting and restraining qualities, interests and desires, which one finds either in one's hereditary endowment or in one's social environment. Thus the third factor being a dynamism of conscious choice is a dynamism of valuation. The third factor has a fundamental role in education-of-oneself, and in autopsychotherapy. Its presence and operation is essential in the development toward autonomy and authenticity. It arises and grows as a resultant of both positive hereditary endowment (especially the ability for inner psychic transformation) and positive environmental influences. (pp. 178-179)

5–1–3–1–3. Dynamic and emergent. As described above, in ideal development, the third factor becomes dominant over hereditary and social influences. Dąbrowski (1973) noted that the development of the third factor is itself a process:

The third factor rarely appears in a "ready-made" form. We work it out slowly and, gradually through inner struggles, through difficulties of affirmation and negation, until the time when our decisions are controlled by the synthetic "inner voice" and the growing role of the inner psychic milieu in the direction of the ideal of personality. (p. 79)

5–1–3–1–4. Expression of the third factor. The third factor is often active during childhood and puberty and in protracted, "higher level" maturation. Dąbrowski said the common route of maturation leads to a "premature" integration of mental structures based on "the desire to gain a position, to become distinguished, to possess property, and to establish a family" and that this premature maturation stifles or may even extinguish the influence of the third factor (Dąbrowski, 1964, p. 57). In individuals who display overexcitability and psychoneuroses, maturation is prolonged and integration is delayed, thus allowing the third factor to fully develop. This period is also characterized by disintegration and, through its role in valuation, the third factor is a basic component of the disintegration process.

5–1–3–1–5. Evaluative role in developing autonomy. As mentioned in the introduction, Dąbrowski (1996) said that the third factor plays a critical role in the process of valuation—the process:

of conscious choice by which one sets apart both in oneself and in one's environment those elements which are positive, and therefore considered higher, from those which are negative, and therefore considered lower. By this process a person denies and rejects inferior demands of the internal as well as of the external milieu, and accepts, affirms and selects positive elements in either milieu. (pp. 38-39)

Ultimately, the third factor "determines the direction, degree, and distance of man's development" (Dąbrowski, 1964, p. 53). Dąbrowski (1964) elaborated that:

Because of the third factor the individual becomes aware of what is essential and lasting and what is inferior, temporary, and accidental both in his own structure and conduct and in his exterior environment. He endeavors to cooperate with those forces on which the third factor places a high value and to eliminate those tendencies and concrete acts which the third factor devalues. (p. 53)

The descriptions of the third factor offered by Dąbrowski sound much like what we might think of as one's conscience. For example, the third factor perceives and compares higher and lower levels, both within oneself—one's feelings, one's thoughts and one's innate drives—and also in the external environment, as expressed through cultural norms and values, and social patterns. The third factor, acting as a dynamism, motivates the individual to choose and affirm the higher over the lower. The critical role played by the third factor in the creation and shaping of one's hierarchy of values is clear—"The shaping of a free, independent and authentic person is unthinkable without activation of this specifically human ability" (Dąbrowski, 1970b, p. 25).

5–1–3–2. Self-awareness and self-control

These dynamisms focus upon self-awareness, especially of one's personal identity as a continuum from past to present and as projected into the future. Awareness of the distinction of the self from the external environment and from others is an important developmental element. In addition, an awareness of one's activities and the impact they have on others, and on the environment, are also important. Awareness of the self is characterized by feelings of uniqueness and appreciation for one's own character, abilities, and traits. Self-control is an initial dynamism by which an individual exerts inhibition over those elements that he or she determines to be lower or inappropriate. Self-control is eventually replaced by a higher order dynamism, the disposing and directing center, that eventually becomes the master controller of one's activities.

5–1–3–3. Education-of-oneself

The third factor contributes to creating an individualized developmental program that calls upon an individual to take responsibility for his or her growth. One must seize one's fate, taking it into one's own hands. A large part of this process is creating and seeking out experiences and knowledge that one feels are suited to and in keeping with one's developmental program. Education becomes a self-directed enterprise by which the individual actively and consciously takes responsibility for his or her educational curriculum. Education-of-oneself (self-education) involves a dualism of subject-object with subject in that part of the self which teaches and object in that part that is taught in oneself.

5–1–3–4. Autopsychotherapy

In conjunction with the dynamism education-of-oneself, autopsychotherapy becomes an indispensable component of an individual's developmental plan. Development creates a great deal of both external and internal conflict and tension that initially contribute to neurotic and psychoneurotic symptoms. With higher development, an individual can use autopsychotherapy to manage and cope with this tension and transform the energy of these conflicts toward self-perfection. As with education-of-oneself, autopsychotherapy involves a dualism of subject-object—that part of the self that helps, and of object, that part which is helped in oneself.

Mendaglio (2017) offered an insightful summary:

> Autopsychotherapy and education-of-oneself are interrelated forces. Autopsychotherapy is conceived of as a process of education-of-oneself. Through autopsychotherapy individuals

essentially deal with psychological distress by using their own resources. When confronted with crises, individuals use self-therapy to deal with anxieties and tensions associated with them. Moreover, distressful situations are not only dealt with, but also they are transformed into opportunities for enhancing personal development. Education-of-oneself is the dynamism by which individuals identify or produce strategies to direct their personal development. In essence, individuals create or select existing self-help activities that will contribute to their development. Through regular reflection on daily experience and influenced by a hierarchy of values, individuals consciously direct their personal growth. (p. 10)

Personality acts as a template for individual development, laying out a set of goals (the personality ideal) and the courses of action needed to achieve them. The nascent personality is a strong force in determining the direction of self-education and autopsychotherapy.

5–1–3–5. Inner psychic transformation

Inner psychic transformation was Dąbrowski's term for the basic process of developmental change, a process allowing mental structures to transcend their original psychological and biological type. At lower levels, stimuli are largely processed automatically and often responded to reflexively. With all of the developmental dynamisms in play, a stimulus can be interiorized and reviewed and reflected upon in various ways prior to a conscious and deliberate reaction taking place. For the highest levels, Dąbrowski (1970b) said, "nothing is taken from the outside that would not be moulded by the dynamism of inner psychic transformation. Similarly, nothing leaves the inner psychic milieu without the active participation of this dynamism" (p. 74). In particular, reflexive and rote reactions and habits become scrutinized in relation to one's hierarchy of values and personality ideal. Reactions become a conscious expression of oneself, one's values and one's character. In this process, the third factor and consciousness play large roles. In addition, retrospection is used to review past reactions and evaluate their appropriateness, while imagination is used via prospection to evaluate what future reactions ought to be and to anticipate what impacts they may have.

5–1–3–6. Subject-object in oneself

Dąbrowski (1973) made the point that traditionally an objective attitude towards the environment is widely advocated and praised while a subjective approach towards oneself is widely accepted. Dąbrowski suggested that objective and subjective reality are equally important. Traditionally, we are encouraged to see others objectively and we naturally accept seeing ourselves subjectively. Dąbrowski said that by using the method of "subject-object," a more complete and deeper understanding and insight into oneself and into others can be achieved. In this method, one approaches oneself as object and approaches others as subjects. In exercising the distinction between subject and object in oneself, an individual develops identification and empathy. It is the subject within oneself which shapes and the object within oneself which is shaped. Once empathy and identification develop, the individual can distinguish that which is "I" versus that which is "not I" (a distinction not possible at the level of primary integration). Seeing oneself objectively helps us to see others subjectively. The ability to utilize subject-object is fundamental to understanding the authentic relationship between oneself and others and is critical in developing empathy.

Three stages of subject-object are illustrated using the relationship between student and teacher:

1. **Basic:** Subject and object remain independent, largely unrelated "individuals." Subject—I am the student. May have limited self-awareness. Object—You are the teacher. I recognize your role as my teacher and passively learn material as it is offered.
2. **Midrange:** Role reversal between subject and object creates a new type of relationship allowing a more objective view of the self and a more subjective understanding of the other.

Subject—I am the student. I have increased self-awareness and an introspective focus allowing me to reflect upon myself objectively and identify my strengths, weaknesses, my higher and lower drives, and my fundamental personality characteristics. I am beginning to objectively articulate my own unique learning needs.

Object—You are the teacher. I can put myself "in your shoes" and subjectively see your learning objectives and your selection of available methodologies. I can then better understand how to communicate my learning style to you to ensure the most efficient learning atmosphere possible. Together we can create a collaborative learning relationship. However, the curriculum you offer is still largely set by the educational system and your interpretation of it.

3. **The highest level:** Subject-object as a developmental dynamism. The subject (the observer) and the other (the observed) are both present in the same inner psychological milieu, allowing an ongoing, objective self-examination and self-exploration. For purposes of our student/teacher illustration, at the highest level the role of teacher is assumed by the individual. Self-education takes precedence. Subject—I am the student. Object—I am my own teacher. I am well aware of my learning styles and I can autonomously create the learning atmosphere that best suits me. I can identify my own learning goals, aims and objectives—I know what I need to learn, and I can seek out the information, knowledge and experience I need. At this level, a sense of understanding the higher and lower drives within one's personality allows one to become aware of and control the direction of one's development. The uniqueness of one's essence is realized, leading to an appreciation, respect, and understanding of the unique essence of other individuals. As a dynamism, subject-object is the basis of self-education, autopsychotherapy, and personality ideal, providing the foundation for advanced personality growth and personality shaping.

5–1–3–7. Empathy and identification with oneself and with others

Dąbrowski differentiated syntony from empathy. Syntony is being able to feel something in common with others, often with little appreciation for what is going on. This may be expressed in a feeling of camaraderie or an identification of oneself with the "we" of a group. Syntony may be expressed in group situations; for instance, when several people begin to cry at a funeral, an individual may also begin to cry even though he or she may not have had close feelings for the deceased. Syntony may be positive or negative. An example of a lower negative syntony would be the individual who joins in mob violence based on syntonic identification "with the action going on." At higher levels, syntony may be seen as an expression of a group cause, for example, to join in a peaceful group protest. Identification with others allows for deeper feelings of syntony with more consciousness of the overall situation and a deeper understanding of the feelings of others. At the highest levels, these feelings become an expression of empathy. Identification with oneself and self-knowledge and awareness of one's past emotional reactions and an appreciation for one's past suffering allows an individual to use subject-object to deeply understand how others are feeling and to empathize with them. This also creates a strong and deep desire to help others who are undergoing similar feelings, situations, or similar developmental challenges. In contrast to primitive feelings of superiority and control over others, an attitude of helpful humility develops, reaching out to assist others as one can.

5–1–3–8. Hierarchization

In his lectures, Dąbrowski would emphasize that the only real solution to problems is to find vertical answers through comparisons between higher and lower options and alternatives. The key element in growth is hierarchization, a process of ordering conflicts into higher and lower categories that opens a vertical channel. Dąbrowski (1996) emphasized the importance of hierarchization: "When this channel is not open, as in unilevel disintegration, the tensions lead to severe psychosomatic illness, psychosis, or suicide" (p. 35). Hierarchization is a broad and relatively undifferentiated dynamism.

5–1–4. Dynamisms characterizing secondary integration

5–1–4–1. Feeling and attitude of responsibility for oneself and for others

Self-awareness and self-control lead to a feeling of increased responsibility for one's self, including one's thoughts and actions, both in relation to one's own life and in relation to one's impact upon others. When other people are experienced as objects, they are perceived as "things," often as interchangeable as physical objects. When others are experienced as subjects, they are each recognized as individuals with a unique inner life that must be understood and respected. A sense of one's own uniqueness and gifts creates awareness that others are equally unique and gifted. A deep sense of connection with others is expressed through a feeling of responsibility when others are in need. These feelings are especially intense when friendships or loving relationships are involved.

5–1–4–2. Autonomy and authentism

Autonomy is the dynamism of inner freedom, signaling one's independence from the influence of one's lower drives and from the influence of the environment. Authenticity and authentism express one's inner truth—one's personality ideal—reflecting a unified hierarchy of values expressed through a high degree of integration of thought, emotions, and actions. The forces of development, autonomy, and authenticity help an individual to consciously and deliberately associate him- or herself with the highest levels of his or her personality ideal. Dąbrowski (1970b) outlined four aspects of authentism: The first was a confidence that one is going in the right direction toward achieving one's personality ideal. The second involved a universality of inner growth characterized by a balanced and holistic development of personality. The third was an appreciation, awareness, and understanding that one is unique—that one's character and mental functions are "unchangeable, irreplaceable and unrepeatable." Finally, authentism included an awareness of one's empathy. Through autonomy and authenticity an individual "separates his independent and affirmed self from the stereotyped, rigid, routine-ridden self, which was subject to primitive urges. The authentic self can thus be distinguished within the whole of man's mental structure" (Dąbrowski, 1970b, p. 78).

5–1–4–3. Disposing and directing center on a high level

The disposing and directing center is a coordinating and organizing dynamism that governs the overall activity of the psyche.

The disposing and directing center expresses different features at different levels of development. At the level of primary integration, it is biologically determined and characterized by the expression and satisfaction of the primary drives. In unilevel disintegration there is a multiplicity of disposing and directing centers reflecting contradictory and conflicting dynamisms, goals, and emotions—many "wills" are at play, much like the situation described by James in his description of various selves (see Section 2–1). In spontaneous multilevel disintegration, there are still various disposing and directing centers: "each representing antagonistic levels of the inner structure: those which are determined by primitive drives and those which are closer to the emerging personality" (Dąbrowski, 1970b, p. 79). At the level of directed multilevel disintegration, the disposing and directing center begins to unify into a single supreme center to become a meta-controlling agent of development. The forces of the primitive drives are no longer felt. In the final phase of development, at secondary integration, the disposing and directing center reflects the personality ideal and eventually becomes synonymous with one's personality.

5–1–4–4. Personality ideal

Initially, in primary integration, images of the personality ideal are imitations, usually of public figures such as movie stars or athletes. During multilevel disintegration, higher aims emerge and become differentiated from lower ones. These higher aims are the raw material of the personality ideal. With development, a multiplicity of aims, values, and goals becomes increasingly interrelated and converges into a single image of the personality ideal. Eventually, the personality ideal becomes the source of the strongest creative dynamisms propelled by the instinct of self-perfection (Dąbrowski, 1970b, p. 89). The ongoing quest for self-perfection becomes synonymous with the quest to attain the personality ideal and to achieve the highest levels of personality development. "The personality ideal is the moving force of all that contributes to the full development of personality" (Dąbrowski, 1970b, p. 80).

The universality of the construct of personality ideal is seen in this quote from a Persian psychoanalyst, A. Reza Arasteh (1974/2008):

Having had an image of such a better life, the awakened

person becomes a seeker and values this image above all else. Motivated by it, he longs for it, becomes concerned with it and directs his efforts toward attaining it so as to become one with it. He becomes competitive, but only with himself, for competition with one's self constitutes perfection. (p. 14)

A visual representation is helpful to see the relationships between dynamisms, instincts, and factors. Figure 2, below, summarizes the interrelationships between various dynamisms (not all dynamisms are shown). This chart also presents the levels of the dynamisms and the second and third factors. The third factor is shown as both a factor and a dynamism. There are no dynamisms at the level of primary integration. A chart appearing in (Dąbrowski, 1970b, p. 66) inspired the figure and the dynamisms are detailed in Dąbrowski (1970b, p. 65).

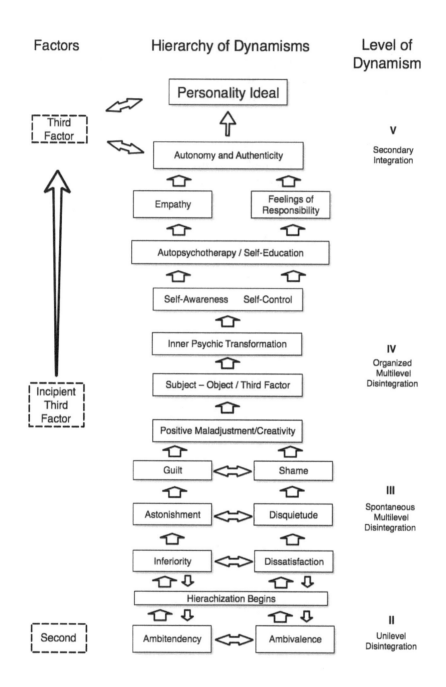

Figure 2. Hierarchy of Dynamisms

5–2. THE INNER PSYCHIC MILIEU

The construct of the inner psychic milieu was introduced to describe a "complex of mental dynamisms characteristic for a given individual" (Dąbrowski, 1970b, p. 62). Dąbrowski (1972b) said these dynamisms may interact on one level or on several levels and may interact synergistically with or antagonistically to each other:

> The establishment of the inner psychic milieu on a higher level and of an increasingly more human attitude towards the external environment requires the stimulation of higher functions and the inhibition of lower functions. This involves many kinds of sensitivity and excitability, numerous inner conflicts, emergence of multilevel inner forces, which can be called the dynamisms of the inner psychic milieu. (p. 62)

Dąbrowski (1970b) went on to describe four kinds of inner psychic milieu. The primitive milieu is integrated on a low level and lacks any major developmental dynamisms. No conflicts are present and self-consciousness is absent or severely limited. In the disintegrated milieu, there is a loosening of the structures and functions. This can occur during periods of strong emotion or conflict, and it is evident in periods of developmental crisis. All of the essential dynamisms are present. This type of milieu is found in individuals experiencing the process of positive disintegration and is a fundamental component of advanced growth. Many of the dynamisms operating at this level have previously been considered pathological. The third type is the inner psychic milieu on the level of secondary integration. This milieu is a hierarchical, well-organized structure. The major developmental dynamisms now have relaxed and have been replaced by a higher order of new dynamisms. The fourth type of milieu Dąbrowski described was a pathological milieu, either representing an integrated or disintegrated character.

5–3. EMOTION IN DĄBROWSKI'S THEORY

5–3–1. A brief review of emotions in a general context

The study of emotions in philosophy and psychology has traveled a circuitous route. One traditional approach to emotion began with Plato and his division of the immortal soul and mind from the ephemeral, earthly body. This dualistic philosophy essentially split emotion into psychic feelings and bodily responses.

Plato described a chariot pulled by two horses. One is white, well-bred, honor-loving, spirited, and well-behaved. The second, however, a dark horse symbolizing irrational passions and bestial appetites, had to be controlled by the whip of the charioteer (who symbolized reason). This image evolved into a broad eulogizing of reason and a damnation of the passions, reaching an apex in Cartesianism—the philosophy of René Descartes (1596-1650) and his complete separation of the mind from the corporeal body. Dualism subsequently influenced Immanuel Kant (1724-1804) and psychological theory, in particular, through the works of William James.

The second traditional approach to emotion was based upon Aristotle's belief that in order to know something, we need to understand both what it is made of and its function. Knowing the physiological basis of an emotion is only half of the story; we also must understand the function of the emotion. Aristotle also introduced the notion that it is the observer's beliefs that lead to emotions—it is not the snake on the trail that scares a person; it is the person's belief that the snake will bite that creates the fear. Aristotle also understood that emotion was situationally specific; i.e., seeing a snake behind a glass panel would not elicit fear; instead it may elicit pleasure from seeing the beauty of the snake. This example illustrates how one's beliefs about the perceived object, as well as the object's function in the particular context in which it is seen, combine to form an emotion (Power & Dalgleish, 2008).

The Platonic tradition and its perception of emotion as irrational had a profound impact in placing emotion at the bottom of the hierarchy of human functions. "Emotion often seemed a 'dirty word in science,' regarded as inferior to reason and indeed as a 'lower animal' heritage interfering with higher cognition" (Levine & Jani, 2002, p. 384). For example, Charles Darwin studied emotion extensively (Darwin, 1872) and "argued that emotions were vestiges of our evolutionary history and, like the appendix in the gut, were no longer of evolutionary value" (Power & Dalgleish, 2008, p. 2). In another example, Dai and Sternberg (2004) make the case that intellectual functioning should be considered along with the motivational and emotional mechanisms involved, but also noted that this integrated view "does not imply that motivational and emotional issues are more important than or as important as cognitive processes and mechanisms" (p. 29). Remnants of this negative view can still be seen in the notion that the ability to successfully control and regulate emotion underpins a number of psychological, social and health outcomes (Goldin, McRae, Ramel, & Gross, 2008).

Over the last few decades our view of emotions has drastically reversed and a new era in emotional research largely prevails (e.g., Damasio, 1994; LeDoux, 1996). "The dominant view now is that emotions are functional and purposive and have high evolutionary value in social mammals such as ourselves" (Power & Dalgleish, 2008, p. 2). This introduction will present a brief survey of the study of emotion to provide a context for Dąbrowski's important contribution. For a comprehensive review one can consult Hacker (2018).

American psychological approaches to emotion essentially began with William James. Based on his approach to psychophysiology, James proposed an unusual construction of emotion. As Lowry (1982) pointed out, common sense would suggest that emotion is an experience that precedes and, in turn, *causes* some behavior to occur. However, James (1884) proposed just the opposite—if one meets a bear in the woods, one will have a perception of the bear and will turn and run—the *action* of running away (the emotional reaction) produces sensations and for James, these sensations are what constitute the felt emotion: "We feel sorry because we cry, angry because we strike, afraid because we tremble and not that we cry, strike, or tremble, because we are sorry, angry, or fearful, as the case may be" (James, 1884, p. 190). Emotion is constructed from a series of more basic physiological processes—emotion is a sensation—a sensation created by the bodily changes produced by the behavior of crying or of running away. Thus, our feeling of an emotion is a slave, occurring in response to our physiology and behavior. Our feelings are produced by and are inseparably linked to our habitual physiological reactions and behaviors. This mechanistic and constructivist approach dominated the early American scene, easily dovetailing into the behaviorist approach that soon followed.

Charles Darwin (1809-1882) made the other primary contribution to research on emotion (Hess & Thibault, 2009). Darwin studied the expression of emotion, especially in the face, and concluded that the process of natural selection and evolution applied to expressive behavior and to emotion, creating a link between animal and human behavior. Darwin's thesis was that the expression of emotion was a warning system designed to make other individuals aware of one's state and intentions. Darwin (1872) was one of the first to use photography as a method of research, specifically looking for evidence of innate recognition and reaction to expressions of emotions, particularly in the face. Ekman (2007) is a major contributor to research on the facial analysis of emotional expression.

In introducing a symposium on personality and emotion, Larsen (2000) noted that a PsychINFO database search revealed significantly more entries for the keyword "emotion" than for "cognition." However, Larsen's summary is quite revealing when he describes the interaction between emotion and personality theories. Numerous examples exist in which emotion is considered as an input or output (or both) of the personality or conversely, where "personality figures prominently as a director, moderator, or instigator of the emotional system" (Larsen, 2000, p. 651). Only one article, by Gasper and Clore (2000) suggested an influence of emotion on decision-making:

> Individuals high in attention to emotion tend to perceive their affect as generally relevant and to use it in their judgments, whereas individuals low in attention to emotion tend not to focus on affect and not to perceive it as relevant to affect his judgments. (p. 709)

The authors also emphasized that attention to emotion differs significantly among people.

An important review of emotion and cognition was provided by Phelps (2006) who concluded that the classic division between emotion and cognition is unrealistic and that emotion and cognition appear to be interrelated at all stages of stimulus processing. Phelps concluded that a complete understanding of cognition must require a consideration of emotion.

Dąbrowski was primarily influenced by British and European approaches, in particular by John Hughlings Jackson and Jan Mazurkiewicz. Hughlings Jackson developed a sophisticated understanding of language as an expression of brain function. As Robinson (2006) summarized: Language either conveys the content of our intellectual processes (the basis of aphasia that Hughlings Jackson and, subsequently, Freud wrote about), or language expresses feelings. Hughlings Jackson went on to suggest that emotional expression is distinct from language and that a brain lesion could disrupt emotion without distorting language functions (Robinson, 2006). Specifically, Hughlings Jackson observed that severe deficits to the left hemisphere could occur in a patient who was still able to communicate emotions verbally, leading to the suggestion that the right hemisphere was involved in emotional functions.

Jan Mazurkiewicz linked emotions with instincts and "considered instincts to be subcortical, mnemonic, hereditary activities. Human instincts are manifested only by components of the emotional tendencies which are the reason for purely emotional reactions" (Kokoszka, 2007, p. 14). In an approach reminiscent of Dąbrowski's dynamisms, emotional tendencies were seen as the source of psychic energy. As Kokoszka pointed out, this energy played an important role in development, allowing the individual to rise above the level of a purely reactive "reflexive machine" and allowing him or her to express autonomy through voluntary behaviors.

Mazurkiewicz considered feelings a dynamic phenomenon representing an individual's subjective appraisal of the value associated with a perception, sensation or thought (Kokoszka, 2007). In this approach, any kind of behavior thus stimulates a feeling, either positive or negative, that represents the subjective value assigned to the behavior by the individual involved.

Constantin von Monakow (1853-1930), the prominent Russian and Swiss neurologist, was the first to advance this idea. Von Monakow suggested that an individual would always show a characteristic reaction to stimuli, either in terms of approach ("klisis") or avoidance ("ekklisis"), thus reflecting the basic value orientation of the individual (Dąbrowski, 1964b). Readers unfamiliar with von Monakow may find this construct more familiar as "approach and avoidance" (Elliot, 1999; Elliot & Covington, 2001). Carver (2006) and Carver, Sutton and Scheier (2000)[22] reviewed models of approach-avoidance and the idea that emotion acts as an important motivation underlying human behavior. These ideas are subsequently seen in Dąbrowski's theory, wherein emotions are essentially equivalent to values and emotional reactions reflect the value orientation of an individual.

Mazurkiewicz also suggested that emotions on higher levels inhibit and suppress tendencies and instincts from lower levels (Kokoszka, 2007). Feelings from the newer, higher levels (à la Hughlings Jackson) are stronger than those from lower levels, particularly when originating in the cortex, which displays a higher level and speed of excitability. In this way, the cortex acts as a "multiplicator of incoming excitements" (Kokoszka, 2007, p. 16). This phenomenon is demonstrated in everyday life when individuals control their instinctual impulses based upon their higher feelings. This line of thought was quite a radical approach when contrasted with the majority viewpoint that the cortex was a passive signal relay device and that emotions were simply vestiges from our animal past.

It is helpful to take a closer look at two significant contributions to understanding emotion that created a new view and new appreciation of the role of emotion. Antonio Damasio (1994) presented a detailed analysis arguing that reason does not stand isolated; rather, feelings and emotions are interwoven with reason, and several brain subsystems, both at low levels and high levels, cooperate in the formation of reason. Damasio said, "At their best, feelings point us in the proper direction" and concluded, "the lowly orders of our organism are in the loop of high reason" (p. xiii).

Damasio also proposed that some of the critical brain circuits of emotion are found in the prefrontal cortex and in the brain areas that integrate body signals, showing that feelings "are just as cognitive as other percepts." Feelings allow us to be in touch with the biological reaction of our organism and sense the various body states reflecting states of pain or pleasure. Damasio boldly concluded that feelings comprise the human soul or spirit. Finally, Damasio elaborated the important role of the body in providing basic information required for brain representations—the body and brain function in continual interaction.

Damasio, a neurologist, showed that emotion intersects with reasoning and decision-making in the ventromedial prefrontal cortex. In addition, several other brain regions contribute to a collection of systems that ultimately involve reasoning, emotion and the processing of body signals. Damasio (1994) summarized his position:

> The picture I am drawing for humans is that of an organism that comes to life designed with automatic survival mechanisms and to which education and acculturation add a set of socially permissible and desirable decision-making strategies that, in turn, enhance survival, remarkably improve the quality of that survival and serve as the basis for constructing a person. (p. 126)

We can see from the above quote that we are still a long way from Dąbrowski's position of placing emotion in a critical management role in collaboration with the force of autonomy—the third factor.

Joseph LeDoux (1996) contributed an important work on emotion and suggested that there are many emotional systems in the brain each having "evolved for a different functional purpose and each which gives rise to different kinds of emotions" (p. 21). LeDoux collected evidence to support his position that information may be processed through two different pathways, a "high road" which involves cognitively identifying and analyzing stimuli before making an appropriate emotion, and a "low road" that bypasses analysis and leads directly to an emotional response. For example, when walking in the woods, one may glimpse "a snake" on the path. This stimulus is processed on the "quick and dirty path," initiating an immediate response to step back. At the same time, information is relayed to the visual cortex and other cortical processing centers where, over the course of a few seconds, a detailed analysis of the visual cues takes place. Based upon this cortical input, the initial reaction may be continued or cancelled. If the "snake" turns out to be a piece of old rope, our initial reaction will have been wasted, but this "better safe than sorry" approach is ultimately life-saving on the occasion that it does turn out to be a real snake. LeDoux (1996) noted that the pathways connecting the cortex with the amygdala are far greater in primates and he speculated that this might allow the cortex to gain more control over the amygdala and therefore allow humans to increase their control over their emotions. Alternatively, this increased connectivity could also signal increased liaison and cooperation between cognition and emotion.

An alternative, dual-process model proposed that, contrary to popular thinking, emotion does not directly cause behavior; instead, emotion merely shapes behavior through a complex feedback system (Baumeister, Vohs, DeWall, & Zhang, 2007). The authors (Baumeister et al., 2007) left little doubt as to the secondary status of emotion:

> Decisions made during emotional states tend to neglect important information, including probabilistic information. Given these drawbacks, evolution would likely have phased emotion out of the human psyche if direct causation of behavior were its main function (because people would be better off without emotion). (p. 195)

The authors concluded that emotion is part of an adaptive, flexible, and reactive feedback system that guides an individual's "cognitive apparatus" in learning how to navigate the complex situations that arise in modern social life.

A more balanced approach between emotion and cognition is illustrated by Blair and Dennis (2010). The classification of von Monakow, described above, is emphasized and put into a contemporary context; the category of emotional approach activates the behavioral activation system (BAS) while emotional avoidance activates the behavioral inhibition system (BIS) (Gray & McNaughton, 2003). The authors note that "emotional responses rapidly signal potential harm or benefit in relation to well-being and thus serve to prioritize certain cognitions and actions," and this interface is adaptive (Blair & Dennis, 2010, p. 18). The authors pointed out that the balance between emotion and cognition "refers to the processes by which cognition 'controls' emotions, or emotions 'control' cognitions but also reflects how feedback-driven interactions solve the fundamental challenge of effectively adapting to and shaping environments" (Blair & Dennis, 2010, p. 18).

One has to look hard for contemporary material that takes the position that the emotions play a dominant role in personality; however, such material exists. For example, Magai and Haviland-Jones developed the thesis that our lives are profoundly shaped by our emotional experiences and that "affect or emotion itself is the creative and organizing force behind all mental life" (Magai & Haviland-Jones, 2002, p. 7). In their interesting book, *The Hidden Genius of Emotion*, the authors suggested that emotion does more than simply provide energy to the cognitive system (Piaget's view); rather, emotion organizes thoughts, memories and perceptions and is a decisive aspect in determining one's unique personality. The authors took a dynamic systems theory approach and described first-order personality change—gradual shifts and adjustments. They went on to cite Tomkins's idea that the goal of complex living systems is not equilibrium but emotional variation and that "turbulence" leads to instability and second-order change. The latter approach is associated with crises that lead to growth. In times of crisis an individual's emotional organization is recruited to assist in managing the situation. Magai and Haviland-Jones (2002) went on to describe a situation quite reminiscent of Dąbrowski's disintegration:

> Conditions do exist where traumatic events can cause significant emotional upheavals and introduce destabilization. Once experienced, strong emotions, previously unexperienced due to psychological defense, may cause such a fundamental sense of disorientation that old patterns of thinking and relating are disrupted. In the wake of these novel experiences, the edge of chaos has been reached providing the opportunity for significant life change. Whether it is used creatively and adaptively for personality growth or provokes disintegration is a matter that persons resolve uniquely. But it is the occasions of intense mood changes that challenges personal identity and introduces instability. (p. 470)

In an approach that echoes Dąbrowski, the authors described how personality emerges from self-awareness by the way that people are motivated in the world and by their value structure.

On the other hand, the authors also emphasized the uncontrollable and random quality of life that both prevents absolute prediction and creates new opportunities for creativity. It is interesting to speculate how these intriguing and challenging approaches could evolve in the future—could positive disintegration and multilevelness merge with a dynamic systems approach, like the one described here, to yield the next qualitative step ahead in our theorizing about personality?

5–3–2. A brief review of emotions and moral judgment

The general context for this discussion is moral psychology. Excellent reviews of the topic are available (e.g., Doris, 2010; Haidt, 2013; Nadelhoffer, Nahmias, & Nichols, 2010; Sinnott-Armstrong, 2008-2014; Wiegmann & Osman, 2017; Voyer & Tarantola, 2017). Selected works on the role of emotions in morality and moral judgement will now be considered.

Lawrence Kohlberg (1927-1987) developed a theory of moral development that dominated the field in the 1970s (Gibbs, 2014; Zizek, Garz, & Nowak, 2015). Kohlberg essentially extended the Piagetian approach to cognitive development and Piaget's view of emotion. Flynn (1995) succinctly summarized the role Piaget assigned to emotion:

> Humans are best understood from a cybernetic perspective where learning is characterized as a mechanical and purely cognitive structuring of information devoid of any emotional content. The role of emotions in all of this lies in their capacity as a motivating force setting in motion further adaptive human interactions with the environment. Emotions, in themselves, have no intrinsic value but act merely as an external force capable of driving the cognitive mechanisms of which the learning machine is composed. (p. 367)

It should therefore come as no surprise that Kohlberg did not consider emotions an important part of moral development.

Things changed considerably in the 1980s as critiques of Kohlberg began to accumulate, and various authors, notably Jerome Kagan (1984), provided a "moral-emotional correction" to the situation (Haidt, 2003b, 2007). The Kohlberg era had come to an end (Krebs & Denton, 2005).

One of the standard instructions given to a jury is not to let any emotions of sympathy influence its judgment (Feigenson, 1997, quoted in Pizarro, 2000). Pizarro (2000) reviewed the traditional stance that emotions are antagonistic to making moral judgments. Pizarro (2000) suggested "emotions reflect our pre-existing concerns, such as our moral beliefs and principles . . . [and] can actually aid reasoning by acting as a centralizing agent, focusing our attention and our cognitive resources on the problem at hand" (p. 358). Pizarro (2000) went on to examine the role of empathy "because it seems the clearest candidate for being a truly moral emotion" (p. 359) in making moral judgments and is the first necessary step toward ensuring that our behavior reflects our moral principles and beliefs.

A review of the role of moral emotions was published by Tangney, Stuewig and Mashek (2007). The authors noted:

As the self reflects upon the self, moral self-conscious emotions provide immediate punishment (or reinforcement) of behavior. In effect, shame, guilt, embarrassment and pride function as an emotional moral barometer, providing immediate and salient feedback on our social and moral acceptability. (p. 347)

In an example of emotional-cognitive interaction, individuals can also use their imaginations to anticipate their emotional reactions, thus learning to cognitively control their moral choices and behavior.

Jonathan Haidt (2007) reviewed research on moral psychology and suggested that four basic principles are germane. The first is intuitive or affective primacy, an approach based upon the work of Robert Zajonic implicating two basic brain systems: an ancient, automatic and rapid system of affects; and an evolutionarily newer and slower cognitive system. Haidt (2007) said:

Zajonc's basic point was that brains are always and automatically evaluating everything they perceive and that higher-level human thinking is preceded, permeated and influenced by affective reactions (simple feelings of like and dislike) which push us gently (or not so gently) toward approach or avoidance. (p. 998)

These theories generally see emotion as at the foundation of human morality. It is now understood that these emotional building blocks are millions of years old in our evolutionary heritage and therefore it is not likely that cognitive and language-related abilities, only appearing in the past hundred thousand years, would suddenly take over control of these well-established emotional brain circuits. Haidt also reviewed two cognitive processes involved—moral intuition, a rapid automatic evaluation that is often affect-laden, and moral reasoning, a post-hoc process whereby an individual consciously searches for evidence to support his or her initial intuitive reaction.

Haidt's second principle was that moral thinking is for social doing—this principle suggests that "moral reasoning is like that of a lawyer or politician seeking whatever is useful, whether or not it is true" (Haidt, 2007, p. 999). Thus, one needs to be careful what one does. However, it is even more important what people think an individual did, and therefore one needs to be able to frame their actions in the most positive light. To this end, Haidt (2007) pointed out that people "readily invent and confidently tell stories" to explain their behaviors. In this context, moral reasoning is like the press secretary to an important politician.

Haidt's third principle was that morality binds and builds. Morality constrains individuals, linking them together to produce new groups with new properties. One's moral behavior contributes to a positive reputation which, in turn, promotes cooperation from others—Haidt cited the example of the importance of reputation in using websites such as eBay and Amazon: "Humans attain their extreme group solidarity by forming moral communities within which selfishness is punished and virtue rewarded" (Haidt, 2007, p. 1000).

Principle four was that morality is about more than harm and fairness, the usual two attributes of interpersonal behavior that Western research has considered. Haidt (2007) expanded this by adding three variables derived from cross-cultural research; ingroup-outgroup dynamics and the importance of loyalty; authority and the importance of respect and obedience; and intuitions about sanctified physical and spiritual purity and the importance of avoiding a carnal lifestyle. Haidt's (2007) conclusion, quoted here in its entirety, summarizes the state-of-the-art:

> People are self-interested, but they also care about how they (and others) treat people and how they (and others) participate in groups. These moral motives are implemented in large part by a variety of affect-laden intuitions that arise quickly and automatically and then influence controlled processes such as moral reasoning. Moral reasoning can correct and override moral intuition, though it is more commonly performed in the service of social goals as people navigate their gossipy worlds. Yet even though morality is partly a game of self-promotion, people do sincerely want peace, decency and cooperation to prevail within their groups. And because morality may be as much a product of cultural evolution as genetic evolution, it can change substantially in a generation or two. For example, as technological advances make us more aware of the fate of people in faraway lands, our concerns expand and we increasingly want peace, decency and cooperation to prevail in other groups and in the human group as well. (p. 1001)

Work on neurophysiology demonstrated the significant role played by the emotional centers in moral cognition. Young and Koenigs (2007) reported that the activity of the ventromedial prefrontal cortex (VMPC), as measured by functional magnetic resonance imaging (fMRI), has revealed that emotions are not only engaged during moral cognition, but after considering patients with impaired function, emotions, particularly those mediated by the VMPC, appear to be critical in human morality.

Neuroscience as a platform for moral behavior is the basis of the framework of Patricia Churchland (2011). Ethics (morality) is shaped by four brain process dimensions: (1) caring; (2) recognition of others' psychological states; (3) problem-solving in a social context; and (4) learning social practices. Her book, *Braintrust: What Neuroscience Tells Us About Morality*, is a first look at how a neurobiological perspective may contribute to understanding human moral values. Churchland stated, "mammals are motivated to learn social practices because the negative reward system, regulating pain, fear, and anxiety, responds to exclusion and disapproval, and the positive reward system responds to approval and affection" (p. 16). A basic function of the nervous system is to ensure the self-maintenance and survival of the self, essentially to seek relief from fear and to avoid pain. The same systems can be used to explain how caring is extended to other individuals including close kin and affiliates.

Thagard (2010) presented another broad approach linking brain science to "philosophical issues about knowledge, reality, morality, and the meaning of life" (p. xii). Thagard's (2010) claim was that these issues can be best informed by scientific evidence and, in particular, by neuroscience. At the root of our wisdom concerning what matters in life, and why it matters, are our cognitive and emotional abilities.

Bloom (2017) noted that moral decisions are powerfully influenced by empathy, but he believes the outcome of these decisions is often detrimental. He developed the case that the world would be better off if moral decisions were made on the basis of conscious and deliberate reasoning. Bloom (2017) concluded:

> Our attitudes about the rights of women, homosexuals, and racial minorities have all shifted toward inclusiveness. Most recently, there has been a profound difference in how people in my own community treat trans individuals—we are watching moral progress happen in real time.
>
> But this is not because our hearts have opened up over the course of history. We are not more empathic than our great-grandparents. We really don't think of humanity as our family and we never will. Rather, our concern for others reflects a more abstract appreciation that regardless of our feelings, their lives have the same value as the lives of those we love. (pp. 329-330)

5–3–3. Emotions in Dąbrowski's approach

Dąbrowski's approach to emotion is fairly complicated, mainly because he labeled a number of various psychological functions as emotions. We have seen that Dąbrowski defined dynamisms as emotions. He also talked about values and emotions interchangeably.

Following his professor Mazurkiewicz, Dąbrowski also viewed instincts as emotions. Essentially, anything that is a source of psychic energy can be considered an emotion.

Emotion, through approach and avoidance, plays a critical role in establishing an individual's values—what one is attracted to and what one is repulsed from. In turn, this attraction-avoidance paradigm reflects the basic character and personality of the individual.

Dąbrowski (1996) pointed out that developmental theories were based on a long and rich tradition of cognition studies and that emotional development had been neglected. Anticipating Magai and Haviland-Jones (2002), Dąbrowski (1996) called for a general theory of human development that includes and accounts for both cognitive and emotional development and that allows for emotional development to play a dominant role in shaping development. Dąbrowski (1970b) said that our "ultimate direction and control is at every level located in the emotional function rather than the intellectual" (p. 9). Dąbrowski (1996) made it clear that "human development must also include emotional development because emotional factors are crucial in shaping the transition from human animal to a human being" (p. 7).

For Dąbrowski, the whole process of development through positive disintegration is focused on emotion. "The most obvious aspects of positive disintegration occur in the sphere of feeling" (Dąbrowski, 1964b, p. 12). In this disintegration of the highest levels, Dąbrowski (1964b) described how the emotions could be mixed, revalued and stratified:

> releasing new managing dynamics and subordinating previously existing forms. Under the influence of positive disintegration, will and intelligence are separated from each other and become independent of basic impulses. This process causes the will to become more "free" and the intelligence to change from a blind instrument in the service of impulses to a major force helping the individual to seize life deeply, wholly and objectively. In the further development of personality, intelligence and will are again unified in structure, but at a higher level. (p. 13)

This is an important quotation because it contains the fundamental idea that an initial constellation of relationships, such as among will, intelligence, and the basic impulses, can be "released," allowing intelligence to form new connections with higher emotions under third factor direction and thus no longer to be the slave of basic impulses. This is a stark example of how disintegration operates—it literally allows existing relationships among psychological structures to be broken and consciously rearranged. These changes can be summarized succinctly: in primary integration, intelligence and other mental functions are controlled by primitive drives or by rote social conformity; in secondary integration, mental functions are guided by higher emotions, which synthesize intellectual and emotional and volitional components. Thinking and feeling meld into a co-determinant structure displaying mutual determination and ongoing developmental transformations (Dąbrowski, 1973).

The theory of positive disintegration is based upon the premise that the level of organization displayed by an organism is an index of development. As discussed above, development must be seen from an evolutionary point of view because many features of development do not occur automatically in the course of ontogenetic development. For example, the level of emotional function seen here is not solely a function of ontogenetic growth; it is a function of "other factors" that may or may not come to fruition. Therefore, a high degree of cognitive development does not ensure a high degree of emotional development.

For Dąbrowski, the development of values/emotions is a prominent component of development in general but no more or less so than the component of positive disintegration. All of these aspects contribute to an individual's personality development, hence Dąbrowski's emphasis on the theory of positive disintegration as a theory of personality and its development.

Dąbrowski directly equated values with emotions and made values an indispensable part of development. Dąbrowski (1972b):

"Psychoneurotic experiences" by disturbing the lower levels of values help gradually to enter higher levels of values, i.e. the level of higher emotions. These emotions becoming conscious and ever more strongly experienced begin to direct our behavior and bring it to a higher level. In this way, higher emotions play a dynamic role in our development and give meaning to our life. As new and higher values the higher emotions slowly begin to shape our "new harmony" after the collapse of the primitive harmony of lower level. The problem of value is essential and emerges sooner or later in each case of psychoneurosis. (p. 3)

Dąbrowski (1972b) said:

There is a strict relationship between emotional functions and the functions of the autonomic nervous system. So-called psychoneurotic disorders are, therefore, emotional perturbations occurring on different levels of the nervous system. Almost always they involve the excitation or inhibition of frontal centers. (p. 40)

Dąbrowski (1964b) cited the idea of Pierre Janet that emotions have a disintegrating effect, especially on the autonomic nervous system:

Emotions play a vital role in the psychic life of man. According to Pierre Janet, they have a disintegrating influence upon the mind: "Every emotion acts in a dissolving way upon the mind, diminishes its capacity of synthesis and renders it weaker for a certain time." On the other hand, it is well known that certain feelings, such as love, are elements that mobilize people, particularly children. (p. 99)

Janet associated the strength of a trauma and its resultant disintegrating effects with "vehement emotions" and with the intensity, duration and repetition of trauma (e.g., van der Kolk, Brown, & van der Hart, 1989). Dąbrowski classified Janet's position as negative disintegration and contrasted this adevelopmental situation with his alternative—positive disintegration, whereby, in individuals who display developmental potential, emotional disruptions play a critical role in stimulating development and creativity.

5–3–4. Emotional intelligence

It makes sense to mention emotional intelligence in a work on Dąbrowski because his emphasis on becoming aware of emotion in oneself and its importance as a motivating and change factor in one's personality development was a parallel theme in the presentation of emotional intelligence. The first formal mention of the term *emotional intelligence* came in two articles published in 1990 (Mayer, DiPaolo, & Salovey, 1990; Salovey & Mayer, 1990). A number of reviews of emotional intelligence are available (e.g., Ackley, 2016; Barchard, Brackett, & Mestre, 2016; Davis & Nichols, 2016; Fernández-Berrocal & Checa, 2016; Hogeveen, Salvi, & Grafman, 2016; Joseph & Newman, 2010; Mayer, Caruso, & Salovey, 2016; Mayer, Roberts, & Barsade, 2008; Petrides et al., 2016; Schulte, Ree, & Carretta, 2004).

Salovey and Mayer (1990) described emotional intelligence as:

> a set of skills hypothesized to contribute to the accurate appraisal and expression of emotion in oneself and in others, the effective regulation of emotion in self and others and the use of feelings to motivate, plan and achieve in one's life. (p. 185)

The authors further defined emotional intelligence as a subset of social intelligence "that involves the ability to monitor one's own and others' feelings and emotions, to discriminate among them and to use this information to guide one's thinking and actions" (Salovey & Mayer, 1990, p. 189). The person with emotional intelligence has achieved at least a degree of positive mental health.

Daniel Goleman, a journalist, popularized the construct of emotional intelligence in a best-selling book of the same name published in 1995. Goleman (1995) described "abilities such as being able to motivate oneself and persist in the face of frustrations; to control impulse and delay gratification; to regulate one's moods and keep distress from swamping the ability to think; to empathize and to hope" (p. 34). Goleman (1995) presented the five main domains of emotional intelligence:

1. Knowing one's emotions (self-awareness and

recognizing feelings as they happen).
2. Managing emotions (the ability to handle feelings in an appropriate way).
3. Motivating oneself (marshaling emotions in the service of a goal).
4. Recognizing emotions in others (empathy and social awareness).
5. Handling relationships (skill in managing emotions in others). (p. 43)

An important framework incorporating emotional intelligence, called the Reinforcement Sensitivity Theory (RST), describes three brain systems that are responsible for individual differences in sensitivity, in particular, for reward, punishment, and motivation (e.g., Bacon & Corr, 2017; Corr, 2004, 2008; Walker & Jackson, 2017; Walker, Jackson, & Frost, 2017). The details of this complicated and interesting theory are peripheral to the purpose of this discussion; the interested reader is referred to Corr (2008) for an overview.

5–4. THE HIERARCHY OF VALUES

As the process of multilevel disintegration begins and the individual starts to observe a differentiated, vertical perspective of life, he or she naturally begins to sort things into higher and lower categories. Dąbrowski referred to this critically important developmental phenomenon as *hierarchization* and, in a fashion similar to third factor, hierarchization emerges as an active process or force that acts to emphasize these vertical differentiations. All subsequent development is based upon the operation of this process of hierarchization.

Initially, at the level of unilevel perception, no conscious hierarchization is seen. In an approach somewhat reminiscent of Maslow's, Dąbrowski described the operation of a hierarchy of needs representing the basic neurophysiological functions of the organism. These are closely related, if not equivalent, to the lower primitive instincts. As multilevel perception develops, an individual consciously perceives something that is "higher" and imagines him- or herself behaving in this way. Thus, Dąbrowski said that as an individual becomes aware of the higher, he or she could use his or her imagination to construct a prospective hierarchy of aims, goals or ideals. Essentially, this early hierarchization represents a "wish list" of what the individual sees as higher and wants to emulate. These imagined and prospective nascent values provide ideals and goals for the individual to strive towards, eventually becoming shaped and formed into a clearer and more concrete hierarchy of values (and ultimately the personality ideal). As the individual achieves and maintains behavior that increasingly conforms to these values, inner conflict subsides and a feeling of internal harmony increases, signaling the incremental transition to secondary integration. The hierarchy of aims continues to act as an extension of the hierarchy of values to provide an ongoing sense of "what ought to be." Major life goals or distant goals may be held as lifelong quests in the "hierarchy of what will be."

One of the most important milestones of development is the emergence of the hierarchization of values. Initially, our value structures are heavily determined by our socialization and there is little differentiation of values. The experiences of positive disintegration create grave doubts: existential feelings of angst and hopelessness and perhaps even suicidal feelings over the meaning and sense of life. These experiences challenge and eventually overwhelm the ability of our socialized values to explain and cope with life, often creating a feeling of disconnection. Feelings shift from relying upon external solutions to a neophytic sense of self-reliance. Slowly, there is recognition of multilevelness—of new, higher possibilities both in our view of external life and in our sense of our inner psychic milieu. We see in ourselves the possibility of a new, different, and higher way. The development of this vertical axis of values and feelings creates a dynamic motivation to explore these higher possibilities. The hierarchy of values first appears at the level of spontaneous multilevel disintegration. As development continues, dynamisms such as self-responsibility, self-awareness, and self-control become active, allowing the individual to move into the phase of organized or self-directed multilevel disintegration and thus take conscious direct control over his or her development. Individual values result from our unique experiences and development. Dąbrowski (1967) described the feeling of something "new" stemming from the emerging personality, specifically from the emerging hierarchy of values.

As we can see, values were central to Dąbrowski's (1970b) basic approach to development:

> To each level of mental development, there is a corresponding level of value experience. Mental development of man and the development of a hierarchy of values are, in fact, two names for the same process. One cannot separate the two. (p. 98)

Dąbrowski (1970b) emphasized that this hierarchy is independent from the value hierarchy created by cultural and social forces:

> The basic assumption of the theory of positive disintegration is that there is an empirically observable development of the capacity to make value judgments and to establish an autonomous hierarchy of values, distinguishable and independent from the hierarchy conditioned by cultural factors. (p. 120)

The vertical, hierarchical structure of values is a critical component as development requires that we be able to distinguish higher values, needs and goals—"what ought to be"—from lower ones—"that which is." We must begin to crave and explore for higher values, seek to adjust to the image or idea they embody, and reject lower levels of behavior and reality, and in the process become positively maladjusted to the lower aspects of life (see Yankov, 2017). For Dąbrowski (1967), the developmental solution is always in an upward direction:

> Without the feeling of a hierarchy of values above us and without an emotional attitude of esteem for these values, there would be no yearning for an ideal and, consequently, no action of dynamisms permitting the discrimination of various levels within our inner environment. (p. 27)

As development culminates at the highest levels, the hierarchy of values merges with and essentially becomes equivalent to the individual's personality ideal. For the individual, this new self-determined hierarchy of values/personality ideal becomes the standard by which one judges one's self. Dąbrowski (1970b) also suggested that this hierarchy could also represent a standard for societies as well.

As we have mentioned, Dąbrowski felt that because differences among levels can consistently be described and measured, they should therefore be considered objective. Through a careful examination of a concrete act, it is possible to ascertain its underlying emotions and the level it represents, and in this way, we can arrive at an objective description of valuation. The lives of eminent personalities give us further evidence and "serve as an empirical verification of the correctness of [the] hierarchy of values" (Dąbrowski, 1970b, p. 107). Thus, Dąbrowski felt that value judgments and the hierarchy of values represent objective and non-arbitrary phenomena that can be used as experiential markers of advanced development, not merely acting as philosophical constructs or guidelines. In addition, Dąbrowski (1970b) observed that at high levels of development, there is strong agreement in moral and value judgments and individuals at high levels tend to share the same values. It was Dąbrowski's position that the study of human development would reveal an objective hierarchy of authentic human values. Dąbrowski (1970b) provided an elegant summary:

> The road towards an independent authentic hierarchy of values is certainly very difficult, but it must be made clear that there is no other safe method open to man, because even the best system of moral norms does not work in practice, if its assimilation is not authentic and does not involve genuine inner psychic transformation. (p. 120)

5–5. PSYCHOLOGICAL TYPES

I will not offer a detailed review of the psychology of personality traits; however, as an introduction, I will mention a few seminal sources. One of the most influential and earliest works was by Jung (1926). Jung's theories were the foundation of a popular approach to trait testing, the Myers-Briggs Type Indicator (MBTI) (e.g., Haas & Hunziker, 2006; Wilde, 2011). In 1957, Timothy Leary published an influential book on the interpersonal dimensions of personality, *The*

Interpersonal Diagnosis of Personality. Leary's work laid the foundation for circumplex models (Plutchik & Conte, 1996). In the last 20 years, the five-factor model has become very popular (e.g., John & Scrivastava, 1999; McAdams & Pals, 2006; McCrae & Costa, 2003; Widiger, 2017; Widiger & Costa, 2013). The circumplex model and the five-factor model have also been amalgamated (e.g., Bäckström, Larsson, & Maddux, 2009; Hofstee, de Raad, & Goldberg, 1992; Woods & Anderson, 2016). For an excellent overview of the psychology of personality traits see Matthews, Deary, and Whiteman (2009).

Dąbrowski used the expression "psychological type" in two contexts. In the first context, psychological type refers to the initial, innate psychological type that one is born with. Part of this approach was based upon Carl Jung's (1875-1961) extravert and introvert classification. In addition, Dąbrowski also referred to several specific personality types, including the cyclic type, schizothymic type, schizoid type, tetanoid type, dysplastic type, intuitive type, masculine and feminine type and so forth. For Dąbrowski, these psychological types represented "the totality of individual, psychobiological, constitutional qualities determining the behavior of an individual with regard to himself and his environment" (Dąbrowski, 1970b, p. 179). Through the process of positive disintegration, the biological life cycle (the "normal" developmental stages) and one's initial psychological type are surpassed and transformed. As development and multilevelness occur, the "drawbacks and limitations of the constitutional psychological type" are brought to light and undergo transformation through inhibition and elimination: "Mental health is accompanied by some degree of ability to transform one's psychological type in the direction of attaining one's ideal" (Dąbrowski, 1964b, p. 116). In addition, Dąbrowski advocated that it was wise for the individual to cultivate and develop his or her opposite type, yielding a more balanced and integrated personality structure. For example, an extravert should try to inhibit his or her outgoing behavior and to develop traits of introversion.

The second context pertaining to psychological type was encapsulated in Dąbrowski's approach to development, leading to the following psychological types (Dąbrowski, 1970b, p. 179).

5–5–1. The primitively integrated type

One's mental structure is dominated by primitive drives that utilize intelligence as a tool toward achieving ends advocated by primitive instincts and emotions. Development is constricted and occurs within the biosocial cycle of life.

5–5–2. The positively integrated type

This type is characterized by the completion of the process of positive disintegration and the resultant reintegration in a secondary level reflecting a new organization and harmonization. Personality reflects a unique hierarchy of values and a fully developed inner psychic milieu.

5–5–3. The positively disintegrated type

A loosening and disintegration of one's psychological structures characterizes this type. A primary feature is the operation of developmental dynamisms.

5–5–4. The chronically disintegrated type (developmentally neutral type)

In this type, a permanent disintegration occurs that does not develop into either negative disintegration or into secondary integration. These individuals lack the developmental forces required to propel them into secondary integration.

5–5–5. The negatively disintegrated type

This type is characterized by a disintegration leading to a "mental illness with unfavorable course and prognosis" (Dąbrowski, 1970b, p. 180). Its primary characteristic is a lack of developmental dynamisms.

5–6. CHAPTER SUMMARY

This chapter described the core of Dąbrowski's developmental approach. The engine of development was represented by the numerous and intricate structures that Dąbrowski described, in particular by the dynamisms and by the inner psychic milieu—the collection of internal developmental features unique to a given individual. The dynamisms representing the fuel or energy of development were described, as were the different dynamisms associated with each level of development. In addition, the developmental instincts were integrated into the discussion, reflecting the important interaction of the dynamisms and instincts in the developmental levels. The role of emotions in the theory was introduced by a general overview of emotions in psychology. Emotion as the basis of moral judgements was then considered, leading to a discussion of emotions in Dąbrowski's theory and then culminating in an examination of emotional intelligence. The hierarchy of values was described. The chapter concluded with an examination of psychological types as described by Dąbrowski. Chapter Six will provide important insights into the strong philosophical roots and rationales that formed the foundation of Dąbrowski's thoughts and that tie together the many constructs he presented.

6

THE FOUNDATIONS OF
DĄBROWSKI'S APPROACH

Dąbrowski was widely read in, and influenced by, philosophy. This chapter will specifically focus on major themes seen in the works of Plato, Kierkegaard, and Nietzsche as they relate to Dąbrowski's work.[23] Among Dąbrowski's other significant influences were Spanish philosopher Miguel de Unamuno (1864-1936), French philosopher Henri Bergson (1859-1941) and German philosopher Karl Jaspers (1883-1969); however, it is beyond the scope of the present work to fully discuss the influence of these three philosophers.

In summary, Dąbrowski incorporated and synthesized several important traditional philosophical constructs into his theory—including ideas from Plato, Kierkegaard, and Nietzsche. This chapter will explore these philosophical aspects.

6–1. PLATO AND MULTILEVELNESS

When I was a student of Dąbrowski's, I asked him what I should read to give me a background to his approach. He replied, "Plato." Dąbrowski explained that during his life, he had seen vast extremes in human behavior, from very primitive violence and cruelty, to the other extreme of heroism and self-sacrifice. He said that to encompass these polar extremes any psychological theory had to use multiple levels incorporating qualitatively different descriptions—he could not conceive that these opposing poles could be on a continuum differing only quantitatively. Plato's work described a four-level approach to reality (Gould, 1969). Therefore, Dąbrowski (1964b) initiated a paradigm shift in thinking about psychology and psychological development by introducing the multilevel approach.

In applying a multilevel, Platonic-like description of reality to psychology, Dąbrowski developed a hierarchical model that incorporated two basic levels of sensory perception; 1) imagination and cognitive (intellectual) features and 2) emotional function. The former represent the lowest levels of function, the latter represents the highest levels. This differentiation is reminiscent of Thesleff's (2002) "two level model" that summarized Plato's lower human level—the world of the body and the senses—versus the higher divine level, characterized by the world of the soul and an unseen, unchanging and unified world. These two contrasting levels (the human versus the divine) are opposites but have some degree of overlap and coexistence, although in this coexistence, the divine level dominates the human level.

In Plato's description of the levels of existence, lower level attempts to describe existence involve *mere* opinions, shadows or inadequate copies of the higher, more authentic, and truer ideal Forms. For example, if an individual draws a right triangle, regardless of his or her artistic ability or mathematical precision, it will represent only one individual's flawed opinion or less-than-perfect copy of the more real, ideal, and divine Form of the right triangle as described by the mathematical theorem attributed to Pythagoras. In contemporary philosophy, this universal, ideal triangle, defined by a mathematical formula, does not exist in space or time—it is an abstract object that one must conceive—one can do this because souls are born with memories of the Forms. In a similar way, socialization produces mere mass copies of personalities, personal identities, social roles, expectations and so forth. The alternative is for one to discover "the higher path" and to imagine an ideal Form for oneself and then to subsequently shape and create one's own unique personality in the image of this ideal. As one proceeds to live by the values of this unique personality, one approaches the individual idealized Form of oneself to the extent that this is possible.

Dąbrowski's multilevel description of development shares several aspects in common with Plato's approach. For Plato, lower levels were associated with limited consciousness and with crude, simple or mistaken perceptions (Santas, 2006). Plato was famous for the complexity of his mathematical description of reality, but he also made his approach readily accessible in his allegory of the cave, as illustrated in Figure 3. "The Cave is a parable to illustrate the degrees in which our nature may be enlightened or unenlightened" (Fogelin, 1971, p. 378). I present a bare narrative of the allegory and a basic illustration in Figure 4. More in-depth treatments are available (e.g., Ferrari, 2007; Hall, 1980; McCabe, 1992; Plato, 1991, 2004; Santas, 2006; Wright, 1906).

The stage is set (paraphrased from Plato, 2004):

Socrates: Imagine human beings living in an underground, cavelike dwelling, with an entrance a long way up that is open to the sunlight and as wide as the cave itself. They have been there since childhood, with their necks and legs fettered, so that they are fixed in the same place, able to see only in front of them, because their fetter prevents them from turning their heads around. Light is provided by a fire burning far above and behind them. Between the prisoners and the fire, there is an elevated road stretching. Imagine that along this road a low wall has been built—like the screen in front of people that is provided by puppeteers, and above which they show their puppets.

Glaucon: It is a strange image you are describing, and strange prisoners.

Socrates: They are like us. I mean, in the first place, do you think these prisoners have ever seen anything of themselves and one another besides the shadows that the fire casts on the wall of the cave in front of them? . . . All in all, then, what the prisoners would take for true reality is nothing other than the shadows of those artifacts.

Glaucon: That's entirely inevitable. (p. 208)

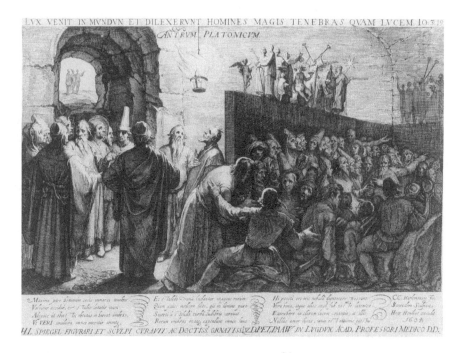

Figure 3. *Plato's Cave* by Jan Saenredam[24]

Thus, unbeknownst to the group, perceived life is simply a low-level illusion, a procession of shadow box images projected on the wall. This shadow play is contrived by the politic of the day and delivered by puppet masters (representatives of the state educational system) who manipulate shadow puppets on a wall to portray life, as they want it to be perceived.

At some point, a prisoner breaks free and sees his or her predicament (paraphrased from Plato, 2004):

Socrates: And if someone dragged him by force away from there, along the rough, steep, upward path, and did not let him go until he had dragged him into the light of the sun, wouldn't he be pained and angry at being treated that way? And when he came into the light, wouldn't he have his eyes filled with sunlight and be unable to see a single one of the things now said to be truly real?

Glaucon: No, he would not be able to—at least not right away.

Socrates: He would need time to get adjusted, I suppose, if he is going to see the things in the world above. At first, he would see shadows most easily, then images of men and other things in water, then the things themselves. From these, it would be easier for him to go on to look at the things in the sky and the sky itself at night, gazing at the light of the stars and the moon, than during the day, gazing at the sun and the light of the sun. (p. 209)

For those who do stumble into the sunlight, life now takes on a completely different perspective; now in the sunlight, one can see truth and knowledge—for Plato, the Form of the Good. One realizes that the life seen in the cave was an illusion and there is a qualitative paradigm shift in perception toward seeing reality.

Plato recognized that the prisoner's impulse will be to stay in the sunlight and look for opportunities to further ascend, so he described the duty of the prisoner who has "seen the light"—he or she must return into the cave and help enlighten the remaining prisoners. Further individual enlightenment must wait until the last prisoner is freed from the cave. Unfortunately, in transitioning from the bright sunlight back into the dimly lit cave, the prisoner is temporarily blinded and flails around to discover his or her way. The remaining prisoners hear a wild story about the surface that they can barely comprehend, and, fearing that this returning prisoner has gone mad, they react by killing the enlightened messenger.

As Plato described (paraphrased from Plato, 2004):

Socrates: If the time required for readjustment was not short, wouldn't he provoke ridicule? Wouldn't it be said of him that he had returned from his upward journey with his eyes ruined, and that it is not worthwhile even to try to travel upward? And as for anyone who tried to free the prisoners and lead them upward, if they could somehow get their hands on him, wouldn't they kill him?

Glaucon: They certainly would.

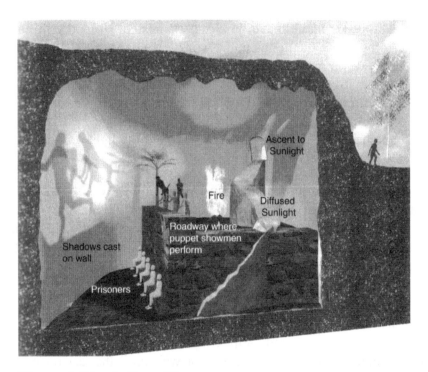

Figure 4. Plato's Cave Diagram
(a depiction commonly found on the Internet by an anonymous author)

Plato then explained that the journey into the sunlight is the soul's journey to the discovery of truth and enlightenment. Education does not help us achieve enlightenment—it only imparts *knowledge*; rather, each of us already has the potential within us to become enlightened.

Using a process of self-insight, self-realization, self-actualization (Teloh, 1976) or, what Plato called self-mastery (C. Taylor, 1989), one can discover true *wisdom*, becoming a philosopher-king, one who will use wisdom—the Form of the Good—to better society.

Individuals at the level of primary integration in Dąbrowski's model share much in common with the lot of Plato's prisoners. For Dąbrowski, the average person passively accepts socialization, endorsing day-to-day reality with little critical question or review. The well-socialized person lives by imitation, following externally prescribed roles with limited consciousness and expressing little individuality or authenticity. At the level of primary integration an individual learns *knowledge* through education and may excel but will ultimately lack *wisdom* because socialization and conventional education prevents the individual from self-mastery—the discovery of true wisdom and enlightenment. In Dąbrowski's terms, self-mastery must be achieved largely through self-education and autopsychotherapy.

Dąbrowski emphasized that higher levels differ on both quantitative and qualitative dimensions when compared to lower levels. Psychology commonly recognizes quantitative differences; for instance, intelligence is commonly differentiated into levels on the basis of differences in test scores. However, Dąbrowski perceived that advanced development displays another important aspect: at some point, major qualitative differences appear—for example, the basic perception of reality is literally different for individuals at the highest levels compared to persons at lower levels. Qualitative differences become an important descriptive feature; they starkly differentiate advanced development from lower-level function, thus providing an evidentiary basis for the classification of personality and development.

6–2. ESSENCE AND EXISTENTIALISM

Dąbrowski coined the term "existentio-essentialist compound" to describe his unusual synthesis of two traditionally disparate philosophical views of human character: one reflecting the essentialist approach of the Platonic tradition, and the other a more modern existential approach found in the works of Kierkegaard and Nietzsche (among others). Dąbrowski considered the inherent essence of a person's character as the initial foundation of development. However, Dąbrowski observed that in the usual course of development, individual essence often remains submerged, as individuality and autonomy are effectively overpowered by socialization and group conformity. Advanced growth involves a disintegration of this initial lower-level integration to create opportunities for the discovery of one's true essence, leading to self-insight and a series of conscious and volitional, day-to-day existential choices. These existential choices subsequently shape and refine one's raw essence to ultimately create a unique and autonomous personality.

Dąbrowski (1972b) believed that an individual's genetics are important contributors to his or her eventual development. One possesses an inner essence composed of the central qualities and traits of one's personality. However, this essence is not strictly fixed; rather, it exists as a potential that may or may not be developed or expressed. In addition, this essence may be positive and act to enhance development, or it may be negative and act to limit development. It may also include a broad spectrum of general features, including influences from our animal ancestry, as well as uniquely authentic human traits expressed individually.

The expression of this individual essence is not a given. Dąbrowski (1973) believed that personality must be achieved—constructed through a series of individual, conscious choices that distinguish characteristics that are "more myself" from characteristics that are "less myself." As development progresses, insight and self-awareness emerge. At a certain point "the individual becomes aware of what is his own 'essence'; that is to say, what are his aims and aspirations, his attitudes, his relations with other people" (Dąbrowski, 1973, p. 109; see also McGraw, 1986). The individual constructs a personality ideal based upon this initial essence, along with his or her imagined possibilities, dreams, and aspirations. As the image of the personality ideal becomes increasingly clear, the individual can compare and contrast this ideal with his or her initial essence. Based upon vertical, multilevel comparisons, he or she makes conscious and volitional choices about what to emphasize and what aspects to inhibit. In this way, the full and final expression of one's character reflects both the essence of who one initially is, as well as the ongoing existential choices that one makes.

In addition to "character" or inner essence, Dąbrowski also described several other innate factors that play critical roles in determining the developmental trajectory of an individual. These include the creative instinct; the instinct toward self-perfection; dynamisms—the combination of drives and emotions that provide the energy for development; and finally, the constellation of factors that he referred to as developmental potential.

We can summarize Dąbrowski's "existentio-essentialist" approach by saying that the individual must become aware of his or her unique traits—essence—and subsequently make volitional existential choices to shape and denote this essence to fully express an individualized personality ideal. Dąbrowski made it clear that "essence is more important than existence for the birth of a truly human being," and he went on to say, "There is no true human existence without genuine essence" (Cienin, 1972, p. 11). Recognizing the unique contributions of essence, developmental potentials, and existential choices, and understanding how these factors interact, provides us with a powerful new insight into understanding development.

It is interesting to note that Maslow also advanced the idea of the mutual contribution of essence and choice. For Maslow, one's inner nature has two components, one reflecting a species-wide identification—a largely hereditary intrinsic instinctoid[25]—and the other reflecting the unique traits of the individual. Maslow (1968, p. 193) explained that one grows into adulthood partly by the "discovery, uncovering and acceptance of what is 'there' beforehand" (one's inner nature) and partly through the ongoing choices the individual makes, constituting "his own project." Authentic selfhood is being able to hear "the impulse-voices within oneself" and getting in touch with what one really wants to do and what one is really fit to do. Once one gets in touch with this, growth becomes an "endless series of daily choices and decisions in each of which one can choose to go back toward safety or forward toward growth. Growth must be chosen again and again; fear must be overcome again and again" (Maslow, 1966, p. 22).

6–3. THE AVERAGE PERSON AS AUTOMATON

It is useful to consider some critical milestones in the development of psychology that promoted the view of the individual as animal-like or robotic.

In comparing animals and humans, Lowry (1982) noted,

The great insight of the eighteenth century was that they are not radically different. We may speak of man as being more complex or more highly organized—but that is all, for it is only a difference of degree, not of kind. (p. 52)

William James published *The Principles of Psychology* in 1890. Lowry noted that James was torn between a mechanistic view that emphasized the role of habit and instinct, essentially making animals and humans automata—James found it hard to refute the automatic response nature of reflexes and habits—versus the existential and ethical implications that this view raised. In addition, James made the "fatal assumption" that the higher centers act passively, like a telephone switchboard, simply taking in and passing along stimuli but contributing no new processing—activities being blindly directed by the nervous system's built-in automatic mechanisms (Lowry, 1982). This view stands in stark contrast to the approach suggested by Hughlings Jackson at around the same time and later by Mazurkiewicz. These views emphasized that the basis of intelligence was produced by the coordinating and synthesizing capacity of the cerebral cortex.

It is sometimes difficult to imagine that for half a century psychology was dominated by behaviorism, largely founded on the work of John B. Watson (1878-1958). This quotation from Watson (1913) set the stage:

> Psychology as the behaviorist views it is a purely objective experimental branch of natural science. Its theoretical goal is the prediction and control of behavior. Introspection forms no essential part of its methods, nor is the scientific value of its data dependent upon the readiness with which they lend themselves to interpretation in terms of consciousness. The behaviorist, in his efforts to get a unitary scheme of animal response, recognizes no dividing line between man and brute. The behavior of man, with all of its refinement and complexity, forms only a part of the behaviorist's total scheme of investigation. (p. 158)

Reading the above, it should come as no surprise that Watson was famous for saying:

> Give me a dozen healthy infants, well-formed and my own specified world to bring them up in and I'll guarantee to take any one at random and train him to become any type of specialist I might select—doctor, lawyer, artist, merchant-

chief and, yes, even beggar-man and thief, regardless of his talents, penchants, tendencies, abilities, vocations and race of his ancestors. I am going beyond my facts and I admit it, but so have the advocates of the contrary and they have been doing it for many thousands of years (John B. Watson, 2016, The twelve infants quote, para. 2).

B. F. Skinner (1904-1990) redefined behaviorism in 1938 by emphasizing the methodology of tracing the functional relations between observable stimuli in the environment and organisms' observable responses to them, a phenomenon he referred to as operant behavior. Behaviorism had a pervasive influence on psychology and also received considerable support from many diverse areas; for example, from business (Watson became an executive in the advertising industry) and in the government. Skinner's book, *Beyond Freedom and Dignity*, was written with a grant from the National Institutes of Mental Health. In fact, behaviorism still appears to have a loyal following in some quarters. For example, in 1985, Zuriff attempted to revitalize behaviorism:

> The fundamental questions concerning the nature of psychology have not been answered, nor is it obvious that progress is being made. Instead, certain recurrent themes are discussed, debated into a numbing stillness and dropped unsettled, only to reappear years later in a different guise and under a new terminology. Therefore, the behaviorist of 1920 may have much of relevance to say to the modern psychologist formulating a conceptual framework for psychology. (p. 5)

Many factors, both within psychology and society at large, likely contributed to the paradigm shift against behaviorism. Certainly one major factor was the publication of Maslow's *Motivation and Personality* in 1954, marking the beginning of the "third force" in psychology (as Maslow himself coined it) and signaling, for all intents and purposes, the beginning of the end of the second force—behaviorism.[26] Moss (2001) also noted the contributions of several others to the rise of the third force, including Kurt Goldstein (1878-1965) who emphasized both biological and psychological self-actualization, as well as Andras Angyal (1902-1960), who provided a holistic approach to personality, including the idea that health and neuroses were opposing forces, both organized and vying for supremacy. If neuroses dominate, the path for the expression of healthy systems is blocked. Additional contributors included Henry Murray (1893-1988), known for his emphasis on the healthy personality; Gordon Allport, who emphasized the idea of conscious and deliberate becoming; and Gardner Murphy (1895-1979) who presented an organismic biosocial view of personality development which moves through the stages of undifferentiated wholeness, differentiation, and finally to integration.

Ludwig von Bertalanffy (1901-1972)[27] made another important contribution to the revolution against behaviorism. Bertalanffy was the founder of General Systems Theory, the idea that an organism can best be understood as a system of self-organization that develops in a progressive series of higher levels of differentiation, organization, and complexity. Dąbrowski endorsed Bertalanffy's dismissive view of psychology, which Bertalanffy presented in his 1967 book, *Robots, Men and Minds.* Bertalanffy (1967) said that psychology was dominated by a positivistic-mechanistic-reductionistic approach epitomized in the robot model of man. He was critical of a social structure that promoted mental "health" under the guise of responding to external demands in socially expected and sanctioned ways while simply creating an endless stream of "robopaths" (as he called them). "Robot psychologists" have helped provide modern psychology with "tricks to turn human beings into subhuman automata, or into a mob screaming for destruction of a supposed enemy or even of themselves; it is just a question of routine techniques used by any car dealer or television advertiser" (Bertalanffy, 1967, p. 13). Modern psychology has cancelled any difference between animal and man "for the anthropomorphic view of the rat, American psychology has traded in a rattomorphic view of man" (Koestler, 1964, p. 560, as cited in Bertalanffy, 1967, p. 15). According to Bertalanffy, this amounts to a functional decerebralization of human beings. Bertalanffy's (1967) solution was to create a new construction based upon the human as an active personality system and to provide an alternative to the robotization of man in psychology by aspiring toward a humanization of science.

Lewis Yablonsky (1972) also used the term robopath to describe the plight of modern man. Yablonsky, a criminologist, was concerned over the growing dehumanization of people—to the point where they often appear as mere zombies. When people play out roles as insincere actors, experiencing pre-programmed emotions with little or no real compassion or sympathy for anyone, the outcome is often an epidemic of violence. Robopaths are socially dead, robot-like people who display Kierkegaard's "sickness unto death" (Yablonsky, 1972, p. 7).

Presenting a contrary position, White (1996) suggested that to choose a robotic mentality might act as a defense against total disintegration and insanity. White (1996) said: "To some degree we all have a tendency to dehumanize ourselves even if this is only manifested by the desire to be statistically 'normal'" (p. 40). Echoing Maslow's views, White (1996) also cautioned us about trying to achieve ideals—"Once I have attained my ideal, then what?" In trying to pursue one's ideal, White feared that the creative impulse could be stifled before it has a chance to express itself.

6–4. THE AVERAGE PERSON AS "BEING ASLEEP"

A common theme in psychological literature is the observation that the average person "is asleep at the switch" and persistently functions at a low level of awareness/consciousness. As we saw above, Plato was probably the first to clearly articulate this idea. Plato described a hierarchy of increasing awareness and consciousness; at the lower levels, individuals are quite unaware of their surroundings and see an imperfect and indirect representation of reality—as it is presented to them by their social and cultural milieu—illustrated in the allegory of Plato's cave. At the highest levels, the divine levels, an individual becomes conscious—emerging into the light—and is able to perceive a more accurate, and more direct, version of everyday reality.

Pierre Janet's hierarchical description, presented in Chapter Two, was similar to Plato's but with a more psychiatric orientation. At the highest level, the individual is fully conscious ("living in the moment") and perceives reality with an energetic vitality and accuracy. At the lower levels, consciousness is dulled, energy is depleted, and perceptions of reality become disjointed and inaccurate.

T. S. Eliot provided an image of waking unconsciousness in his poem, *Four Quartets*. Eliot (1944) wrote:

> Or as, when an underground train, in the tube, stops too long
>   between stations
> And the conversation rises and slowly fades into silence
> And you see behind every face the mental emptiness deepen
> Leaving only the growing terror of nothing to think about.
> (p. 19)

Ormsby (2006) noted that in Eliot's description, terror is not the result of "having nothing to think about"; instead it is the product of having to think about nothing. This condition seems to be pervasive in our modern world, where people complain of being tremendously busy and exhausted from thinking so much but, in reality, spend most of their time having to contemplate and plod through nothing but a trivial, external, and meaningless reality.

In another startling image, Saint-Exupéry (1939) observed a train full of workers, somehow reduced to mere lumps of clay, now no more than machines performing manual labor. He asked what kind of "terrible mould" could have produced these effects—"as if they had gone through a monstrous stamping machine?" Saint-Exupéry (1939, p. 305) lamented a small child on the train, "a Mozart murdered," as he too "will be shaped like the rest by the common stamping machine" and with the death of his individuality, so too will die a little bit of the human race.

In examining the limited consciousness of the average person, it is useful to examine the work of Georges Ivanovich Gurdjieff (c. 1866-1949). Gurdjieff, an Armenian mystic, developed a system of thought that emphasized an integrated, systemic, and balanced approach to development, encompassing body, mind, and emotions. Gurdjieff's student, P. D. Ouspensky (1878-1947), popularized the approach as the "Fourth Way" (Ouspensky, 1971). Gurdjieff (1969) described various states of consciousness and contrasted the subjective nature of our dreams while sleeping with the average person's experience of being awake, suggesting that the two states were quite similar. Most people go through life in a sort of waking sleep state where accurate perceptions of reality are obscured by an uncontrollable stream of egocentric thoughts, emotions, desires, and images from the imagination, leading to robotic, machine-like behavior. In its worst manifestation, physically awake but otherwise asleep individuals act as machines in carrying out the directives of their society (for example, going off to fight a war). Gurdjieff's answer to this situation was to admonish the individual to fully "wake up."

Dąbrowski recommended the Gurdjieff primer written by Ouspensky, *The Psychology of Man's Possible Evolution* (1945/1973). This slender volume described personal development while reflecting the essential ideas presented by Gurdjieff. In it, Ouspensky outlined four possible states of consciousness: sleep, the waking state, self-consciousness, and objective consciousness. The average person lives in the first two states which are similar to each other. Ouspensky (1945/1973) said:

> Sleep . . . does not disappear when the second state arrives, that is, when man awakes. Sleep remains there, with all its dreams and impressions . . . dreams become invisible exactly as the stars and moon become invisible in the glare of the sun. But they are all there, and they often influence all our thoughts, feelings, and actions—sometimes even more than the actual perceptions of the moment. (p. 32)

The third state Ouspensky (1945/1973) described, self-consciousness, appears only in glimpses or rare flashes.

> We can say that man has occasional moments of self-consciousness leaving vivid memories of the circumstances accompanying them, but he has no command over them. They come and go by themselves, being controlled by external circumstances and occasional associations or memories of emotions (pp. 21-22).

In another description of the third state, Ouspensky, (1945/1973) said:

Self-consciousness is a state in which man becomes objective towards himself and objective consciousness is a state in which he comes into contact with the real, or objective world from which he is now shut off by the senses, dreams and subjective states of consciousness. (p. 35)

In the state of self-consciousness, we can come to know the full truth about ourselves. In the fourth state, objective consciousness, we can attain truth about everything and study the world at large the way it really is. Unfortunately, Ouspensky (1945/1973) believed "objective consciousness is a state about which we know nothing" (p. 34).

Ouspensky emphasized that the differences between higher and lower levels are greater than we can imagine and went on to say that "you can understand other people only as much as you understand yourself and only on the level of your own being" (Ouspensky, 1945/1973, p. 107). This classification is reminiscent of Dąbrowski's unilevel and multilevel divisions.

Gurdjieff's call to "wake-up" was again popularized by Charles Tart (1937-). Tart (1987) gave a modern context to the idea that the average person is going through life asleep, essentially in a robotic trance. Tart's model proposed that we do not perceive reality as it literally is; rather, each of us has an individual experience based upon our own unique biological, psychological and sociological makeup. This "consciousness as-we-experience-it" is heavily influenced by society and culture. Tart observed that culture plays the role of hypnotist and induces a "consensus trance," leading the average individual to focus on a semi-arbitrary, narrow reality defined and prescribed by culture. Tart encouraged people to wake up from this trance and to embrace the full individual experience of reality. Tart (1987) offered a succinct description from the point of view of culture, saying:

It is far better if your everyday mind, the habitual, automatized way you think and feel, is shaped to reflect the culture's consensus beliefs and values. Then you will automatically experience the right perceptions and interpretations and so it will be "natural" to act in the culturally appropriate way, even when there are no agents of social coercion around. (p. 88)

This automaton-like state reflects the "cultural consensus trance." Tart reviewed Gurdjieff's methods for waking up from this trance; a first and most important step is to simply pay more attention to one's self—to become aware of one's own automatic reactions.

Another critical part of Tart's solution lies in recognizing an important lesson from Buddhist philosophy: that compassion and empathy are highly evolved emotions which, for Tart, need to be integrated with our intellectual and instinctive intelligences to yield a more conscious, more aware, and more sensitive interaction with others and the world.

Colin Wilson's description of "Faculty X" is pertinent to this discussion. Wilson (1971) said:

When you are deeply asleep, you have no consciousness. When you are very tired, your consciousness is like a dim light that hardly illuminates anything. When you are wide awake and excited, consciousness seems to increase in sheer candlepower. Its purpose is to illuminate reality, to reach out into its recesses, and thus to enable us to act upon it and transform it. It is obvious that our basic aim should be to increase its candlepower. When it is low, reality becomes "unreal"; as it becomes stronger, reality becomes "realer": Faculty X. (p. 60)

Wilson presents Faculty X as an ordinary, but generally untapped, potentiality of everyday consciousness and goes so far as to say that it is the key to the future of the evolution of the human race. Wilson's (1971) description is succinct for our purposes:

When I am half asleep, my sense of reality is restricted to myself and my immediate surroundings. The more awake I am, the further it stretches. But what we call "waking consciousness" is not usually a great deal better than sleep. We are still wrapped in a passive, sluggish daydream. But this is not because there is some natural limit to consciousness, but only because we remain unaware that it can be stretched. We are like dogs who think they are on a chain when in fact they are free. (pp. 61-2)

A major implication of these descriptions of a hierarchy of consciousness is that people will vary widely in their attention and perception of reality based upon their inherent psychological attributes. Not everyone will be able to see the vertical contrasts of reality—for some, the depth of their "cultural trance" is too great and their level of reality functions (Plato and Janet) too low.

In summary, to combine several metaphors: many people are unable to rise above the common, social, and cultural reality of life—a reality that hypnotizes most people, producing a robot-like trance. For many, the "pressure" of consciousness and psychological tension is too low to permit the development of an autonomous consciousness—to wake up and independently create an "individual" view of reality.

6–5. SOCIALIZATION SQUELCHES AUTONOMY

In describing primary integration, Dąbrowski noted that behavior is commonly organized in the service of self-satisfying instincts and impulses. Social roles are often acted out and manipulated in order to achieve ego-satisfying goals. Many people are charismatic and strong, often taking on leadership roles in society. Unfortunately, even when attaining social positions of responsibility, some of these individuals continue to act in egocentric and self-satisfying ways, with little appreciation of the damage they may be doing to themselves or to others, or for their social duties. As the Dalai Lama (2017) observed:

> Under the sway of self-centeredness from time immemorial, you have brought yourself only harm and suffering. Now take control of this misplaced attitude and destroy it. If your mind does not comply, the only thing you can do is destroy your self-centered attitude. (p. 50)

Images of the "psychopath" as a suit-wearing, "win-at-any-cost" businessperson, or of the self-justifying politician, come to mind (Babiak & Hare, 2006).

Our educational and political system (Plato's puppet masters) is predicated upon creating and encouraging highly able and competitive individuals who can excel in the "dog-eat-dog" business and political world. That society develops and so esteems these "winners" "indicates that the society itself is primitive and confused" (Dąbrowski, 1970b, p. 118). Dąbrowski was further concerned that definitions of mental health based upon an individual's adjustment to prevailing social norms do not represent authentic human development or function. Adjustment to a society that is itself "primitive and confused" is adevelopmental and holds one back from discovering individual essence and from exercising choice in shaping and developing one's self—Dąbrowski's criteria for mental health (Dąbrowski, 1970b).

6–5–1. Kierkegaard's crowd

Dąbrowski was not the first to be concerned with the negative impact of socialization on human authenticity. Kierkegaard expressed similar concerns, saying that reliance on social roles and church doctrines prevent the individual from real action. McDonald (2014) summarized Kierkegaard's position, saying:

> Kierkegaard's central problematic was *how to become a Christian in Christendom*. The task was most difficult for the well-educated, since prevailing educational and cultural institutions tended to produce stereotyped members of "the crowd" rather than to allow individuals to discover their own unique identities. (section 2, para. 1)

The crowd robs the person of individual responsibility. As Kierkegaard (1962) explained:

> A crowd—not this crowd or that, the crowd now living or the crowd long deceased, a crowd of humble people or of superior people, of rich or of poor, etc.—a crowd in its very concept is the untruth, by reason of the fact that it renders the individual completely impenitent and irresponsible, or at least weakens his sense of responsibility by reducing it to a fraction. (p. 112)

Kierkegaard described two modalities that could lead to the experience of despair, the first being relinquishing one's true self through an identification with socialization. Nielsen (2017) succinctly described how Kierkegaard viewed the individual who experiences the modality of "the despair of not willing to be oneself," who is spiritless, and is merely "a talking-machine":

> Spiritlessness describes a special relationship that an individual has with the world and with the self. In this understanding of the world, the individual experiences the world as already constituted. This also means the individual associates with immediate possibilities and remains unaware of the potential and the possibilities embedded in existence. The individual identifies with existing standards to obtain self-knowledge and primarily evaluates him- or herself through achievement and functionality. Thus, the object of self-knowledge is how the individual lives up to the functional standards offered by various institutions, such as the state, the nation, the workplace, and so on. (pp. 7-8)

Kierkegaard observed that society effectively blocks the development of individuality; society provides a myriad of objects the individual can identify with (e.g., a job) that create security and distraction, thereby protecting the individual from having to face his or her real self, and thus avoiding the experience of true personal despair.

In Kierkegaard's second modality, an individual experiences a despair that arises from being willing to be oneself. As Kierkegaard (1941) said, "The self is its own lord and master, so it is said, its own lord, and precisely this is despair" (p. 111). Kierkegaard went on to explain that "by closer inspection one easily ascertains that this ruler is a king without a country, he rules really over nothing" (p. 111). Kierkegaard concluded: "So the despairing self is constantly building nothing but castles in the air, it fights only in the air" (p. 111).

There is no pre-existing deeper self for one to discover or bring forth.

Kierkegaard's (2017) explanation for the creation of the self was comprised of several key elements, including the complex relationship between the self and faith:

> Personality is not a sum of doctrines, nor is it something immediately accessible; personality is conjugated only on the

basis of itself, it is a Clausum, [an enclosed space], an αδυτον, [innermost sanctuary] a μυστηριον; [mystery] personality is a ["]that within,["] hence the word persona (personare) is telling: it is that within, that to which a person, himself a personality, must relate believingly. Take the two most passionate lovers who have ever lived; even if they are, as the expression goes, one soul in two bodies, they nonetheless can never go beyond the one person believing that the other loves him or her.

The concept of faith rests in this purely personal relationship between God as personality and the believer as *existing* personality. (pp. 437-438)

An individual usually experiences the present as a seamless continuity. Kierkegaard observed that occasionally one will become fully conscious in an instant. In this sudden break from continuity, an individual takes part in real life—a Kierkegaardian process Nielsen (2017) called self-sufficient individuality.

I can illustrate a sudden break from my own life experience. While learning to fly, during my first solo flight, I looked at the seat beside me and saw that it was empty. I was immediately struck by the awareness that I was alone in the airplane and that my life was in my own hands now—I alone now had to land this airplane. I suddenly became aware of the choice facing me and felt the uncertainty and angst over the possibility that I could *choose* not to land, but to crash instead. I did decide to land and, before my next flight, paused for a moment to bolster my faith that I would make the same decision again. Of course, my instructor expected me to simply carry out my training to land the plane safely (by unconscious rote if necessary). Had I simply landed my first flight without experiencing the internal realization of my existential choice, I would never have had this moment of self-awareness, the momentary uncertainty and dread, or the subsequent feeling of self-determination, self-accomplishment, and subsequent self-satisfaction of successfully landing.

Kierkegaard and Dąbrowski would say that in making the conscious choice to land the airplane, I had taken responsibility over my life as an individual and in doing so, at least for that moment, I had chosen my own authentic path. In Kierkegaard's terms, the sudden but fleeting occurrence of experiencing a moment of real-life and its attendant consciousness creates existential anxiety—we become aware that there is *more*. Once we become aware of a door, we wonder what is behind it and whether we should choose to open it or not. We are torn by the choice—is it a mistake to open the door? Or, is the mistake to leave the door closed? While many try to deny the existence of the door and its attendant choices, the only true solution is to become fully conscious of reality and live with the dread and anxiety associated with our freedom to choose. "In anxiety we experience ourselves as the owners of our existence and its possibilities, that is, we experience our freedom" (Obsieger, 2017, p. 179). This freedom includes the day-to-day choices that generally seem so innocuous that we don't even notice them, as well as the occasional moments when we consciously confront our mortality— moments when we engage in real life.

Kierkegaard said that these choices are critical in creating a self: "A man possesses his own self as determined by himself, as someone selected by himself" (as cited in Dąbrowski, 1967, p. 36). To accept, manage, and surmount anxiety, and to follow through in making each choice based upon one's own values and faith, demonstrates and reaffirms one's human authenticity.

In a position similar to Dąbrowski's, Kierkegaard differentiated the vertical comparison of the lower, actual situation versus the higher alternative of what is possible—a possibility one may glimpse during a sudden break from continuity. As Dąbrowski (n.d.c) said, "We may say that Kierkegaard hated his (lower) self and his physical defects, but loved his ideal self on a higher level. His ideal self is presented in the courageous knight; it was this possibility that he loved in himself" (p. 208). Dąbrowski gave the example that Kierkegaard realized he could not marry Regine Olsen and orchestrated the end of their relationship because their conceptualizations of the ideal marriage were different.

In summary, instead of defining oneself based upon external social mores and roles, Kierkegaard suggested that the only true freedom for an individual is the heavy responsibility of being able to and having to, choose oneself—to construct oneself, one's beliefs and one's values through the successive decisions that one makes in day-to-day life (e.g., Hannay & Marino, 1998; Kaufmann, 1956). This day-to-day process of "acting and making decisions" is "guided by [the] individual's moods, sudden impulses, and loose thoughts" (Nielsen, 2017, p. 10). Stokes (2015) provided a synopsis: "the Kierkegaardian self is always a created self, a self that finds God as the ultimate 'criterion' for its own self-actualization and Christ as its prototype for emulation"[28] (p. 15).

6–5–2. Nietzsche's herd

Nietzsche was even more critical of the role played by society, suggesting that all schemes of morality are simply dogmas of the day representing "herd moralities" that prevent individuals from developing their own values by averaging mores "to the middle and the mean" (Nietzsche, 1968, p. 159). The morality of the herd reflects a homogenization, where the group mean now dictates values and ideals, representing the place where the numerical majority finds itself.

Reflecting the positions of Kierkegaard and Dąbrowski, Nietzsche described how adopting mores derived from socialization suspends the individual from the need to review his or her individual value assumptions and the accompanying responsibility to develop an individual, autonomous morality. The individual becomes content to simply conform and loses any internal motivation to develop him- or herself. Using the analogy of a camel, an unquestioning beast of burden, Nietzsche suggested that the average person learns to kneel and accept the expectations and duties imposed by society, reacting with fear and guilt if he or she fails to do so. In particular, Nietzsche rejected religion, suggesting that belief in religion absolves the individual of the responsibility of self-development.

6–6. EXEMPLARS OF ADVANCED DEVELOPMENT

In contrast to primary integration, advanced development is characterized by more complex (but less well organized) structures that now become subordinate to a new master—individual autonomy—characterized by self-control, full self-consciousness, and the creation of an internal value structure that comes to direct behavior. Dąbrowski contrasted individuals exemplifying primary integration with persons capable of empathy and self-reflection—for example, individuals like Abraham Lincoln, Socrates, and Gandhi. Such individuals consciously place the needs of others ahead of their own needs, and they lead by example. This group represents the higher end of the developmental continuum, and their secondary integration reflects Dąbrowski's autonomous force of third factor, reflecting self-definition, self-determination and the growth and expression of "one's own forces"—the criteria Dąbrowski used to define mental health (Dąbrowski, 1973, p. 39).

Contrasting the socialized individual, Plato, Kierkegaard, and Nietzsche also presented descriptions of the advanced individual, and each emphasized self-control, self-responsibility, and self-determination. Plato described three levels of individual function corresponding to three levels of the soul: (1) the worker class, corresponding to the "appetite" of the soul (from the waist down); (2) warriors who are strong and brave, corresponding to the "spirit" of the soul (the heart); and (3) the governing class, characterized by intelligence, rational thought, self-control, and love of wisdom. Ultimately, only a few individuals represent the governing class, a class corresponding to the "reason" aspect of the soul (essentially the head). These philosopher kings develop through the discovery of ideal Forms, Plato's ultimate level of reality.

For Kierkegaard, the discovery of one's mortality triggers one's consciousness and signals the activation of true existence. Although very critical of religious dogma, Kierkegaard emphasized a faith-based approach in which true selfhood requires being willing to take a leap of faith and to choose the self that one truly is, risking despair in not being able to achieve this ideal.

> Faith is the most important task to be achieved by a human being, because only on the basis of faith does an individual have a chance to become a true self. This self is the life-work, which God judges for eternity" (McDonald, 2014, section 5, para. 2).

Unfortunately, in everyday life, normality hides the true reality of being; however, when pushed to the edge of a cliff (or when realizing that one is alone in an airplane) one tends to see ordinary life and one's role in it from a new, clearer perspective.

Part of our developmental task is to try to see ourselves more objectively. Both Kierkegaard and Dąbrowski suggested that most people view themselves too subjectively and relate to others too objectively. One of Dąbrowski's key developmental features is subject-object in one's self: "a process of looking at oneself as if from outside (the self as object) and of perceiving the individuality of others (the other as subject, i.e., individual knower)" (Dąbrowski, 1972b, p. 305). This perceptual shift allows one to develop insight into one's mental life in order to better understand and critically evaluate one's self.

Kierkegaard described a theory of the stages or spheres of existence, comprising three spheres of selfhood from which the individual may choose, each characterized by its own unique worldview (e.g., Grøn, Rosfort, & Söderquist, 2017; Hannay & Marino, 1998; Ugochukwu, 2012). The lowest, aesthetical sphere is illustrated by the sensuality and hedonism of a Don Juan. This level is subhuman, because the same forces that control animals also govern us. Today, this level may be illustrated by the selfishness of the "dog-eat-dog," "cutthroat" businessperson who values profits and deal-making above all else. As mentioned above, this corresponds to Dąbrowski's primary level of integration. In order to break out of this inauthentic existence, the individual must embody Kierkegaard's (1987) famous either/or: "It is for freedom, therefore, that I am fighting (partly in this letter, partly and chiefly in myself), for the time to come, for Either/Or" (p. 176). The individual must either accept his or her lower self or consciously decide to will an end to the old self and to move forward "in a movement from state to state. Every state is posited by a leap" (Kierkegaard, 1980, p. 113).

The next sphere, the ethical, is characterized by ethical and moral responsibilities as expressed in a commitment to self-perfection, attaining one's ideals, and in honoring commitments to others. Like Dąbrowski, Kierkegaard was less concerned with which ideals are chosen than with the process—the autonomy employed in establishing one's ideals.

The final, religious sphere, involves a vertical leap—this time a personal leap into an infinite abyss. One does not come to know God through belief in ideas or through the reasoning of the intellect; one comes to know God through making an eternal leap in faith. In making this final leap, the individual also finally constructs him or herself. This moment highlights the responsibility of self-construction. One is initially filled with angst, anxiety and dread. This anxiety reflects the realization of the burden of making eternal choices, but it also reflects the exhilaration and the freedom of being able to choose. Each choice is frozen in time as it carries forth into eternity. However, one's past choices do not hamstring an individual—each new moment is another opportunity to choose again and thus alter one's course. The self is constructed through repeated avowals of faith—that is, the self continually relates to itself and to faith as its creative power through the day-to-day choices one makes along with the ongoing leaps of faith that these choices demonstrate. Individuals attaining this high level of development are rare; Kierkegaard called them "knights of faith." Ironically, as Hanson (2017) noted,

> Kierkegaard of course never used the phrase "leap of faith," but the leap is a common figure for the sort of movement that faith requires—a leap involves commitment, passion, risk, and resolute courage. But the knight of faith's most impressive feat is not the leap itself but the ability to leap with every step, to make his walking a series of leaps, in such a way that nobody notices he is leaping at all, and for him the movement, though learned, practiced, and disciplined, is now as natural as putting one foot ahead of the other. (p. 111)

For Kierkegaard, this process of self-creation produced an authentic individual value structure culminating in authentic human acts; thus, to make this final leap is to become an authentic human. Ultimately, for Kierkegaard, the sum of our choices, values, personality, and acts will stand to be judged by God.

Like Kierkegaard, Nietzsche also began with a severe critique of moral dogma and of the role of religion. Nietzsche (2001), using the voice of a madman, proclaimed, "The madman jumped into their midst and pierced them with his eyes. 'Where is God?' he cried; 'I'll tell you! *We have killed him*—you and I! We are all his murderers'"

(p. 120). Nietzsche asked us to imagine a Godless world where we are free to create—where we must create—our own moral ideals, thus emphasizing immediate and concrete responsibility for our actions in the day-to-day, here-and-now world. To achieve this, the individual must resort back to the innocent state of the child to allow new creations: "For the game of creation, my brothers, a sacred 'yes' is needed: the spirit now wills his own will, and he who had been lost to the world now conquers his own world" (Nietzsche, 1966, p. 27).

In describing human development, Nietzsche presented a hierarchy of three outcomes: At the lowest level is the "last man," composed of the herd or slave masses and reflecting content, comfort-seeking conformers who display no motive to develop the self. The middle level, the "higher man," is an individual who must be more and who must write his or her own story. Finally, Nietzsche (1961) described an ultimate role model for the ideal human as the *Übermensch*, a term he frequently used, which is commonly translated as "superman" but can also be translated as "overman" or "hyperman."[29] Nietzsche acknowledged that this standard might be unrealistically high to achieve for most people.

We have already mentioned the analogy of the camel that Nietzsche used to describe the masses. In a transformation, similar to Plato's prisoner discovering the sunlight, a few of Nietzsche's "camels" come to question the status quo and transform themselves into lions seeking to capture freedom and autonomy. Nietzsche used a lion to symbolize the higher man, noting that it takes the might of a beast of prey to steal freedom away from the dogma of socialization—the "thou shalt"—the idea that others tell us what we must believe, what we must accept as truth, and what we must do (and our corresponding love of, and blind compliance to, these external rules). The lion must kill the dragon of the "thou shalt" to create an opportunity—the right to pursue new values and a freedom for new creation.

At the highest level, the lion must be transformed into a child so as to create new values. Not yet having been acculturated, and with no sense of the "thou shalt," the child is innocent and without guilt. The superhuman/child thus represents a new model of individuality—"the spirit now wills its own will, the spirit sundered from the world now wins its own world" (Nietzsche, 1961, p. 55). Nietzsche described the individual's will to power as the need to become more, the will to act in life and not merely react to life. In a description reminding us of Dąbrowski's third factor, the will to power is not power over others but the feelings of creative energy and control over oneself that are necessary to achieve self-creation, self-direction, and the expression of individual creativity. The individual uses his or her will to power to reject, re-evaluate, and overcome old ideals and moral codes, and to create new ones. Nietzsche (1961) said that this is a continual process of self-overcoming by which superhumans take control of their genealogies and write their own stories. Members of the herd have their life stories written for them.

It is interesting to note that Nietzsche (2007, p. 32) also foreshadowed the third factor when he described what he called the organizing idea. Nietzsche described this as an emerging force that "begins to command," building towards one's goals and purpose. In the organizing idea, Nietzsche also included a reevaluation of values and the creation of a "hierarchy of capacities."

6–7. DISINTEGRATION IN THE PROCESS OF DEVELOPMENT

Nietzsche's description of human development, delivered through a character named Zarathustra, mirrored Dąbrowski's. Zarathustra descends from a mountaintop cave, where he has spent 10 years seeking wisdom. He passes a man who had previously known him, and the man comments that Zarathustra has changed; he has become the enlightened one—a child. At the first village he sees, Zarathustra stops to watch a circus tightrope walker and then begins to speak to the assembled crowd, who assumes he is part of the circus act (Nietzsche, 1966):

> *I teach you the overman.* Man is something that shall be overcome. What have you done to overcome him? . . . You have made your way from the worm to man, and much in you is still worm. Once you were apes, and even now, man is more ape than any ape. (p. 12)

Using the analogy of the tightrope walker, Zarathustra explains that we are a rope, a bridge connecting the animal and superman. To develop, one must cross this rope, risking the fall into the abyss below while moving away from animal and toward superhuman. The crowd rejects Zarathustra's story and he warns that: "You higher men, learn this from me: in the market place no one believes in higher men. And if you want to speak there, very well! But the mob blinks: 'We are all equal'" (Nietzsche, 1966, p. 286). The people in the mob have accepted their roles and collective definitions from their cultural milieu. For the mob, there are no higher men; all stand equal before God.

As we have seen, Nietzsche's solution was to try to shift the derivation of mores and values from an external locus—by declaring God dead (or, more specifically, by declaring the *idea* of God dead), to an internal locus—creating the opportunity for the individual to exercise autonomy in creating his or her own values. This shift will also spark the desire to release one's higher potentialities and resurrect and free the higher man: "God died: now *we* want the overman to live." (Nietzsche, 1966, p. 287).

Unfortunately, the mob reacts to Zarathustra in much the same way that Plato's prisoners welcome back the enlightened messenger; Zarathustra is considered either insane or simply a fool. Nietzsche (1966) described how Zarathustra lamented his reception:

I will teach men the meaning of their existence—the overman, the lightning out of the dark cloud of man. But I am still far from them, and my sense does not speak to their senses. To men I am still the mean between a fool and a corpse" (pp. 20-21).

Just as Plato's prisoners unquestioningly derive their values from their shadow play, Nietzsche's mob uncritically takes the ideals of "good and evil" from the cultural and religious conventions of the day. Nietzsche calls on us to resist the impulse to submit to this "slave morality" and to "undertake a critique of the moral evaluations themselves" (Nietzsche, 1968, p. 215). Zarathustra tells us that the superhuman must overcome his or her acculturated self and apply the will to power to a momentous new creativity—to building a truly autonomous self. Thus, superhumans move beyond "good and evil" through a deep reflection on their own basic instincts, emotions, character traits, and senses; they go on to develop their own individual values for living, analogous to the hierarchy of values and personality ideal described by Dąbrowski. Emphasizing the need to create one's own values, Nietzsche (1968) said: "Fundamental thought: the new values must first be created . . . we shall not be spared this task!" (p. 12). Nietzsche emphasized that the process of value creation and the new values must not be prescriptive: "'This is *my* way; where is yours?'—thus I answered those who asked me 'the way.' For the way—that does not exist. Thus spoke Zarathustra" (Nietzsche, 1966, p. 195).

Again, reflecting Dąbrowski's approach, the shift to a superhuman perspective involves a qualitative change in the way one views life. The "here and now" takes on a new perspective. Life is not lived for the promise of some better future (for instance, a reward in heaven). Rather, every second of life is now seen and valued for its intrinsic worth and contribution to our existence. In contrast to Kierkegaard's God as the eternal and ultimate judge, by eliminating God, Nietzsche (1966) calls on the individual to become his or her own judge. After creating a new value structure and self, Nietzsche's superhuman must now take on the responsibility of ultimately becoming the judge of himself or herself:

> Can you give yourself your own evil and your own good and hang your own will over yourself as a law? Can you be your own judge and avenger of your law? Terrible it is to be alone with the judge and avenger of one's own law. (p. 63).

This developmental process represents the rebirth of man and the creation of new, human, life-affirming values in this real and finite (temporal) world. These new beliefs reflect our intrinsic will to be more and our ability to transcend, to constantly overcome our old self, and to create a new self and new works. In summary, Nietzsche said: "*To make ourselves*, to *shape* a form from various elements—that is the task! The task of a sculptor! of a productive human being!" (quoted in Parkes, 1994, p. 159).

Nietzsche described the chaos and hardship involved in self-creation, including the need to overcome seven personal "devils" on the way to personality development (Nietzsche, 1966). Reminiscent of Dąbrowski's personality ideal, the superhuman develops a clear, internal view of his or her "calling" that now must be followed and applied through self-mastery. The will to power is involved in this development in two stages. First, social morality (analogous to Dąbrowski's second factor) is used to gain control over nature and the "wild animal" within us (Dąbrowski's first factor). Subsequently "one can employ this power in the further free development of oneself: will to power as self-elevation and strengthening" (Dąbrowski's third factor) (Nietzsche, 1968, p. 218). One must overcome the external, lower elements of oneself to achieve the ideal, representing the higher elements of oneself—to "*become who we are*—human beings who are new, unique, incomparable, who give themselves laws, who create themselves!" (Nietzsche, 2001, p. 189).

It is important to emphasize that when Nietzsche and Dąbrowski discuss ideals, they are not suggesting a prescriptive approach where exemplars and their ideals should be emulated by others. The individual is not encouraged to emulate or desire to become like an external ideal. As Nietzsche (1968) said, "All ideals are dangerous" (p. 130). Instead, the impact of becoming aware of ideals, and of observing exemplars setting and achieving their own ideals, helps one see the possibility of achieving one's *own* ideal. One also sees the general process of advanced development through the creation of an individualized, personal ideal of the self, reflecting one's essential character traits—aims, goals, values and so forth. The only ideal to emulate is the ideal one creates for one's self.

Nietzsche (1966) equated the quest for personality development with an individual's attempt to cross an abyss in order to give birth to the overman. "Man is a rope, tied between beast and overman—a rope over an abyss. A dangerous across, a dangerous on-the-way, a dangerous looking-back, a dangerous shuddering and stopping" (Nietzsche, 1966, p. 14). This journey is predicated on internal crises: "'I say unto you: one must still have chaos in oneself to be able to give birth to a dancing star. I say unto you: you still have chaos in yourselves" (Nietzsche, 1966, p. 17).

Nietzsche related an individual's potential to develop to the richness and intricacy of his or her emotion, cognition and volition (the will to power). The more potential a person has, the more internally complex he or she is: "The higher type represents an incomparably greater complexity . . . so its disintegration is also incomparably more likely" (Nietzsche, 1968, p. 363). Lower forms of life and people of the "herd type" are simpler, and thus, the lowest types are "virtually indestructible," showing few noticeable effects of the impact of day-to-day life (and none of the suffering that characterizes the superhuman) (Nietzsche, 1968, p. 363). Nietzsche's view nicely dovetails with the hierarchical approaches to neurophysiology of Hughlings Jackson and the views of Dąbrowski.

Nietzsche went on to describe a general, multilevel, developmental disintegration—suffering leads to a vertical separation, allowing the "hero" to rise up from the herd. This uplifting leads to "nobility" and, ultimately, to individual personality—attaining one's ideal self. This vertical separation finds one alone, away from the security of the masses and, for Nietzsche, without God for company or comfort: "The higher philosophical man, who has solitude not because he wishes to be alone but because he *is* something that finds no equals: what dangers and new sufferings have been reserved for him" (Nietzsche, 1968, p. 514). Nietzsche (1966) made clear the need to disintegrate, saying: "You must wish to consume yourself in your own flame: how could you wish to become new unless you had first become ashes!" (p. 64). A state of extreme vulnerability and over-reactivity (equivalent to Dąbrowski's overexcitability) characterizes this transition: "I love him whose soul is deep, even in being wounded, and who can perish of a small experience: thus he goes gladly over the bridge" (Nietzsche, 1966, p. 16). The seed must die for the plant to grow.

The capacity to endure solitariness, and to experience and overcome suffering, are key traits of the superhuman. Nietzsche proposed that happiness is not the result of satisfaction, rather, it is the ongoing mastery of small obstacles placed in one's way. He concluded that "the feeling of pleasure lies precisely in the dissatisfaction of the will" and that "the happy man" is "a herd ideal." (Nietzsche, 1968, p. 370). Further, day-to-day dissatisfaction of one's drives acts as "the great stimulus to life" and is the basis of pleasure.

Nietzsche (2001) attributed all human enhancements to suffering and said that one's path to self-creation always leads through one's own hell. Unhappiness, tension, and suffering must be endured, persevered, interpreted, and even exploited by the soul, thus cultivating strength, inventiveness and courage. Nietzsche (1968) foreshadowed Dąbrowski's realization that disintegration permeates our existence and leads to new insights, strength and development:

> Thereupon I advanced further down the road of disintegration—where I found new sources of strength for individuals. We have to be destroyers!—I perceived that the state of disintegration, in which individual natures can perfect themselves as never before—is an image and isolated example of existence in general. (p. 224)

Nietzsche's words are reminiscent of Dąbrowski's own. For example, Dąbrowski (1964b) said: "Crises are periods of increased insight into oneself, creativity and personality development" (p. 18). In another passage Dąbrowski (1970b) said: "We are human inasmuch as we experience disharmony and dissatisfaction, inherent in the process of disintegration" (p. 122). Finally, Dąbrowski (1973) said:

> Every authentic creative process consists of "loosening," "splitting" or "smashing" the former reality. Every mental conflict is associated with disruption and pain; every step forward in the direction of authentic existence is combined with shocks, sorrows, suffering and distress. (p. 14)

Physical illness may also play a major role in this transformation; as Nietzsche said, he was "grateful even to need and vacillating sickness because they always rid us from some rule and its 'prejudice'" (Nietzsche, 1989, p. 55). Suffering many serious, life-long health issues himself, Nietzsche defined health not as the absence of illness, but rather by how one faces and overcomes illness—"illness makes men better" (Nietzsche, 1968, p. 212). Nietzsche said he used his "will to health" to transform his illness into autonomy. It gave him the courage to be himself. In a practical sense, it also forced him to change his lifestyle—changes that facilitated a lifestyle more suited to his personality and to the life of a philosopher.

6–8. FOUR MAJOR THEMES

A review of the major philosophical foundations of Dąbrowski's theory has illustrated four major themes. First, a multilevel framework is vital for understanding the complex and broad variety of phenomena represented by psychology and development. A weakness of traditional approaches has been a reductionistic and simplistic view that cannot account for the wide disparity observed between the lowest and highest behaviors or the subtleties of development. Tremendous individual differences exist between people—differences that require a multilevel approach to understand. Although the multilevel model presents its own challenges, it is a much more realistic reflection of human reality, and Dąbrowski refined and applied it as a critical component of his full-fledged theory of personality development.

Second, Dąbrowski presented a unique view of the philosophical antecedents of development that combined elements of the essential approach to human character with those of existentialism in a new framing he called the existentio-essentialist compound. This approach charges the individual with the responsibility of becoming aware of his or her individual essence and subsequently shaping and refining one's personality in a process of literal self-creation.

Third, each author we examined presented an illustration of the socialized person. Plato's prisoners, the crowd of Kierkegaard, Nietzsche's mob, and Dąbrowski's primary level all illustrate individuals dominated by and adhering to an external system of social mores and standards. Each clearly shows how adherence to an external standard robs the individual of the opportunity for growth and blocks the development of true individuality and autonomy. Each author also described a higher form of development that involved overcoming this external adherence and achieving autonomy. These authors also described certain conditions and limitations to this process. For example, Plato made it clear that breaking free and making the journey out of the cave is the exception to the rule. Similarly, Kierkegaard made it clear that not everyone can face the abyss, manage the anxiety and dread, and make the leap(s) of faith necessary to achieve higher individual development—his knight of faith. Nietzsche also noted the hardships involved in making the transformations of the self required to first become the higher individual and ultimately the superperson.

Dąbrowski developed the construct of developmental potential to describe the possibilities of individual growth. Dąbrowski observed that not everyone can achieve the ultimate level of secondary integration characterized by a self-created, autonomous personality. All of the authors are clear that exemplars of advanced development exist, and they hold them out to us as general role models of development, illustrating the possibility, as Dąbrowski liked to say, and the process, but not advocating for the content of advanced growth.

Finally, each author emphasized the struggle involved in confronting the status quo and the tremendous anxiety, even the dread, that results. Nietzsche wrote at length about the need for the individual to disintegrate in order to create opportunities for growth. Foreshadowing Dąbrowski, Nietzsche placed the subsequent task of development squarely on the shoulders of the individual, including the tasks of creating an individualized value structure and a unique idealization of the self that will become the guidepost for individual growth. As we have seen, Dąbrowski made disintegration the central element of the developmental process and elaborated its features from a psychological point of view.

While Dąbrowski's approach may be radical within contemporary psychology, as this chapter has illustrated, it is certainly not radical as a philosophical approach to human nature or psychological development. Dąbrowski's ideas represent the logical extension and application of several major philosophical approaches, highlighted above. Dąbrowski combined these philosophical elements—including multilevelness, the discovery and shaping of essence into personality, and the developmental role of positive disintegration—into a unique systematic approach that is a new paradigm for philosophy, psychiatry, psychology and related disciplines, such as education, to better understand personality and its development.

6–9. CHAPTER SUMMARY

Chapter Six placed Dąbrowski in a philosophical context showing that his theory is a logical extension of previous mainstream philosophy in several key aspects. Utilizing Plato's early description of a multilevel reality and the importance of essence, along with the emphasis on self-creation and self-responsibility of the existentialist philosophers, Dąbrowski combined both perspectives and presented a new approach—the existentio-essentialist compound. The taken-for-granted harmony of the average individual reflects a rote endorsement of social mores and values with little or no conscious reflection. For Dąbrowski, this harmony mirrors a primitive state of development where no unique, individual personality yet exists. Development rests upon waking up and becoming aware—thus realizing a broader, deeper reality, analogous to the prisoner in Plato's cave escaping into the sunlight. This new reality brings contrasts between higher and lower levels into focus and creates feelings of alienation and frustration with the social status quo, often leading to intense questioning and eventually to disintegration. This disintegration philosophically marks the birth of a new individual and the beginning of the process of self-creation of his or her unique personality.

7

DĄBROWSKI IN CONTEXT

7–1. THE ROLE OF SUFFERING AND SUICIDE
IN DEVELOPMENT

The vital role played by experience, crisis, and suffering in personality development has not always been appreciated, even by Dąbrowski's supporters. While attending a conference on Dąbrowski, one of the presenters came up to me and shook his head: "All of this talk about suffering! Why can't we just have growth without suffering?"

A long philosophical tradition has associated the "need to suffer" with the opportunity to grow (e.g., Davies, 2012). Both from religious and philosophical schools of thought, the message has been that life's pain is a necessary part of learning that challenges us to rise above, to find more strength, to reach inside and to discover one's character. Pain and unhappiness play vital roles in validating a person's experience and in providing benchmarks to better appreciate life. Pain has been considered a motivation for the search for meaning in life (Frankl, 1959/1985) and in personal creativity and growth (Morris, 1991). As we will see below, the field of psychology is again recognizing the role of crises in development through research on posttraumatic growth.

From Dąbrowski's perspective, overexcitability is inextricably linked to crisis and suffering and, in turn, with personality development. Overexcitability can intensify negative experiences and may be extremely upsetting as human suffering, injustice, and sorrow are brought into the forefront of one's awareness and experience. This may overwhelm a person emotionally and/or experientially (Gendlin, 1962) and may lead to depression, breakdown or even suicide. Yet, the intense experience of emotional overexcitability can also compel a person to discover the unique and personal sense and meaning of suffering in his or her life, and thus to derive direction and meaning from the experience. To paraphrase Frankl, there is meaning in life and there is meaning in suffering; we can discover the two are linked (Frankl, 1959/1985).

Young-Eisendrath (1996) noted:

> Coming from the elite ranks of medicine, biology and sometimes even psychology is an almost uniform lack of interest in the value of suffering. Instead the focus is on avoiding or eliminating it. This strategy tends to increase our worst fears—that pain and suffering are intolerable and useless. (p. 187)

Young-Eisendrath advocated that suffering must be accepted and made sense of in order to achieve an understanding of the meaning of suffering both within our own lives and within the larger human context. Deriving this meaning will also make one aware of the transition from suffering to compassion.

7–1–1. The tragic sense of life

Spanish philosopher Miguel de Unamuno and his 1921 work, *The Tragic Sense of Life*, were major influences on Dąbrowski. The tragic sense of life recognizes that rationality has distinct limits in being able to understand life, and in particular, tragedy and suffering. Human understanding can only go so far in pursuing the truth of existence, and we are left to grapple with a significant degree of irrationality underlying existence. Unamuno (1921) sets the stage:

> Since we only live in and by contradictions, since life is tragedy and the tragedy is perpetual struggle, without victory or the hope of victory, life is contradiction. The values we are

discussing are, as you see, values of the heart, and against values of the heart reasons do not avail. (p. 14)

And the most tragic problem of philosophy is to reconcile intellectual necessities with the necessities of the heart and the will. For it is on this rock that every philosophy that pretends to resolve the eternal and tragic contradiction, the basis of our existence, breaks to pieces. (pp. 15-16)

There is something which, for lack of a better name, we will call the tragic sense of life, which carries with it a whole conception of life itself and of the universe, a whole philosophy more or less formulated, more or less conscious. (p. 17)

Life is fundamentally unintelligible; however uncomfortable and anxiety provoking this irrationality may be, it is inescapable in the human psyche.

Unamuno framed the tragic sense of life as a mode of experience not defined by external events but instead by the internal meaning and interpretation one gives to events. In this way, a phenomenological approach to understanding tragedy and life is emphasized, characterized by a balance of rationality versus the recognition of irrationality in the quest to understand life (Rubens, 1992). Suffering is an inexorable part of life, a subjective individual experience. As Solomon (1999) said:

What counts as suffering—what makes someone suffer—may well vary enormously from case to case, from individual to individual. But suffering as such is a part of every life and, as tragedy, it is not just suffering. As tragedy, I will argue, it has meaning. What gives meaning to suffering is what it is philosophy's job to investigate. (p. 115)

Unamuno (1921) believed that one had to make a commitment of faith in order to make sense of life—by making commitments one can give meaning to suffering. Unamuno (1921) explained that suffering leads to consciousness and awareness of one's self:

Suffering is the path of consciousness and by it living beings arrive at the possession of self-consciousness. For to possess consciousness of oneself, to possess personality, is to know oneself and to feel oneself distinct from other beings and this feeling of distinction is only reached through an act of collision, through suffering more or less severe, through the sense of one's own limits. . . .

And how do we know that we exist if we do not suffer, little or much? How can we turn upon ourselves, acquire reflective consciousness, save by suffering? When we enjoy ourselves we forget ourselves, forget that we exist; we pass over into another, an alien being, we alienate ourselves. And we become centred in ourselves again, we return to ourselves, only by suffering. (p. 115)

Rationality can interfere with this process, for instance, by dissolving such meaning in cynicism. For Unamuno, one must rebel against reason and passionately come to believe what one cannot believe rationally. As Solomon (1999) said, "The meaning of life is to be found in passion—romantic passion, religious passion, passion for work and for play, passionate commitments in the face of what reason 'knows' to be meaningless" (p. 116). This creates an unresolvable struggle between one's emotions and values, and one's rationality, a struggle characteristic of the authentic human. Unamuno (1921) made it clear that affect plays the dominant role: "Man is said to be a reasoning animal. I do not know why he has not been defined as an affective or feeling animal. Perhaps that which differentiates him from other animals is feeling rather than reason" (p. 3).

Unamuno (1921) said that as we choose our reactions in the face of the stressful events that occur in our lives, we create ourselves:

Suffering is the substance of life and the root of personality, for it is only suffering that makes us persons. And suffering is universal, suffering is that which unites all us living beings together; it is the universal or divine blood that flows through us all. That which we call will, what is it but suffering? (p. 205)

Unamuno (1921, pp. 205-206) lamented people who fall into an "apparent happiness" and "fall asleep in habit, near neighbor to annihilation." The alternative is to choose to confront and grapple with suffering.

Clearly, Unamuno saw himself as an agitator in helping people to confront the tragic sense of life: "My painful duty," Unamuno once said, "is to irritate people. We must sow in men the seeds of doubt, of distrust, of disquiet and even of despair" (Barcia & Zeitlin, 1967, p. 241). "My aim is to agitate and disturb people. I'm not selling bread; I'm selling yeast" (Unamuno quoted in Tillotson, 2010, p. 23).

7–1–2. Suicide: Surviving authentic development

For almost 60 years of his professional career, Dąbrowski's number one concern was suicide occurring among psychoneurotics. He explained that his concern originated during his master's studies when his best friend committed suicide. His doctoral dissertation in the Forensic Medicine Department at the University of Geneva in 1929 was an examination of the conditions leading to suicide (Dombrowski, 1929[30]; Kobierzycki, 2000). This section will provide a synopsis of some of the challenges presented by suicide in general and in the context of Dąbrowski's theory and I will also illustrate some of the important points with personal examples.

My interest in suicide was stimulated personally: When I was 21, and he was 52, my father committed suicide. There was no note, and this was unexpected and inexplicable. During my psychology studies, I had the opportunity to read quite a bit about suicide. Later in my career as a psychologist in a prison, I saw many suicidal people, many of whom eventually committed suicide, some while in custody under observation, some after release. We generally had 10 people a day under observation, every day. I had a chance to deeply observe these people and understand some of the dynamics involved in their lives.

7–1–2–1. Suicide is complicated

Suicidal ideation, suicidal and self-harm behaviors, and suicide are extremely complex phenomena related to a host of recognized risk factors that can be classified into three main groups: health factors (mental and physical, including substance abuse disorders and chronic conditions); environmental factors (e.g., traumatic life events, prolonged stress, weak support systems, and suicidal role modeling); and historical factors, including a history of abuse, previous self-injurious behavior/suicide attempts, and/or family history of suicide behaviors (Risk factors and warning signs, n.d.). Common mental health risk factors include depression, bipolar disorders, and eating disorders. Many intriguing, but often ambiguous, risk factors are increasingly being implicated, including genetic and biological factors (Roy & Dwivedi, 2017). To illustrate, research estimates that 10% of suicides may be attributable to the effects of severe infection and/or inflammation (e.g., Brundin, Bryleva, & Thirtamara-Rajamani, 2017; Brundin & Grit, 2016; see also Brundin et al., 2016; Jokela, Virtanen, Batty, & Kivimäki, 2016; Lund-Sørensen et al., 2016; O'Donovan et al., 2016; Priya, Rajappa, Kattimani, Mohanraj, & Revathy, 2016). Karpinski et al. (2017) presented a causal hypothesis which linked intellectual overexcitability with physiological over-reactions, causing immune and inflammatory dysregulation. Young women (15-30) using hormonal contraception have been found at higher risk for suicide attempts and completed suicide (e.g., Brent, 2018; Skovlund, Mørch, Kessing, Lange, & Lidegaard, 2017). A final illustrative example is the discovery that a protein involved in neurogenesis and synaptic plasticity is found to be persistently lower in the blood of individuals (in this research, in women) who have attempted suicide in the past (Kudinova, Deak, Deak, & Gibb, 2017). Kudinova et al. (2017) concluded this protein, brain-derived neurotropic factor (BDNF), has the potential to be used as a biomarker for future suicidal behavior.

There is no one theory that adequately accounts for suicide. Recent publications on suicide are diverse and helpful: (e.g., Bertini, 2016; Brent, Poling, Goldstein, & Poling, 2011; Chehil & Kutcher, 2012; Courtet, 2016; Cutcliffe, Santos, & Links, 2013; Ditum, 2017; Franklin et al., 2017; Goldblum, Espelage, Chu, & Bongar, 2015; Goldsmith, 2017; Hatcher, Crawford, & Coupe, 2017; Jobes, 2016; King, Foster, Rogalski, & Rogalski, 2013; Klonsky, May, & Saffer, 2016; Michel & Jobes, 2011; Miller et al., 2017; Mishara & Kerkhof, 2013; Murphy, 2017; Ngwena, Hosany, & Sibindi, 2017; Nock, 2014; O'Connor & Pirkis, 2016; Pompili, 2018; Wasserman, 2016; Worchel & Gearing, 2010; World Health Organization, 2010, 2014).

In terms of treatment, a recent study shows there is little proof that treatment with antidepressant medications prevent suicide attempts or completed suicide, and there is controversy over whether such medications may actually increase the risk of suicide attempts and suicide (Braun, Bschor, Franklin, & Baethge, 2016). Research on the effectiveness of therapy in preventing suicide is limited but generally promising (e.g., Miloseva, Milosev, & Rihter, 2016; Rudd et al., 2015; Winter, Bradshaw, Bunn, & Wellsted, 2013). Data support the efficacy of psychotherapies such as cognitive behavior therapy (CBT) and dialectical behavior therapy in suicide prevention (Zalsman et al., 2016), although it should be noted that long-term psychoanalytic psychotherapy provided substantially better results than counseling or CBT in treating major depressive disorder (Fonagy, 2015; also see Shedler, 2015). Rudd et al. (2015) concluded that "effective treatment of risk for suicidal behavior does not require complete remission of a psychiatric diagnosis or symptom severity but rather the development of core skills in the areas of emotion regulation, interpersonal functioning, and cognitive restructuring" (p. 447).

In terms of assessment of suicidal risk, it appears that prediction is unrealistic. Underscoring this is the fact that after 50 years, no satisfactory risk assessment tool has been developed that can successfully predict suicidal outcome (based on research looking at patient populations) (Large, et al., 2016; see also Bridge, Horowitz, & Campo, 2017; Franklin et al., 2016; Quinlivan et al., 2016). Assessment is primarily dependent upon the willingness of the client to disclose his or her feelings and intentions.

Dąbrowski associated risk of suicide with the strength of overexcitabilities and the intense emotions they produce. With our brief overview of suicide complete, we will now consider how intense experiences create vulnerability to suicide.

7–1–2–2. Dynamisms and overexcitability create intense experiences

Strong dynamisms and overexcitability create an experience of the world that may often be emotionally overwhelming. To illustrate, one day when I was going to work (I would have been about 30) I saw a bird had flown into a tree and fallen dead on the sidewalk in front of me. I was instantly overwhelmed with a feeling of wanting to kill myself. I felt lost. I felt like I wanted to fall down on the ground; I wanted to run away; I wanted to pull my teeth out. Later that day, I was shocked and confused at how I had felt and the ideas that had popped into my head. Where did they come from? What did they mean? Did other people have these strange reactions? Knowing the theory of positive disintegration helped me process these feelings by offering a context in which to understand them. I was not crazy. I was not losing control of reality. I understood these feelings and strange ideas as a reaction to, and reflection of, my strong sensitivities and overexcitabilities. Yet, I was left with the question of how to live and manage life without having these overwhelming feelings destroy me. What was I to learn from them? How could I use my sensitivities and strong reactions in a positive way in life? How could I turn such a strange experience into something I could learn and develop from? And most important, how could I help others who have similar reactions?

Psychoneurotics experience strong feelings of inferiority and self-criticism *toward oneself.* "The feeling of inferiority toward oneself . . . arises from the greater self-awareness and the self-examination that occur in multilevel disintegration" (Dąbrowski, 1964b, p. 45). This feeling reflects a disparity between who one "is" and who one "ought to be" and often occurs when one feels one has let oneself down, when one secretly knows that one could have done better—made a better choice—or that one should have stopped oneself from some behavior.

The psychoneurotic rarely asks for help because of his or her strong tendency to internalize psychic conflicts and psychological experiences. This leads the psychoneurotic to try to handle things him- or herself. Because the psychoneurotic is characterized by an emphasis on his or her inner psychic experience, emotions may not be exhibited overtly, and obvious signs of depression, anxiety, and angst may not be seen.

The inner experience of the suicidal psychoneurotic may become an unrelenting overexcitable state of angst and depression leading to psychological exhaustion. If the individual does not choose to share his or her inner experiences, I think it is often impossible to adequately assess suicidal potential.

Psychoneurotics face strong challenges and often have trouble coping with the realities of life; as challenging or overwhelming experiences accumulate, sometimes a suicidal life trajectory is created (Goldston et al., 2016). As one experiences the evil that can be perpetuated by people, as one sees the unfairness and harsh cruelties of life, an accumulating feeling of loss and dread can become overwhelming. This, combined with the angst of knowing that one can rarely intervene to change things, often creates feelings of helplessness and desperation. These feelings may accumulate to the point where a person comes to vehemently reject what is and develops the feeling that he or she can no longer live in this world. In such cases, suicide may become an inevitable endpoint of this long trajectory—culminating in an overwhelming need "to have a break" or seek a respite from life—"like taking a vacation from life out of desperation."[31]

7–1–2–3. Suicide is different at different levels

Dąbrowski described the very different motivations and intentions of suicide at different levels (1996, pp. 118-119). At the lowest level, suicide is often a desperate attempt to flee a difficult situation or to escape responsibility, liability or punishment. Examples might include murder of a spouse followed by the suicide of the perpetrator, or suicide as an act of revenge against someone.

At the second level, suicide is often a by-product of the chaotic emotions and reactions that one experiences during the "ship without an anchor" crises of unilevel disintegration. Alcohol and drug related suicides are common at this level. Acting out through self-mutilation or suicide attempts is often a mechanism for dealing with unbearable tension. Dąbrowski (1964, p. 7) said that the second level was the most intense period of crisis and that a person would either have to regress back to the familiar, rigid structures of Level I (what the person is trying to escape from), advance ahead, or risk suicide or psychosis.

At the third level, spontaneous multilevel disintegration, Dąbrowski described suicide as the result of a deep identification with the suffering of the world—an existential despair. Here the individual feels developmentally stuck and is overwhelmed with feelings of existential despair or loneliness. Conflicts are "between the 'lower self' and the 'higher self,' between the forces of negation and the forces of affirmation. Not infrequently very intense conflicts lead to suicide or even psychosis" (Dąbrowski, 1996, p. 37).

At the level of directed multilevel disintegration, the individual takes an active and conscious role in his or her development. In the pursuit of growth, Dąbrowski, writing under his pseudonym, said: "Self-perfection is always a partial suicide. A developing instinct of life must cooperate with the instinct of death because it is the death instinct, which eradicates brutish impulses and the remainder of disintegrating negative structures" (Cienin, 1972, p. 39). Actual suicide becomes less likely. "There are existential, philosophical, and transcendental conflicts. The danger of suicide or psychosis is nil. The powers of conflict are looked upon as positive; they are in the service of personality and its ideal" (Dąbrowski, 1996, p. 37).

At the fifth level, secondary integration, there are no inner conflicts. Here, empathy may be expressed in suicide as a heroic act—for example, to give one's life to save another. It may also be an active, voluntary submission to the law, as shown by Socrates. Suicide may represent acceptance of death by facing critical health conditions without taking treatment. Suicide may be a social protest (the self-immolation of Buddhist monks). Suicide may facilitate a conscious departure to "other dimensions," as portrayed at the end of the movie *Crouching Tiger, Hidden Dragon* when the character Jen Yu leaps from the bridge (Kong, Li-Kong, & Lee, 2000).

7–1–2–4. Some dilemmas of suicide

I have found that counselors and other healthcare providers are often uninformed about suicide and lacking in empathy to deal with suicidal individuals. I've heard it said, "He couldn't have been suicidal! I would have seen it." This kind of attitude often leads to a therapist being shocked at the suicide of a student or client. It must be understood that suicidal individuals often do not want others to know how they are feeling and will become skilled actors at hiding their emotions. For example, in a hospital setting, some 80% of patients who committed suicide denied having suicidal thoughts or intentions in their last communication before dying (Nock, 2016). What we need to realize is that any client, even any person next to us on the bus, can be suicidal, and that we must eliminate arrogant "but-I-would-have-seen-it" orientations. Our training and experience do not give us a crystal ball; the fact is that if the individual in front of us does not want to disclose, we are basically in the dark.

So, what are we to do? I think the common answer may be to ask the direct question: "Are you suicidal?" But I think it makes more sense to simply open the door by saying something indirect like, "You know, sometimes when people feel suicidal it helps to talk to someone, so if you ever feel this way, I would certainly be there for you to talk about things."

Case vignette 1

D. was a man about 45 years old, a meticulous, professional cabinetmaker by trade. He explained that he had never experienced happiness—he had been in the throes of a deep depression since he had been a teenager. He was completely lethargic and had a chaotic lifestyle. He would get a good job, do a good job and then simply lose interest and leave. He had no family or friends. He had tried every treatment that had ever been recommended, including ECT. He said being in jail was a benefit as he did not have to think about anything—he simply robotically followed the day-to-day routine. He revealed that he would have committed suicide at least 20 times but could not summon the energy required to go to the cupboard to get the gun. He had brief psychotic experiences—talking to his long dead mother, and also episodes of magical thinking. Once, he got the idea that he could bring his mother back to life by spending time in a field and he spent several days and nights sitting in the field waiting for something to happen. This was the most depressed man I have ever met. He revealed something about his state that I will always remember: he said he could not even imagine what it would feel like not to be depressed.

It was ironic that when I was an undergraduate at the University of Calgary, I spent an entire year wearing gloves—I did not want my

hands to get dirty. I would put them on when I left my apartment, and
took notes with them on, and kept them on until I came back at the
end of the day. Thus, it really resonated with me when I later read
Dąbrowski's (1972b) poem, *Be Greeted Psychoneurotics*, when he
said:

> For you feel the anxiety of the world, and its bottomless
> narrowness and self-assurance. For your phobia of washing
> your hands from the dirt of the world, for your fear of being
> locked in the world's limitations, for your fear of the absurdity
> of existence. (p. xvi)

Sometimes this feeling of being contaminated by the
inauthenticity, corruption, and "dirt of the world" becomes
overwhelming and creates a psychic crisis with no obvious resolution
available.

I believe that if a man were standing in front of me with a gun to
his head, the best thing to say would be: "Listen, I don't want the gun,
and I'm not going to report you. Why don't you put it in your pocket
and let's go have coffee? If you want to kill yourself later, you
certainly have that option, but what's the harm in giving it a little
more time?" I don't subscribe to the idea that there is some magic
question, or observation, or approach that will suddenly provide
insight for the suicidal client alleviating his or her distress. Often an
individual in such circumstances has thought about suicide for days
and days—or years and years—and there is nothing magic or new that
I can say that he or she has not already contemplated. So, what can we
do? I think the only practical approach is to engage the individual as a
fellow human being and be with them in the moment—no lectures, no
grand theories, no paternalistic advice, no deep philosophy, no
patronizing. Suicidal feelings, intentions and behaviors are not simple
problems, and not simply cognitive problems; they arise from
emotional states. These feelings must be embraced and related to with
emotional sensitivity.

As mentioned above, suicide is an extremely complex behavior
and not all suicides involve simply severe depression alone. In many
cases a more complex picture of the emotional state must be
considered. These emotional states may include feelings of

hopelessness, overwhelming pressure (both external and internal), despair, exhaustion, and as Dąbrowski often pointed out, feelings of positive maladjustment and rejection of the world as it is. Positive maladjustment is a strong factor, involving feelings of being out of sync or not fitting in—to be maladjusted to an environment that one morally objects to is generally a positive phenomenon but these feelings call for judicious management when intense.

Suicide is often seen as an individual act—many even characterize it as being a selfish act. On the contrary, suicide occurs in a community and social context and, while it is an individual act, it reflects a complex causality involving both individual and community factors. One cannot judge the individual who commits suicide without also to some extent judging the world in which we live.

Finally, intuitively, it would seem that a complex client would require an equally complex therapist. Unfortunately, I think it is often the case that a client may have a more sophisticated experience and understanding of emotional states, and of suicide, than his or her therapist. Traditionally, the pairing of client and therapist has been a rather random, "hit and miss" phenomenon, although research has demonstrated that the personal views of the therapist are an important variable in delivering therapy to suicidal clients (Neimeyer, Fortner, & Melby, 2001). In a small study, Gurrister and Kane (1978) found that the previous experience of the therapist with suicide (either in their personal history or in their clientele) created significant differences in their perception and treatment of the suicidal client, and paradoxically, those therapists who experienced suicide on their caseload were *less* likely to question the value of the treatment they had provided. A systemic corrective to improving the matching of clients and therapists may be an unrealistic goal at this time. From a Dąbrowskian perspective, the complexity and authenticity of the therapist are important factors. The troubled and overexcitable client potentially represents huge challenges and emotional demands on the therapist. Awareness of therapist burnout and compassion-fatigue in dealing with these clients is critical.

7–1–2–5. Some myths about suicide

There is a strong social stigma against discussing or even

acknowledging suicide. Large institutions like school districts seldom track or research suicide. For example, I asked someone from a large school board how many suicides had occurred in their student body the previous year and she replied, "I have no idea; we don't keep track." In the research community, there is also a stigma associated with suicide. Our knowledge of suicide is limited by these stigmas, and this makes the subject even more nebulous and more difficult to understand. As a consequence, this state of affairs provides fertile ground for myths to arise about suicide.

One such myth is that individuals often attempt suicide merely as a means to attract attention or as an act of manipulation. This may be true in some cases; however, in many individuals who attempt suicide, there is a real, underlying intention to end life, especially in multiple attempters. Recent research emphasizes that a suicide attempt represents more of a lethal risk factor for subsequent suicide than previously thought (Bostwick, Pabbati, Geske, & McKean, 2016). In the jail, we often had offenders with multiple suicide attempts—usually by slashing their arms with razor blades. Ironically, some guards would often relax their observation of these offenders based on the rationale that they were not really serious about committing suicide. In one case, an offender, M., had a razor blade and was taunting the officer standing in front of his cell that he would slash himself. A struggle of wills ensued: the officer taunted back and, unable to risk showing weakness, M. slashed his wrist. The officer calmly walked away leaving others to sound the alarm. Sadly, at a later date, M. died by his own hand. Contrary to the myth that multiple attempters "are not really serious," many of these individuals will go on to die of suicide.

Another myth regarding suicide is that success, achievement, or a high skill set, somehow protects or prevents people from suicide. People often say that individuals who are well qualified at a specific skill or who, for example, do particularly well in school, have "everything going for them, so, why would they want to commit suicide?" For example, "She was too smart to become so overwhelmed and helpless." Again, we do not have access to the thinking or feeling of these individuals, and we cannot judge them based on what we see. An individual may have everything they need from our perspective and yet may feel sad and desperate. So again, we need to assess and understand the suicidal individual on his or her own terms and not interject our own expectations, observations or values. We often hear a unilevel reaction—something like, "Suicide is irrational; she must have been out of her mind or crazy." As Dąbrowski illustrated (and as discussed above), motivations for suicide vary widely and can, in some contexts, even be described as noble and heroic. Each case must be looked at from a multilevel perspective, both in terms of assessment and post-mortem analysis. The suicide completer should not be deified ("he was an angel, and his work on Earth was done") or demonized ("how could he have done this to his family and friends? He must have been a monster!").

Another myth is that suicide is a relatively rare act. Sadly, in Canada suicide is the second leading cause of death in people under 24 years of age at 20% (behind accidents at 38%). In the group aged 25 to 44, some 16% of deaths are by suicide ("The 10 leading causes of death," 2015). In the United States, suicide rates rose 24% between 1999 and 2014; men aged 45 to 64 saw a 43% increase, while girls aged 10 to 14 years accounted for an increase of 200% during the study period (Curtin, Warner, & Hedegaard, 2016). "Suicide in the United States has surged to the highest levels in nearly 30 years, . . . with increases in every age group except older adults" (Tavernise, 2016; see also Caine, 2017; Gibbons, Hur, & Mann, 2017; Olfson et al., 2017a). More people die by suicide in the United States than in auto accidents (Erlich, 2016). For every completed suicide, there are estimated to be 20-30 attempts (Zalsman et al., 2016). Thus, suicide presents a significant and increasing social event.

It is a myth that children and adolescents are not suicidal. Suicidal ideation may be significant much earlier than once thought, starting as young as early-to-middle adolescence (Adrian, Miller, McCauley, & Vander Stoep, 2016). Using surveys conducted on over 500,000 U.S. adolescents in grades 8 through 12, and national statistics on suicide deaths for those aged 13 to 18 between 2010 and 2015, Twenge, Joiner, Rogers, and Martin (2017) reported:

> Depressive symptoms, suicide-related outcomes, and suicide deaths among adolescents all rose during the 2010s . . . . The rise in depressive symptoms and suicide-related outcomes was

exclusive to females. Between 2009/2010 and 2015, 33% more adolescents exhibited high levels of depressive symptoms . . . 12% more reported at least one suicide-related outcome . . . and 31% more died by suicide. (p. 6)

Twenge et al. (2017) found important gender differences; increases in depressive symptoms and suicide-related outcomes were exclusively driven by females:

Between 2009/2010 and 2015, 58% more females scored high in depressive symptoms . . . and 14% more reported at least one suicide-related outcome. . . . The increase in suicide rates among adolescents also appeared among males but was larger among females, rising 65% between 2010 and 2015 . . . and more than doubling between the late 1990s and 2015. (p. 6)

New calls for suicide prevention programs that target younger people are appearing (e.g., Bloch, 2016; Cox & Hetrick, 2017; Hawton, Saunders, & O'Connor, 2012; Schilling, Aseltine, & James, 2016). The complex antecedents seen in children and adolescents emphasize the need for, and challenges of, prevention strategies in this group (Rodway et al., 2016; see also Saunders, 2016). Pharmaceutical treatment of major depression in children and adolescents is an important concern. A recent study found that only one drug out of 14 examined (fluoxetine) was more effective than placebo in this age group and that one drug in particular (venlafaxine) was strongly associated with increasing the risk for suicidal behavior or ideation (Cipriani et al., 2016). "Suicide ranked 10th as a cause of death for US *elementary school–aged children* [emphasis added] in 2014" (Sheftal et al., 2016, p. 2). This very young group of decedents were most likely to have had attention deficit disorder (with or without accompanying hyperactivity) in contrast to early adolescents who were more likely to have had depression (Sheftal et al., 2016).

Finally, I would like to discuss the myth of intervention. While as therapists we can intervene by physically taking a gun away or perhaps locking someone up for 72 hours, ultimately, we are powerless to intervene. This must be clearly understood and acknowledged. The only person who can prevent suicide is the person feeling suicidal. Our role in this prevention is not proximal; at best, it is supportive and peripheral. In addition, no one prevention strategy stands out over another (Zalsman et al., 2016). That being said, prevention programs and strategies need to be carefully considered, implemented and included in evaluative research (e.g., Eggertson & Patrick, 2016; Wasserman, 2016; World Health Organization, 2010; Zalsman et al., 2016).

Often therapists and mental health professionals portray a superhuman image of their abilities. On the other hand, as one trend yields to the next (cognitive behavioral therapy yielding to behavioral activation, etc.), we are told that simpler and cheaper is better: "effective psychological therapy of depression can be delivered without the need for costly and highly trained professionals" (Richards et al., 2016, p. 1).[32] A growing trend shows movement away from face-to-face intervention and toward telemental health services (TMH or e-therapies) (Myers & Comer, 2016). Telemental health services utilize telecommunications technology to deliver services; for example, the use of videoconferencing, interactive Internet sites, cellular telephone applications, and blogs. Computer and Internet-based interventions using computerized CBT (cCBT)—intended to address anxieties and depression in children and adolescents—are reviewed by Stasiak et al. (2016).

7–1–2–6. The role of trauma in suicide

Trauma plays a critical role in mental health and suicide in three primary ways. First, it is well known that trauma in childhood, and especially repeated trauma, is a major risk factor for developing psychopathology including depression, mania, anxiety disorders, and psychosis (e.g., Binder, 2016; Hunt, Slack, & Berger, 2017; van Nierop et al. 2015). Childhood trauma is associated with higher rates of suicide, non-lethal suicide attempts, and non-suicidal self-injurious behaviors in adolescence and adulthood (e.g., Brodsky, 2016; Brown, Armey, Sejourne, Miller, & Weinstock, 2016; Castellví et al., 2017; Klemera, Brooks, Chester, Magnusson, & Spencer, 2017; Souza, Lopez Molina, Azevedo da Silva, & Jansen, 2016).

Second, suicide-related behavior may be precipitated by some overwhelming trauma (van der Kolk, 2014). It is critical to keep in mind that it is the individual experiencing the trauma who defines its impact and, consequently, the intervention indicated. It is a truism that crises are defined in the eye of the beholder.

Third, specific to Dąbrowski, there will be a clear and significant interaction between the developmental level of the individual and the trauma experienced. For example, the same event may be inconsequential to a person at Level I and a major trauma to a person at level III—or vice versa. When thinking about traumatic events, the individual's perception must be considered in the context of his or her level of development and developmental potential. To illustrate, a father and his daughter are walking down the street together. A dog runs out from a nearby yard and is run over. The father comments, "That's what you get for letting your dog run wild." His daughter, conversely, is severely impacted by witnessing this accident. For weeks, she has nightmares replaying what she has seen. She tries to speak to her father about the incident, but he cannot seem to relate to why she is so upset.

Often, the initial trigger of trauma is external, if not immediately obvious. For example, sometimes an apparently innocuous event— like me seeing the dead bird on the sidewalk—may evoke a crisis. Sometimes the impact of an event may be more obvious; for example, the death of a close friend or family member. A triggering event may even be experienced at arm's length; for example, by watching the news, a television show or movie, or seeing an image in a magazine. But rarely is the overriding crisis stimulus external in nature; instead it is our subsequent replay of what we have observed along with our own, ongoing, psychological reactions, that generate the true inner psychological conflicts that push one toward suicide. As Saint-Exupéry described, true horror does not exist in the world of events. "Horror is something invented after the fact, when one is re-creating the experience over again in the memory" (Saint-Exupéry, 1939, p. 78). The psychoneurotic is responding to his or her view of the world and the experiences that he or she has had. The psychoneurotic feels more and cares more; this creates a vulnerability to view things as hopeless. It is further accentuated by the intense sensitivity and overexcitability displayed by many psychoneurotics. This combination of psychological features predisposes self-harm and suicidal thinking. In understanding these qualities in a student or client, one can better understand the foundation of his or her suicidal ideation. Many people say words to the effect that "I just don't understand why *Jane Doe* felt so desperate—why could *Jane Doe* not just enjoy life more?" Such comments illustrate the difficulty the average person (and average therapist) has empathizing with, understanding, and having compassion for the psychoneurotic and the true inner psychic experiences he or she lives with.

7–1–2–7. Self-harm

There is a significant relationship between self-harm and eventual suicide (e.g., Cooper et al., 2005; Hawton, Zahl, & Weatherall, 2003; Owens, Horrocks, & House, 2002; Wilkinson, Kelvin, Roberts, Dubicka, & Goodyer, 2011). Representative publications on self-harm are available (e.g., Butler, 2016; Chaney, 2017; Duffy, 2009; Klemera, Brooks, Chester, Magnusson, & Spencer, 2017; Lockwood, Daley, Townsend, & Sayal, 2017; Mikolajczak, Petrides, & Hurry, 2009; O'Connor et al., 2017; Olfson et al., 2017b; Quinlivan et al., 2016). In assessing future risk of harm behavior after a self-harm event, Quinlivan et al. (2017) suggested that currently available risk scales are so poor at prediction they should not be used at all.

The majority of young people who self-harm do so in a dysfunctional attempt to regulate unpleasant emotions (Mikolajczak et al., 2009). Mikolajczak et al. (2009) found that adolescents with higher trait emotional intelligence (trait EI) were less likely to self-harm, and that trait EI is positively correlated with adaptive coping styles and negatively correlated with maladaptive emotional coping styles (e.g., self-blame), and depression.

Dąbrowski (1937) associated self-mutilation (self-harm) with the release of intense tension. As he explained, unbearable tensions generally lead either to tendencies to injure others or tendencies to injure oneself (Cienin, 1972). The latter reactions often occur in overexcitable individuals who experience a strong emotional shock. Dąbrowski (1937) spoke of self-mutilation and suicide almost synonymously, and certainly as interrelated constructs—suicidal attempts being a manifestation of the deeper self-mutilation process.

7-1-2-8. The role of therapy in suicide

In Dąbrowski's framework, it is the therapist's role to identify the developmental potential of the client and provide the developmental framework of positive disintegration. The therapist must not be prescriptive, as true solutions come only from the client. To a large degree, the therapist must stand to the side and let the developmental process unfold. Clients need to be encouraged and supported in their coping attempts. The focus is not simply on the amelioration of crises; rather, crises need to be understood as necessary experiences on the path to growth. It has been my experience that these clients appreciate an honest discussion of the issues. They don't want to hear grandiosity, platitudes or pontifications. They need to be supported— but also challenged via a clear discussion of the context and consequences of their behavior and of the crisis. The possible developmental benefits and opportunities presented by facing the challenge must be weighed against the risks of self-harm presented.

Self-harm prevention and suicide prevention should be openly discussed, and as Dąbrowski advocated, temporary positive regressions may be suggested if developmental crises become overwhelming. As Dąbrowski (1970b) described, "we may find positive regression in order to rest and relax before attempting new, more authentic and more elevated activity" (p. 52). Positive regressions may be a conscious choice, constituting "a conscious or semiconscious protection of one's own development toward personality through the search for the most proper conditions for its growth" (Dąbrowski, 1970b, p. 177). When emotions are overwhelming one may need a "psychic rest or time off to accommodate an experiential load" (Dąbrowski, 1972b, p. 302). Emotional regressions may involve periods of isolation or immersion in a supportive environment.

Dąbrowski emphasized using a broad range of therapeutic techniques including conventional psychotherapy, medication, meditation, and spiritual guidance. He suggested therapeutic interventions need to be tailored to the developmental level and potential of the individual client. Dąbrowski also used specialized techniques he described as *developmental psychotherapy* (Dąbrowski, n.d.a). Two such techniques are self-education (or education-of-oneself) and autopsychotherapy. Contrary to traditional approaches, the theory of positive disintegration emphasizes placing the responsibility and focus of therapy with the client. Self-education begins when an individual forms an internal picture of a personality ideal—the type of person he or she wants to be. The person feels inferiority because he or she realizes how distant this ideal is from his or her everyday behavior. This vertical conflict creates an attitude towards oneself that emphasizes the need to work out and create one's personality in one's inner life.

Case vignette 2

S. was a commercial painter and had run a successful business. He said that he lost everything—his marriage and children, his house and car, his job—because he was addicted to gambling. He had committed a robbery to finance his gambling. As he put it, although he knew the consequences, he simply could not control himself. S. described descending into a deep, deep hole, and he could not visualize ever being able to control himself or to climb back into life. He was deeply regretful and sorry for the harm done to his family and concluded that suicide was his only avenue remaining. I was unable to reconnect him to any vision of past success or future hope. We had this man in our jail's observation unit, but we felt his situation required hospitalization. The next day at the hospital's forensic psychiatric unit, while under constant observation, he managed to commit suicide.

Self-education goes beyond mere introspection and involves the development of Dąbrowski's construct of subject-object. In its simplest terms, subject-object is the ability to "take an objective look at oneself." Many individuals are afraid to do this. Dąbrowski suggested that the therapist must try to slowly awaken and gradually strengthen the patient's self-reliance and independence. "The patient's ambition should be awakened and his confidence in himself and his therapist should be developed and gradual realization of his own abilities and other values promoted" (Dąbrowski, n.d.a, p. 225). In essence, this gives the individual confidence to face him- or herself.

Dąbrowski (n.d.a) used the idea of a mirror in his therapy. Initially one can think of a physical mirror. We see our physical selves and we can observe changes in our expressions as our moods change. We can observe our physical selves in times of great happiness and, as well, in times of depression or illness. As development of subject-object goes on, the physical mirror becomes psychic. Individuals with imaginational overexcitability can see themselves in their psychic mirror and imagine both retrospective and prospective events. Using subject-object, an individual can imagine him- or herself in the psychic mirror and, for example, imagine the outcomes of actions. Using psychic imagery, the individual can stop or change these behaviors before they are acted on in the real world. The individual can imagine him- or herself as an object leading to the ability to see what needs to be strengthened and what needs to be eliminated in his or her personality ideal. Thus, people can develop themselves using psychic subject-object.

Likewise, an individual can use what Dąbrowski called the psychosocial mirror. He noted that many people see themselves only through the eyes of other people and they live vicariously through the opinions of other people. Often one does not even imagine the necessity of having an opinion of oneself. One can use one's psychic image to develop a vision of how one may appear in the eyes of others, and to develop independent opinions of oneself (Dąbrowski, n.d.a).

Once psychic subject-object is sufficiently developed, the therapist can encourage the individual to make a developmental jump, moving from observing oneself to controlling oneself; effectively taking one's fate into one's own hands, and thus embarking upon autopsychotherapy (Dąbrowski, n.d.a).

Closely related to self-education is autopsychotherapy—an active participation in determining one's character and in shaping one's personality—essentially, planning and implementing therapy on oneself. Autopsychotherapy allows an individual to successfully cope with and manage developmental crises and to maintain his or her mental equilibrium.

In summary, autopsychotherapy is an important part of developing long-term coping skills and personality growth. Combined with self-education, autopsychotherapy becomes a strong developmental force in itself, acting to inhibit lower elements of the self considered contrary to one's personality ideal and expanding elements represented in one's ideal. This approach minimizes the role of the traditional therapist, and long-term therapy with a therapist becomes a contradiction in terms. The direction and help must come from within, not from ongoing "guidance" from an external agent. Unfortunately, it is beyond the scope of this work to fully explore Dąbrowski's approach to therapy.

7–1–2–9. Postvention with those impacted by suicide

I want to end this section with an acknowledgment of the secondary trauma done to the survivors of suicides: the friends, partners, parents, teachers, caregivers, mental health professionals, first responders and others. This trauma is usually not intended on the part of the person committing suicide, but it has significant impacts that are seldom addressed by mental health professionals. Postvention is an approach to dealing with the aftermath of suicide first proposed by suicidologist Edwin Shneidman. "It aims to destigmatize the tragedy of suicide, promote survivor recovery, and strengthen suicide prevention efforts by providing multiple resources to the survivors—including behavioral health, psychosocial, spiritual, and public health services" (Erlich, 2016). There is a continuum of exposure predicated on the relationship between the decedent and the survivor. For example, maximum exposure would occur when the relationship to the suicide completer is as partner or parent; lesser exposure would be expected in relationships like therapist, relative, schoolmate, co-worker, and friend. There is also a continuum of bereavement and trauma seen in survivors that can help inform the need for, and type of, postvention services required (Groff, Ruzek, Bongar, & Cordova, 2016). Consensus guidelines to provide comprehensive support programs for survivors of suicide loss are being developed (Survivors of Suicide Loss Task Force, 2015; see also Linde, Treml, Steinig, Nagl, & Kersting, 2017). Postvention programs are also being specialized for various settings; for example, for firefighters (Gulliver et al., 2016) and secondary schools (Cox et al., 2016; see also

Goldney & Berman, 1996). Postvention can play a major role assisting in mitigating and managing the effects of trauma.

The challenges of trying to understand the motivations of the suicidal person often haunt the survivors. Guilt over countless scenarios is common: "Why didn't she ask for help?" "Could I have done more?" "What could I have done differently?" "Did I make a mistake somehow?" Survivors must understand that however difficult a suicide is for us to comprehend, compassion must be paramount, as the pain and suffering must have been even greater for the person who has passed away. In this context, anger at the victim is inappropriate. The deep challenge of understanding what is seemingly incomprehensible is an existential aspect of life; often, life does not make sense. We can never know the challenges or thoughts or feelings of the person taken by suicide. As much as we want to make sense of his or her motivations, we are usually left frustrated. This becomes a reality of life that we must manage as we move forward with the decisions and challenges that we face in the future.

Finally, survivors have to deal with the social stigma associated with suicide. Sadly, people tend to act differently in interacting with those in grief over a suicide compared to, say, a motor vehicle accident death. There is often silence or even anger expressed to survivors. Again, compassion must be shown even in the absence of understanding.

In summary, Dąbrowski's paramount concern was suicide and self-harm in the psychologically sensitive and vulnerable individual as he or she struggles to develop. This section has reviewed suicide, both in general, and from a Dąbrowskian perspective. We need to be sensitive to the needs of those undergoing developmental crises, especially younger individuals. We need to consider what we can do to better address suicide in students and clients who express psychoneurotic traits and personalities. We can begin by understanding that any one of these individuals could be suicidal at any time. We can greatly improve our understanding of suicide in psychoneurotics by understanding more about their basic personality characteristics and how these traits may predispose a suicidal dynamic. We need to have a more open and honest dialogue among ourselves to learn more about these characteristics and about suicide.

Suicide is among the most complex of human acts. Our analysis and response to suicide must be equally complex. To save one life makes our efforts worthwhile.

7–2. CRISIS INTERVENTION

Sadly, it was a major tragedy that started the modern era of psychological research into the effects of trauma and which essentially initiated the field of crisis intervention. In 1942, the Coconut Grove nightclub in Boston burned, killing 492 people and injuring well over a hundred more, some who later died from their injuries. Erich Lindemann (1900-1974), a psychiatrist at the Massachusetts General Hospital, examined 101 people who were impacted by the fire, focusing upon their readjustment and "grief work." Lindemann's findings were instrumental in establishing expectations about grief, the impact of trauma, and in generating interest in crisis intervention (e.g., Cobb & Lindemann, 1943; Lindemann, 1944).

Jacobson (1980) summarized Lindemann's relevant contributions to crisis theory:

- Lindemann described the normal grief process, including somatic distress, preoccupation with images of the lost one, guilt, hostile reactions often focused on the deceased, and the loss of usual patterns of behavior.
- Lindemann concluded that when the resolution of grief is uninterrupted, a resolution of symptoms occurred within four to six weeks. This four-to-six-week time frame was a crucial window in determining whether grief would be resolved adaptively or maladaptively.
- A major traumatic life event has an immediate and significant impact on psychological functioning with a predictable pattern of responses occurring over a finite length of time.
- For a given individual, it is not clear in advance whether the outcome will be adaptive or maladaptive.

In an excellent paper, Harrison (1965) compared Lindemann's crisis theory with Dąbrowski's construct of positive disintegration.

Harrison explained that in Lindemann's crisis theory:

> The individual's solution of the disturbance will either return
> him to his previous state of equilibrium or will result in a
> "subsequent greater capacity for emotional well-being." If
> integration of the disturbance is beyond the present ability of
> the individual, he will "show non-adaptive solutions and will
> have restored equilibrium at a lower level of integration." (p.
> 8)

Harrison (1965) concluded:

> Workers in the field of mental health will find the papers by
> Lindemann and Dąbrowski stimulating and provocative. One's
> outlook on growth and development, mental health and mental
> illness cannot but be influenced by what these two theorists
> have presented. (p. 13)

Gerald Caplan (1917-2008), a British psychiatrist, worked in
Boston for many years, several as a colleague of Lindemann's; he was
instrumental in following up on Lindemann's observations about
crises. Caplan was interested in community mental health and was
best known for his work on preventative psychiatry and crisis
intervention. Caplan (1961) defined a crisis as:

> provoked when a person faces an obstacle to important life
> goals that is, for a time, insurmountable through the utilization
> of customary methods of problem-solving. A period of
> disorganization ensues, a period of upset, during which many
> different abortive attempts at solution are made. Eventually
> some kind of adaptation is achieved, which may or may not be
> in the best interest of that person and his fellows. (p. 18)

Caplan (1961) saw the ego as developing coping mechanisms
throughout one's life. This coping repertoire is based upon having
faced crises successfully in the past. As well, our coping repertoire
may grow from negative life instances. Caplan explained that we face
two types of crises: the threat of loss and loss itself. He further
explained that the structure of an individual's coping repertoire
determined the type of person he or she is in the face of crisis. Caplan

differentiated "richer personalities" from people with "poorer personalities" and suggested that those with a larger variety of coping mechanisms could handle more crises in more flexible ways: "You can think of personality development as being in certain respects the enriching of the repertoire of social and other coping responses" (Caplan, 1961, p. 41). Caplan emphasized that when a crisis overwhelms an individual's coping repertoire or falls outside of it, the individual seeks some new solution and eventually finds some way to deal with the situation, either good or bad. For Caplan, this resolution should occur within about four to six weeks.

In his view of coping, Caplan (1961) included what he called "psychological work." This work is "switched on, stimulated or initiated" by two phenomena—anxiety or depression: "anxiety is the switch that is turned on by threat of loss [worry work] and depression is the switch that is turned on by actual loss [grief work]" (Caplan, 1961, p. 43). In successfully facing a crisis, an individual simultaneously adapts the external world to him- or herself and as well, makes an internal adjustment to the situation. Through the disequilibrium of the crisis, one adapts to find a new equilibrium, a process that Caplan clearly associated with development.

Caplan (1961) also included the possibility that the outcome may not be positive and in such cases, a new equilibrium is established; however, it is regressed in the direction of a neurosis, as a psychosis or some form of lasting alienation or disintegration. Caplan suggested that a crisis is a vulnerable time and that "a relatively minor force acting for a relatively short time can switch the whole balance over to one side or the other," either towards mental health or "mental ill-health" (pp. 186-187). Interestingly, Caplan said that the individual should not be the reference point of our attention; instead, we should focus on "a field of forces, of the unit of society—whatever the size of it—rather than of an individual patient" (p. 186). Caplan (p. 187) observed the importance of the relationships the patient has with a few key people in his or her life—these relationships may be supportive and tip the balance in a positive direction, or may be destructive, tipping the balance towards illness.

We can use Jacobson's (1980) conclusion as a summary:

The concepts of equilibrium, change, coping and time are

essential to crisis theory. Major changes in the physical, social, or physiological sphere disturb the psychological equilibrium when pre-existing coping fails. New coping restores equilibrium at the same, a worse, or a better level than existed before. (p. 9)

7–3. POSTTRAUMATIC GROWTH

As we have seen above, Caplan (1961) believed that a fundamental assumption of traditional crisis theory is that outcomes may be positive or negative. As psychologists began to study trauma, it became apparent that trauma outcomes could lead to growth. Most of this literature postulates the possibility of growth in outcomes after trauma. Conceptually, the theory of positive disintegration fits within this approach. However, Dąbrowski took the construct one step further: Not only is growth possible after trauma, but trauma is necessary for growth.

Various terms have been used in the literature to describe the positive changes that follow crises. The terms *resiliency, resilience* or *resilient* are usually associated with the idea of a return to the original level of functioning—to bounce back—after a crisis (Newman, 2002); however, the usage of these terms has been ambiguous in the literature (Fletcher & Sarkar, 2013). Other common terms include *stress-related growth* (e.g., Park, Cohen, & Murch, 1996), *thriving* (e.g., Abraido-Lanza, Guier, & Colon, 1998; O'Leary & Ickovics, 1995), *perceived benefits* (e.g., McMillen & Fisher, 1998) and *potentially traumatic events* (PTEs) (e.g., Bonanno, Westphal, & Mancini, 2011). Notably, it was the term *posttraumatic growth* (PTG) (Tedeschi & Calhoun, 1995, 1996) that researchers gravitated to and which has now become the term most widely used to describe this field of study and clinical practice.

Posttraumatic growth is a wide-ranging construct that is still in the early stages of development (e.g., Addington, Tedeschi, & Calhoun, 2016; Arikan, Stopa, Carnelley, & Karl, 2016; Berger, 2015; Blackie et al., 2016; Elderton, Berry, & Chan, 2017; Jayawickreme & Blackie, 2014; Johnson & Boals, 2015; Joseph, 2011; Joseph & Linley, 2008; Morgan & Desmarais, 2017; Patrick & Henrie, 2016; Ramos & Leal

2013; Rendon, 2015; Roepke, 2014; Roepke & Seligman, 2015; Shuwiekh, Kira, & Ashby, 2017; Tedeschi & Calhoun, 2004b; Tedeschi, Blevins, & Riffle, 2017; Tedeschi & Moore, 2016; Weiss, 2014; Werdel & Wicks, 2012; Zoellner & Feeny, 2014; Zoellner & Maercker, 2006). For a recent, concise summary, see Jayawickreme and Blackie (2016).

To date, three broad domains of positive change have been noted throughout the literature (Tedeschi & Calhoun, 1996): First, relationships are enhanced in some way. For example, people describe that they come to value their friends and family more and feel an increased sense of compassion for others and a longing for more intimate relationships. Second, people change their views of themselves in some way—they develop a greater sense of personal resiliency (Bonanno, 2004; see also Kalisch, Müller, & Tüscher, 2014), wisdom and strength, perhaps coupled with a greater acceptance of their vulnerabilities and limitations. Third, people describe changes in their life philosophy, for example, finding a fresh appreciation for each new day and re-evaluating their understanding of what really matters in life (e.g., Joseph, 2011; Joseph, Murphy, & Regel, 2012, p. 317).

Tedeschi and Calhoun (2004a) summarized posttraumatic growth. In this work, the authors described posttraumatic growth as growth beyond an individual's level of psychological adaptation prior to the experience of crisis or trauma, and they offered an overview of the relevant literature on the role of suffering as a vehicle for learning and positive change.

Calhoun and Tedeschi (1998) summarized growth and crisis and included the suggestion that growth may be associated with more crises, not fewer: "Growth may well be more likely to occur as a result of a process that begins with the shaking of the foundations of the individual's assumptive world and a concomitant increase in psychological pain and distress" (Calhoun & Tedeschi, 1998, p. 217).

Calhoun and Tedeschi (1998) called for a shift in perspective to recognize growth as a routine possibility when individuals are faced with major trauma. The authors ended with a speculation on clinical approaches that both respects the negative effects of trauma and presents a positive perspective; they indicated this would be the topic of a future work.

King (2001) examined the relationship between maturity and happiness and found that each may follow its own distinct and independent pathway. Jane Loevinger's (1918-2008) theory of ego development and maturity was used in this research. In Loevinger's approach, a mature person displays a more complex self and takes a more differentiated and integrated view of the world (Loevinger, 1976). King concluded that "difficult life circumstances" (p. 57) provide an opportunity to develop more complex perspectives on life and to grow. King pointed out that the quality of happiness is an important consideration and that "hard-earned maturity can change the meaning and experience of happiness" (p. 54).

Interestingly, King (2001) reported that narrative variables relating to happiness are unrelated to personality development and that variables related to personality growth tend to be independent of levels of happiness:

> When life is easy, so is happiness. When life is difficult, finding a way to be happy may be a greater challenge. Furthermore, being happy may be viewed as only one of the possible valuable outcomes of having difficult life experiences. (p. 56)

One way to achieve happiness may be to avoid thinking about one's losses, although this strategy may also preclude the kind of self-examination necessary for personality growth. One of King's suggestions is that the desire to be happy after a difficult life event may necessitate personality development in order to readjust "one's meaning structures" to conform to one's post-trauma world of experience.

In a comprehensive review of the effects of trauma, sixteen parents who had a son or daughter murdered were selected for interview (Parappully, Rosenbaum, van den Daele, & Nzewi, 2002). The construct of thriving after trauma was examined, and it was found that at times, an individual may surpass his or her previous level of function to yield a "better-off-afterward experience." Parappully et al. (2002) concluded:

The general profile of the transformed survivor that emerged from this study is that of a resilient, competent, compassionate and caring individual, characterized by a benevolent, benign and thankful attitude toward life; shaped by belief systems; strengthened by successful coping with previous tragic experiences; supported by spirituality, friends, family, community and a strong affective bond with the victim; and nourished through self-care. (p. 59)

Parappully et al. (2002) also considered the circumstances and resources involved in a positive outcome and found:

The processes that facilitated the transformation were accepting the tragedy, finding meaning in it, making the personal decision to leave the tragedy behind and move on with their lives and, in a very special way, reaching out in compassion to others. The resources that helped most in this transformation were personal qualities, spirituality, having a continuing bond with the victim, social support, previous coping experiences and self-care. (p. 59)

The authors ended the article with a particularly appropriate quotation (Segal, 1952, p. 199, as cited in Parappully et al., 2002):

It is when the world within us is destroyed, when it is dead and loveless, when our loved ones are in fragments and we ourselves in helpless despair—it is then that we must recreate our world anew, reassemble the pieces, infuse life into dead fragments, recreate life. (p. 60)

Peterson, Park and Seligman (2006) found that recovery from illness or disorder can sometimes be associated with building character strengths that lead to increased life satisfaction once the crisis is resolved; bravery, kindness, and humor were associated with a return to life satisfaction when the stress was physical illness; the appreciation of beauty and love of learning were associated with recovery from psychological disorder.

Continuing our theme, Haidt (2006) discussed three benefits that may arise during posttraumatic growth. The first benefit is that the individual often surprises him or herself when rising to the challenge at hand. This is reminiscent of Dąbrowski's "astonishment with oneself"—"I never thought I could survive that—I really surprised myself." This kind of positive self-realization can be critical in the early stages of an expanding awareness of an individual's deeper and often hidden potentials. The second benefit is a reappraisal of one's relationships, often involving both a cleavage of some, but a major consolidation and strengthening of others. Finally, trauma is often the impetus to review and change one's priorities and philosophies of life, including how one wants to live life and how one should treat others.

Haidt (2006) reviewed and utilized the three levels of personality described by Daniel McAdams (1954-) (McAdams, 1995, 2001). At the first level are basic dispositional traits, where personality research has traditionally focused, including the traits in the five-factor model (Openness, Conscientiousness, Extraversion, Agreeableness and Neuroticism). At the second level are characteristic adaptations; for instance, one's personal goals, values, beliefs, coping mechanisms, and the skills required to interface with one's environment (being a parent, succeeding at business and so forth). Haidt (2006) listed the four categories used to sort characteristic adaptations: work and achievement; relationships and intimacy; religion and spirituality; and generativity (the legacy one leaves behind). McAdams's third level is an overarching narrative story of one's life, integrating one's confabulated memories of the past, perceptions of the present, and dreams about one's future. Haidt (2006) presented the idea that happiness is related to having coherence or compatibility among each of the three levels; for instance, one's intrinsic traits, one's religion, one's work, one's relationships, and one's overall personally conceived and understood life narrative must all mesh into a smooth compatible whole.

Haidt (2006) asked the question: "Must we suffer?" and differentiated a weak and a strong version of "the adversity hypothesis." The weak version, which is well supported by research, indicates that adversity can lead to growth; the strong version states that people must suffer to grow and that "the highest levels of growth and development are only open to those who have faced and overcome great adversity" (Haidt, 2006, p. 141). Haidt noted that adversity and crises create windows of opportunity for an individual to review his or her goals and to make changes in one's priorities. Haidt went on to describe how trauma may shatter one's belief system, forcing one to reassemble the pieces back into a new coherent self.

The impact of trauma and the recovery from trauma can be analyzed using McAdams's three levels, particularly by addressing the question, "Can the changes precipitated by the trauma be integrated into the pre-trauma, coherent structure of one's personality?" If an individual can make changes that contribute to maintaining or increasing the coherence of the three levels, then a positive outcome is more likely. Finally, Haidt (2006) noted that personality change after trauma would be least likely to occur in the basic first level personality traits.

Affective characteristics are important aspects of experiencing trauma. Two major divisions are described. Negative affective personality types (NA) are characterized by the long-term and stable expression of anger, contempt, shame, fear, and depression (Norlander, Bood, & Archer, 2002). These characteristics contrast positive affective personality types (PA), that reflect enthusiasm, activity, control, and commitment. Positive affectivity involves maintaining a positive outlook, higher life satisfaction, and self-confidence (Norlander et al., 2002). Norlander et al. (2002) described four categories: the self-actualized personality (high in PA and low in NA), the high affective personality (high in PA and high in NA), the low affective personality (low in PA and low in NA) and the self-destructive personality (low in PA and high in NA). In a subsequent publication, it was shown that the high affective type displayed the highest ability to thrive after trauma; the self-actualizing and high affective groups showed the most receptivity to change, while the self-destructive group showed the least (Norlander, Schedvin, & Archer, 2005). This study also showed that high positive affect is a necessary condition for developing positive and transformational coping while low positive affect leads to negative coping; finally, the self-destructive type is the most fragile, experiencing the most stress and inability to cope. Low affective types appear to emerge with major impairment but with lower stress levels.

High affective types displayed positive transformational coping that led to thriving (growth); self-actualizing types displayed homeostatic coping leading to resilience; low affect individuals displayed negative transformational coping but leading to survival; and finally, self-destructive types displayed negative transformational coping and succumbing (Norlander, Schedvin, & Archer, 2005).

Kunst (2011) followed up this theme in a study that demonstrated high affective individuals reported the highest levels of posttraumatic growth (self-actualizing individuals only marginally demonstrated posttraumatic growth). This study emphasized that the relationship between PTG and PTSD is unclear and that results supported the view that a degree of negative affect (a certain minimum level of distress) may be necessary to promote posttraumatic growth (Kunst, 2011).

Contrary views also exist. For example, Kast (1987/1990), a Jungian therapist, explained:

Overstimulated individuals are carried away by their emotions: fear, rage, love and other forms of arousal. They get flooded; ego-consciousness is not able to hold the emotion within bounds. Such crises impress us with their "loudness" which makes them recognizable by nearly everyone. Individuals in this condition need to be calmed down and to regain their composure. (p. 20)

It should also be noted that Coyne and Tennen (2010) raised major objections to some of the research and conclusions in the posttraumatic growth literature.

7–4. POSITIVE PSYCHOLOGY

Since 2000, positive psychology has been extremely successful on many fronts, with over 1000 publications, numerous special issues, and handbooks, etc. As well, hundreds of millions of government and corporate dollars have been secured to support research. Many references on positive psychology are available (e.g., Boniwell, 2012; Chaves, Lopez-Gomez, Hervas, & Vazquez, 2017; Cowen & Kilmer, 2002; Csíkszentmihályi & Csíkszentmihályi, 2006; Donaldson, Dollwet, & Rao, 2015; Gable & Haidt, 2005; Garbarino, 2011; Haidt,

2012; Hefferon & Boniwell, 2011; Johnson & Wood, 2017; Linley, Joseph, Harrington, & Wood, 2006; Lopez, 2009; Pawelski, 2016a, 2016b; Pérez-Álvarez, 2016; Rich, 2001, 2017a, 2017b; Sheldon, Kashdan, & Steget, 2011; Snyder & Lopez, 2002; Snyder, Lopez, & Pedrotti, 2010; Tavris 2014; Wong, 2017; Wood & Johnson, 2016).

In the psychological literature, positive approaches can clearly be traced back to William James and his interest in optimal performance (e.g., Froh, 2004; Rathunde, 2001). Over the years, there have been various efforts to measure well-being and happiness (e.g., Davis, 1929; Terman, 1938). Smith (1979) summarized research measuring well-being and happiness from 1945 to 1979 in his review of happiness trends in the United States. Maslow introduced positive psychology in 1954, and, as we saw in Chapter One, Jahoda made a significant contribution in 1958. Psychology was generally unreceptive, and positive definitions were slow to be accepted (Secker, 1998).

At the outset, it is helpful to delineate two basic approaches to happiness. One construct, called *eudaimonic well-being*, began with Aristotle and his suggestion that true happiness is the by-product of a virtuous life and doing what is right and worth doing (e.g., Boniwell, 2012; see also David, Boniwell, & Ayers, 2013; Ryan & Deci, 2001). Aristotle portrayed the realization of one's potential as the ultimate human goal. As Ryan and Deci pointed out, eudaimonic well-being "consists of fulfilling or realizing one's daimon or true nature" (p. 143).

Boniwell (2012) noted that hedonism (*hedonic well-being*) is a second common philosophical tradition often seen in positive psychology today. Hedonism is based upon the idea that the goal of life should focus on reducing pain and discomfort while maximizing happiness over all other considerations—it does not matter what kind of person you are or what kind of life you live as long as you are happy. Expressing a cautionary view, Power (2016) suggested the preoccupation with happiness is a deeply misguided approach and concluded: "Happiness is a simple transitory momentary state so cannot and should not be an endpoint or life goal in itself, for if happiness is pursued you will become one of its many victims, trapped in its blinding illusions" (p. 166). As well, McGuirk,

Kuppens, Kingston and Bastian (2017) empirically demonstrated the downside of promoting happiness as a goal in itself and observed:

> Experiencing failure is a negative emotional experience that is inconsistent with the goal of feeling happy, and leads people to engage in unconstructive, negative, and self-focused thinking on the reasons for their failure. . . . Placing social value on happiness sets up a hard-to-attain goal that is constantly reinforced through popular culture, through advertising, and through the ways in which others who adhere to these norms communicate their own emotional experiences, making that goal hard to abandon. (p. 7)

Waterman (2008) made an important distinction between the two constructs: "Whereas hedonia will arise from getting those things a person wants from *any* source, eudaimonia will be experienced only in connection with a limited set of specific sources, such as activities associated with self-realization and expressions of virtue" (p. 237).

Following Maslow and Carl Rogers, Dąbrowski uses a eudaimonic approach, emphasizing striving to achieve goals and ideals bigger than oneself, personal growth, testing limits and breaking homeostasis, emphasizing autonomy, and the importance of contributing to society.

7–4–1. Maslow and positive psychology

Using a eudaimonic approach, Maslow presented a framework for positive psychology in a chapter entitled, *Toward a Positive Psychology* (Maslow, 1954b, pp. 353-363). He felt that psychology had failed to consider the heights that an individual could attain and he described self-actualized people as examples.

The common practice of studying people with psychological problems and using this data to define mental health (by the absence of symptoms) made no sense to Maslow. Maslow (1954b) suggested that psychology should use "a fully grown, perfectly formed individual with a full development of those characteristics that define the species" (p. 361) as a prototype, both in terms of an exemplar of development for others to emulate and as a research subject in general. "The psychology generated by the study of healthy people could fairly be called positive by contrast with the negative psychology we now have, which has been generated by the study of sick or average people" (Maslow, 1954b, p. 361).

Maslow (1954b) said:

It becomes more and more clear that the study of crippled, stunted, immature and unhealthy specimens can yield only a cripple psychology and a cripple philosophy. The study of self-actualizing people must be the basis for a more universal science of psychology. (p. 234)

In making this plea, Maslow (1954b) elaborated:

Of course, the most pertinent and obvious choice of subject for a positive psychology is the study of psychological health (and other kinds of health, aesthetic health, value health, physical health and the like). But a positive psychology also calls for more study of the good man, of the secure and of the confident, of the democratic character, of the happy man, of the serene, the calm, the peaceful, the compassionate, the generous, the kind, of the creator, of the saint, of the hero, of the strong man, of the genius and of other good specimens of humanity. (p. 377)

Maslow (1954b) said: "Ought a biological species to be judged by its crippled, warped, only partially developed specimens, or by examples that have been overdomesticated caged and trained?" (p. 211). Extrapolating from this position, Maslow felt that we should consider any failure to achieve self-actualization as a form of psychopathology, leading to his suggestion that the "average or normal person is just as much a case [for therapy] as the psychotic, even though less dramatic and less urgent" (p. 370).

Maslow (1954b) also criticized what he felt was a major mistake of psychologists in general:

their pessimistic, negative and limited construction of the full height to which the human being can attain, their totally inadequate construction of his level of aspiration in life and their setting of his psychological limits at too low a level. (pp. 353-354)

In a prescient passage, Maslow (1954b) wrote:

The science of psychology has been far more successful on the negative than on the positive side; it has revealed to us much about man's shortcomings, his illnesses, his sins, but little about his potentialities, his virtues, his achievable aspirations, or his full psychological height. It is as if psychology had voluntarily restricted itself to only half its rightful jurisdiction and that the darker, meaner half. (p. 354)

In this seminal work, Maslow (1954b) also presented a solution to the situation:

If we are interested in the psychology of the human species we should limit ourselves to the use of the self-actualizing, the psychologically healthy, the mature, the fulfilled, for they are more truly representative of the human species than the usual average or normal group. The psychology generated by the study of healthy people could fairly be called positive by contrast with the negative psychology we now have, which has been generated by the study of sick or average people. (p. 361)

7–4–2. Seligman's contribution

Martin Seligman made positive psychology a focus during his 1998 presidency of the American Psychological Association (Seligman, 1999). "The creation of a new science of positive psychology can be the 'Manhattan Project' for the social sciences. It will require substantial resources but it does hold unprecedented promise" (Seligman, 1999, p. 562). Seligman and Csíkszentmihályi followed up in 2000 with a paper introducing a special issue of the *American Psychologist*, devoted to positive psychology (Seligman & Csíkszentmihályi, 2000). In this article, the authors presented positive psychology as a corrective to what they described as the dominant approach of modern psychology: the disease model of human functioning. The authors described three levels of analysis, including the subjective (about valued subjective experiences such as well-being, contentment, hope, optimism, flow, and happiness); the individual level (positive psychological traits such as the capacity for love, vocation, courage, perseverance, forgiveness, spirituality, high talent, and wisdom); and the group level (civic virtues and institutions that facilitate citizenship, responsibility, nurturance, altruism, civility, moderation, tolerance, and work ethic). The contributions of Maslow (1954b) and Jahoda (1958) were not mentioned in the article. Seligman and Csíkszentmihályi (2000) were also critical of the contributions of humanistic psychology as a whole, using the rationalization that these efforts were unscientific and lacking a rigorous research base (a criticism that can now be levelled at subsequent work in positive psychology as well). Medlock (2012) presented a discussion of the relationship between positive psychology and humanistic psychology (see also Elkins, 2009; Rich, 2017a, 2018; Waterman, 2013).Seligman has promoted positive psychology in diverse areas, including psychotherapy, youth development, occupational and workplace psychology, neuroscience, coaching, educational curricula, health, and a major initiative involving the American Army. Seligman sees his efforts trying to teach positive traits and resilience in the American Army as a critical testing ground. "The use of resilience training and positive psychology in the Army is consciously intended as a model for civilian use" (Seligman & Fowler, 2011, p. 85). If successful, these programs will then be implemented "in other very large institutions" (Cornum, Matthews, & Seligman, 2011).

Part of Seligman's agenda is the assumption that most of the traits associated with positive psychology can be learned and therefore ought to be taught in schools (they can be subtly delivered while teaching any subject matter by using "embedding techniques") (Seligman, Ernst, Gillham, Reivich, & Linkins, 2009, p. 305).

It is beyond the scope of this work to fully critique recent developments in positive psychology. For a recent critical review of positive psychology see Wong and Roy (2017).

Suffice to say, I believe Seligman (2002) presents an extremely naïve view:

So positive psychology takes seriously the bright hope that if you find yourself stuck in the parking lot of life, with few and only ephemeral pleasures, with minimal gratifications, and without meaning, there is a road out. This road takes you through the countryside of pleasure and gratification, up into the high country of strength and virtue, and finally to the peaks of lasting fulfilment: meaning and purpose. (p. xiv)

Power (2016) noted positive psychology has focused inordinately on the individual and individual traits and concluded, "so-called positive traits often interact with other aspects of a situation, context or person, and these interactions can reduce or even nullify the supposed positive benefit [of a trait]" (p. 133).

Further, Seligman (1999) presented psychological strength as a panacea, apparently disregarding biological or genetic contributions to mental conditions:

I look to a new social and behavioral science that seeks to understand and nurture those human strengths that can prevent the tragedy of mental illness. For it is my belief that no medication or technique of therapy holds as much promise for serving as a buffer against mental illness as does human strength. But psychology's focus on the negative has left us knowing too little about the many instances of growth, mastery, drive, and character building that can develop out of painful life events. (p. 561)

In summary, Dąbrowski builds on the foundational works on positive psychology by Maslow and Jahoda. A review of developments in positive psychology since 2000 is disappointing, as much of this material appears to be simplistic, reductionistic, and, in Dąbrowski's terms, unilevel. It would be interesting see an in-depth analysis of positive psychology that incorporates Dąbrowski, Maslow, and Jahoda.

7–5. SELECTED APPROACHES TO PERSONALITY DEVELOPMENT

Dąbrowski emphasized that his was a theory of personality development and so it seems appropriate to consider his work in terms of other such theories. Several reviews and general overviews of personality development are available (e.g., Bateson & Martin, 2000; Crago, 2017; Horowitz, 2016; Mascolo & Griffin, 2013; McAdams, 2015; Shaffer, 2009; Simanowitz & Pearce, 2003).

For this discussion, I begin with two well-known approaches: those of Carl Jung and Erik Erikson. I also discuss the work of Reza Arasteh in some detail because it closely parallels Dąbrowski's and because it is scarcely known in psychology today. I conclude this section with introductions to the work of Robert Kegan and self-authorship.

7–5–1. Carl Jung

The most pertinent of Carl Jung's (1875-1961) writings to our discussion is a chapter on the development of personality (1940). There are several significant similarities between Dąbrowski and Jung that will be highlighted.

Jung (1940) took a hierarchical approach to personality and development. He believed that consciousness slowly arises from unconsciousness like an island rises from the sea. Initially we act without really knowing ourselves, but we can reflect upon our actions and, in this way, we can discover who we are. Most of this development takes place from birth to psychic puberty, which occurs at about age 20 for women and at about age 25 for men. The individual psyche rises from a collective psyche. Jung described a hierarchy of five levels through which the individual rises: animal ancestors, human ancestors, one's nation, one's family, and finally, individualization.

Like Dąbrowski, Jung (1940) said that personality is not a given—it is an achievement—a lifelong process of creation involving all aspects of an individual's life:

> The achievement of personality means nothing less than the best possible development of all that lies in a particular, single being. It is impossible to foresee what an infinite number of conditions must be fulfilled to bring this about. A whole human life span in all its biological, social, and spiritual aspects is needed. Personality is the highest realization of the inborn distinctiveness of the particular living being. Personality is an act of the greatest courage in the face of life,

and means unconditional affirmation of all that constitutes the individual, the most successful adaptation to the universal conditions of human existence, with the greatest possible freedom of personal decision. (p. 286)

Jung also advocated an individual personality ideal: "Personality as a complete realization of the fullness of our being is an unattainable ideal. But unattainability is no counterargument against an ideal, for ideals are only signposts, never goals." (Jung, 1940, p. 287).

Personality needs some *cause* to develop, as Jung (1940) said:

Now, no one develops his personality because someone told him it would be useful or advisable for him to do so. Nature has never yet allowed herself to be imposed upon by well-meaning advice. Only coercion working through causal connections moves nature, and human nature also. Nothing changes itself without need, and human personality least of all. It is immensely conservative, not to say inert. Only the sharpest need is able to rouse it. (p. 288)

Volition plays a major role in the process of personality development, in particular in choosing a moral code. As Jung (1940) succinctly said:

Personality can never develop itself unless the individual chooses, his own way consciously and with conscious, moral decision. Not only the causal motive, the need, but a conscious, moral decision must lend its strength to the process of the development of personality. If the first, that is, need, is lacking, then the so-called development would be mere acrobatics of the will; if the latter is missing, that is, the conscious decision, then the development will come to rest in a stupefying, unconscious automatism. But a man can make a moral choice of his own way only when he holds it to be the best. If any other way were held to be better, then he would live and develop that other personality in place of his own. The other ways are the conventions of a moral, social, political, philosophic, or religious nature. The fact that the conventions always flourish in one form or another proves that the overwhelming majority of mankind chooses not its own way, but the conventions, and so does not develop itself, but a method and a collectivity at the cost of its own fullness. (pp. 289-290)

Developing personality is "an uncongenial deviation from the highway"[33] making the quest rare and unpopular; "No wonder, then, that from the beginning, only the few have hit upon this strange adventure" (Jung, 1940, p. 209).

The idea of an individual force or path of development, reminiscent of Dąbrowski's third factor, is encapsulated in Jung's idea of vocation.

Vocation: fatefully forces a man to emancipate himself from the herd and its trodden paths. . . . He must obey his own law, as if it were a demon that whisperingly indicated to him new and strange ways. Who has vocation hears the voice of the inner man; he is *called*. (Jung, 1940, pp. 290-291)

Jung (1940) further develops the analogy of a developmental law:

To become a personality is not the absolute prerogative of the man of genius. He may even have genius without either having personality or being a personality. In so far as every individual has his own inborn law of life, it is theoretically possible for every man to follow this law before all others and so to become a personality—that is, to achieve completeness. (p. 296)

Jung (1940) observed "In so far as a man is untrue to his own law and does not rise to personality, he has failed of the meaning of his life" (p. 301).

Jung called the process leading to authenticity—the progression from the unconscious to the conscious—"individuation" and suggested that it "can be seen at important stages in life and at times of crisis when fate upsets the purpose and expectation of the ego-consciousness" (Bennet, 1966/1983, p. 171). In the normal course of events, individuation leads to a unification and integration of the personality.

Ellenberger (1970) described Jung's approach to development as a lifelong series of metamorphoses; the infant must rise out of a non-differentiated unconsciousness to slowly develop a conscious ego. Jung was not primarily concerned with the first stage of life, up until about the age of 35 to 40. For Jung, the central metamorphosis of human life concerned the midlife crisis, a time when an individual is called upon, sometimes by a neurosis sent as a warning from the unconscious, to re-examine his or her life and to become aware of changes that need to be made to avoid wasting the second half of life. The crucial second half of life "is a period of confrontation with the archetype of the spirit and of the self" (Ellenberger, 1970, p. 711). With individuation, the ego loses its central position in personality and becomes merely another planet revolving around the sun—the self (Ellenberger, 1970). The individual has achieved a comfort with life and with those around him or her and has reconciled death. For Jung, this marks the achievement of wisdom.

It is common for the process of individuation to regress or stall and it is the task of therapy to remove obstacles and to restore the process. Jung emphasized self-regulation and an idea he referred to as a return to the opposite. Perhaps referring to his own creative illness, Jung suggested that at times an individual might experience a spontaneous reversal of a regression (Ellenberger, 1970).

Storr (1966/1983) noted that analysis was a spiritual quest "to come to terms with oneself, to accept oneself and to become, as far as possible, the person which it was intended one should be" (p. ix). In describing Jung's approach to neurosis, Storr suggested neuroses were seen in a positive light because they acted as pointers, letting one know that a re-examination of values and of one's way of life were called for. When confronted with a neurosis, the question is: "Which task is the patient trying to avoid, what difficulty in life is he or she trying to escape?" When successfully resolved, neuroses result in growth as more and more of the unconscious is integrated into the psyche and the self becomes more and more whole.

It is interesting that Jung experienced a long breakdown. Ellenberger (1970) described Jung's "creative illness," a break that lasted some six years. During this time Jung utilized "self-therapy" and "emerged from his psychological experience as a man who had undergone a deep-reaching interior metamorphosis" (Ellenberger, 1970, p. 673).

Society does not encourage the individual to develop consciousness, Jung (1933) said:

> Nature cares nothing whatsoever about a higher level of consciousness; quite the contrary. And then society does not value these feats of the psyche very highly; its prizes are always given for achievement and not for personality—the latter being rewarded, for the most part posthumously. (p. 118)

This throws the responsibility back upon the individual to decide what kind of existence he or she will have. Jung concluded that the common solution was to limit oneself to the attainable and renounce all other possibilities.

Dąbrowski (1972b) said that there was "some similarity" between Jung's theory and his own:

> According to Jung, neurosis resulted from an unsuccessful attempt at solution of vital human problems within oneself. Thus, neuroses are not only results of some pathological causes, but are expressive also of an attempt at a new synthesis of inner contradictions. (p. 235)

While Jung emphasized disagreements with one's self—"man disunited with himself"—as being problematic, Dąbrowski saw this state as critical to the process of development.

Dąbrowski (1972b) was quite critical of Freudian analysis because symbols represent something that has been suppressed and is now a static image, and thus, psychoanalysis is limited to searching for causes. In Jung's model, a symbol is dynamic and may represent the future development of an individual, and this creates a more powerful level of analysis. However, Dąbrowski (1972b) criticized Jung for relying too heavily upon hypothetical assumptions, for being vague and for not being of practical significance. Dąbrowski also criticized Jung for not differentiating levels of mental functions—deficits of theory that prevent an understanding of the developmental path of humans.

Dąbrowski used the vocabulary of analysis when he said: "This path of development is a path of transformation of archetypes into 'neotypes,' of individual unconscious into individual superconscious which contains all the elements of human psychic structure. Naturally such achievements are paid for with suffering, disintegration and psychoneurosis" (Dąbrowski, 1972b, p. 241). Jung believed that the psyche is self-regulating, maintaining itself in equilibrium similar to the homeostasis maintained by the body. Anything that threatens this equilibrium will trigger compensatory mechanisms. Dąbrowski explained that the collective unconscious, as well as the individual subconscious, must be transcended to achieve consciousness and superconsciousness. Thus, a healthy equilibrium cannot exist until secondary integration and this must be achieved by going through considerable disintegration and psychoneuroses.

7–5–2. Erik Erikson

In introducing Dąbrowski's 1964 book, Aronson (1964) presented a brief introduction to the work of Erik Erikson (1902-1994). I will elaborate on Erikson in some detail because his approach has been popular over the years, especially in the context of developmental psychology, and it shares much with Dąbrowski. Aronson summarized Erikson's view of personality growth:

> Erikson sees human growth "from the point of view of the conflicts, inner and outer, which the healthy personality weathers, emerging and re-emerging with an increased sense of inner unity." The solution of each crisis is dependent on the solution of earlier ones. His constructs of ego synthesis and resynthesis in the development of identity are similar to Dąbrowski's constructs of disintegration and secondary integration in personality development. (p. xxiii)

Erikson's (1959) formulation of the stages of personality echoed Dąbrowski's:

> One might say that personality at the first stage crystallizes around the conviction "I am what I am given," and that of the second, "I and what I will." The third can be characterized by

"I am what I can imagine I will be." We must now approach the fourth: "I am what I learn." (p. 82)

Identity is largely an unconscious sense of who one is and of one's contribution to society. Hoare (2002) identified it as "a deep sense of ideological commitment, of knowing what is worth one's fidelity in the expansive social world" (p. 31). In reading Hoare's description, Erikson's construct of identity seems strikingly similar to Dąbrowski's idea of personality ideal. Hoare explained: "Identity's achievement is the hard work of building one's own 'adult' through knowing personal talents, interests and ideological commitments and working to mesh these into a self-image and then an ongoing process of vocational, ideological and personal commitments" (p. 31). In a construct similar to Dąbrowski's descriptions of personality and third factor, Erikson suggested that identity is a rarely attained process which acts to move an individual throughout his or her life—an "integrator" that continually moves one towards "wholeness."

Erikson described the moral adult as:

a rule-driven, judging, right-versus-wrong, reciprocity, quid pro quo person. To Erikson, nearly all adults are moral. Some are also ethical. Ethical adults are principled. They build on their own and others' strengths, give of themselves without expecting a return of favors in kind and avoid judging and controlling others. (Hoare, 2002, p. 71)

In differentiating between the moral and the ethical, Erikson complained that many people are highly moral but are undeveloped ethically, leading to harsh judgments against others. He also described a category of unethical and immoral but did not elaborate this group. In summary, the ideal adult combines morality and ethics.

Erikson presented an ontogenetic developmental stage model involving eight identified stages that unfold as time goes on, analogous to the predetermined stages seen in embryonic development. In general, each stage poses a developmental task that has to be successfully met, yielding a virtue associated with that stage. The challenge of each stage may be repeated in future stages even if the initial challenge was successfully negotiated. Likewise, challenges involving unsuccessful resolutions may also be repeated in the future. Just as virtues will accumulate with each past success, contributing to coping with future tasks, unsuccessful adaptations will carry forward and may hinder future development—or require eventual future resolution.

Each stage involves two aspects, the first focused on the growth of the individual and the second on his or her social relations. Thus, Erikson described a healthy person as one who knows one's self, who knows one's culture and who knows one's role in that culture.

Erikson (1968) reflected on his use of the term *identity crisis* and noted:

> "Crisis" no longer connotes impending catastrophe, which at one time seemed to be an obstacle to the understanding of the term. It is now being accepted as designating a necessary turning point, a crucial moment, when development must move one way or another, marshalling resources of growth, recovery and further differentiation. (p. 16)

The term identity crisis became associated with a normative crisis that is associated with a stage of development. Erikson (1968) concluded:

> Judged by the clinical origin of these terms, then, it would seem reasonable enough to link the pathological and the developmental aspects of the matter and to see what might differentiate the identity crisis typical for a case history from that of a life history. (p. 18)

Erikson continued by noting Freud's discovery that neurotic conflict is much like the "normative" conflicts which every child must pass through as he or she negotiates adolescence, and Erikson concluded that, even though the "symptoms" of adolescent episodes may resemble neurotic or even psychotic symptoms, adolescence should not be considered pathological; rather, these symptoms signal a normative crisis marked by a high potential for growth.

Early crises leave "residues" that are maintained in one's personality and that are "re-resolved" on an ongoing basis. Erikson

(1968) described human development:

> from the point of view of the conflicts, inner and outer, which
> the vital personality weathers, re-emerging from each crisis
> with an increased sense of inner unity, with an increase of
> good judgment and an increase in the capacity "to do well"
> according to his own standards and to the standards of those
> who are significant to him. (pp. 91-92)

As mentioned above, Erikson emphasized that each stage
develops its own unique core crisis. The resolution of this crisis
results in the development or re-emergence of a basic strength, virtue
or quality of the self; for example, hope. Erikson (1968) said each
stage represents an opportunity to develop a significant new
perspective on life:

> Each successive step, then, is a potential crisis because of a
> radical change in perspective. Crisis is used here in a
> developmental sense to connote not a threat of catastrophe, but
> a turning point, a crucial period of increased vulnerability and
> heightened potential and therefore, the ontogenetic source of
> generational strength and maladjustment. (p. 96)

Erikson emphasized the effect early crisis management successes
and failures had on subsequent adult (midlife) development. He
emphasized that as people age, they come to look back at their lives,
reviewing past successes and failures. Some become obsessed over
past mistakes and what went wrong in life, developing depression and
bitterness over their perception of a failed or meaningless life
("despair") while others are able to accept their failures as part of life,
deepen their level of self-acceptance and resolve to learn from their
mistakes ("ego integrity") (Torges, Stewart, & Duncan, 2008). Thus,
in Erikson's model, the adult who can examine his or her history and
come to terms with life regrets facilitates further personality
development, an idea supported by research (Torges et al., 2008).

In summary, Erikson suggested that normal development spans
the lifetime and includes "normal" developmental crises associated
with resolving challenges at each stage of growth. For example,
adolescence involves the challenge of forming an identity that will

guide one's adult years. The "pathology" associated with these crises is connected with one's expected and normal course of development.

Dąbrowski (1972b) clarified that, in contrast to Erikson, positive disintegration is not concerned with crises connected to specific developmental stages. Dąbrowski (1972b) summarized his opinion of Erikson:

> Although Erikson's theory of crises is a very interesting attempt to characterize the various stages of man's development, this position is based exclusively on psychoanalytic dynamisms without sufficient recognition of the influence of heredity, of various experiences in life together with influence from others and especially of autonomous factors in development. (p. 245)

7–5–3. Abdol Reza Arasteh

The Persian psychoanalyst Abdol Reza Arasteh (1927-1992) presented a comprehensive theory of personality development with many ideas in common with Dąbrowski and, like Dąbrowski, his ideas are virtually unknown in psychology today. An expert in Islam and in Sufi mysticism, Arasteh also studied Western approaches to mental health when he taught at Princeton and George Washington University. His major work, *Final Integration in the Adult Personality*, was published in 1965 (Arasteh, 1965b) and republished in a second edition in 1975 (Arasteh, 1975). The theory was illustrated in a major case study of Rumi (Arasteh, 1974/2008). A final work was published in 1980 entitled *Growth to Selfhood: The Sufi Contribution* (Arasteh, 1980/1990).

Arasteh (1965b) delineated three universal developmental stages. The first, "natural" stage consists of basic instincts and corresponds to Freud's id. Enculturation and socialization lead to the second, cultural stage, beginning at about age two. Socialization corresponds to Freud's superego, what Arasteh calls the phenomenal self. However, the socialized individual is only "half born" and is prevented from further growth by the forces of culture. The ordinary demands of social life create a wide range of "false values"—external, socially defined and valued goals and immediate needs that take precedence over one's conscience or self-development. Emphasizing the idea of the partial human, we tend to over-develop ourselves in one particular area, for example by specializing in our careers, and in the process ignore our self-development.

In Eastern thought, the prototype for the third stage final integration is Buddha, whereas in the West, Arasteh submits that it is Socrates. A new sense of identity and of a greater transcendental self arose in the Renaissance and gained momentum in the Age of Enlightenment. Arasteh (1965b) concluded this momentum was lost, and today, fragmented individuals live "within a well-organized society" (p. 85).

In describing final integration, Arasteh pitted socialization against existentialism—one must rise above culture and discover one's true self to become fully mature. This final stage is characterized by individuality and creativity, leading to the cosmic or universal self. The socialized individual is limited to choosing and unable to create, whereas in the transcultural state, one becomes a creator rather than a selector. To detach oneself from traditional values and from one's social self is to become "awakened," to become one's "real self."

Moving from socialization to final integration involves first becoming aware of the conflict between one's social self and one's cosmic self. The individual must embrace this conflict and "strive to develop sufficient strength to stand up against the conventional self, to acquire the mental fortitude to resist undesirable social forces and to set a new standard free of all that which is usually held dear" (Arasteh, 1974/2008, p. 26).

Arasteh (1974/2008) illustrated his approach with several case studies, including one of Johann Wolfgang von Goethe. Arasteh (1972/2008) said that the basic inspiration for his theory came from his study of the Sufi scholar and poet Jalal-e-Din Mohammad Molavi of Rumi (1207-1273):

> Rumi said that a seeker faces two major tasks: to dissolve his present status (*fana*), then reintegrate again; "Unless you are first disintegrated, how can I reintegrate you again?" Disintegration here refers to the passing away of the conventional self, reintegration means rebirth in the cosmic self. (p. 129)

This disintegration (*fana*) from a self-intellect, partial soul and social self, and subsequent rebirth or reintegration (*baqa*), is necessary for "activization of one's totality into the cosmic self." Rebirth is a passing from "I-ness" to a state of universality or "one-ness," a necessary transition to be considered a whole and mature individual.

The Sufi approach to development emphasizes the conflict between inherent forces that can either act to regress an individual to a lower instinctual state or elevate an individual into the cosmic self. These inherent forces are in conflict because older evolutionary instinctual tendencies are now challenged by the appearance of reason in the human psyche. In the Sufi tradition, reason is considered necessary but not sufficient for development. The individual must either rise beyond reasoning to a state of cosmic certainty or risk falling back into uncertainty and instinctual impulses. Therefore, echoing Unamuno, a central task facing the individual is to come to realize that intellect and reason alone cannot resolve the existential dilemmas of life. As Rumi observed, the more developed the intellectual self, the more proud and self-conceited one becomes, thus further distancing one from one's real self.

The duality between the mind (emphasizing reasoning and thinking) versus the heart (emphasizing emotion, insight, and intuition) has been with us for millennia. Arasteh (1965b) believed that this duality reached its apex with Freud and that today, the "ordinary individual" lives in the mind in a fundamentally fragmented state, split off from emotion and intuition. Not everyone is able to come to appreciate this fragmentation. Arasteh said that it takes an "intuitive individual" to appreciate this duality, leading to the realization that reason alone cannot give one certainty and to the discovery that experience and emotion are legitimate avenues of development.

One must allow one's real self to speak and become aware of the possibility of development. The individual can sometimes glimpse a more authentic state of security, but a dominant ego and the social self inhibit growth (Arasteh, 1965b). Under favorable conditions, one's true conscience will challenge the social self and increase one's psychological disharmony. One's real personality ("that which he ought to become") stands in opposition to the "I" and eventually the individual "falls into a state of quest and the object of this search consists of becoming a real self, a thoroughly-born man, a perfect and universal man" (Arasteh, 1965b, p. 157).

The anxiety and stress generated from existential concerns about the nature and purpose of life are the impetus for change: "If a man faces his existential dilemma, then the task becomes, not one of giving three hours a week to a psychiatrist, but entering the state of anxious search, which requires complete concentration and entrance into an 'existential moratorium'" (Arasteh, 1965b, p. 152). As Knabb and Welsh (2009) summarized:

> The act of separation from culture, coupled with anxiety, produces a sort of shedding of the old self in order to make way for a new reality. The anxiety that one experiences is embraced because it serves as a catalyst for change so as to acquire a new object of desire. As a result of the existential moratorium and the acquisition of the new object of desire, the individual gradually experiences a rebirth in totality; this rebirth in totality produces a trans-cultural state of being. (p. 55)

The term *existential moratorium* designates the process of the rebirth of the social individual into the final integration as a trans-cultural human being. This moratorium gives the individual a break from existential anxiety, allowing time to search for new experiences and new values that lead to final integration.

Arasteh's existential moratorium can be compared with Erikson's construct of the *psychosocial moratorium*, the bridge between adolescence and rebirth as a social adult. Erikson described the moratorium as the status of a person who is actively involved in exploring different identities but who has not yet made a commitment to one or another.

Ironically, although Arasteh was trained as a psychoanalyst, he concluded that psychoanalysis limits psychological growth by directing the individual toward social adaptation, the upper limit of analysis. In support of this view, Arasteh (1965b) cited Everett Knight: "The Western individual not only accepts the herd values of his society but he has invented psychoanalysis to prevent him from straying from them" (p. 173). Knight (1960) went on to explain that in cases where a "sensitive or intelligent individual" develops stress or anxiety over the social status quo, this is quickly attributed to the individual being wrong and consequently being neurotic. Effectively marginalized, the insightful individual cannot become a revolutionary for social change. Knight went on to say that even those who may be critical of the values of society—for example, Karen Horney (1885-1952)—end up concluding that it is best for the individual to "conform, to integrate himself with the masses, to accept" (Knight, 1960, p. 65). One needs to learn to role-play and adapt to those he or she interacts with, and in so doing, one becomes a non-entity. "Happiness in our individualistic society has come to consist in being as much like other people as possible" (Knight, 1960, p. 65). As an alternative to psychoanalysis Arasteh developed a therapeutic approach he called *normative psycho-cultural analysis* (Arasteh, 1965a, Arasteh, 1965c, Welsh and Knabb, 2009).

In summary, Arasteh (1975) called for the "disintegration and removal of the social self," leading to an inner metamorphosis and rebirth characterized by a "gradual enlightenment which elevates man above his social self and reintegrates him into the cosmos, thus relating him to the non-human environment" and ultimately culminating in a state of final integration where "he breaks through the boundaries of the unconscious and feels a new harmony with the world," expressed through the claim: "I live, therefore I am." (pp. 142- 143.)

7–5–4. Robert Kegan

Harvard psychologist Robert Kegan (1941-) presented a theory of development based upon Piaget (Kegan, 1982). He used subject-object as the basis to analyze the ongoing tension between the human desire to be part of the social group versus the desire to be independent and autonomous. The theory has six stages of development, each describing a particular subject-object relationship representing how individuals make sense of the world and of themselves. Subject is in essence how we know (the structure of how one knows) and object is essentially what we know (the content of what one knows). Moving from one stage to the next involves a transformation: taking what we were once subject to and making this the object of the next stage.

As Kegan (1982) described:

> All transitions involve leaving a consolidated self behind before any new self can take its place. . . . Every transition involves to some extent the killing off of the old self. The phenomenological side of that cold Piagetian/biological notion of differentiation is repudiation. I must for a time be not-me before I can reappropriate that old me as the new object of a new self. (p. 232)

In this way, development involves a progressive deepening in the understanding of both the self and the world. The developmental stages Kegan (1982) described are presented in Table 4.

Table 4. Kegan's Developmental Stages

#	Name	Age	Subject	Object	Kohlberg	Piaget	Maslow
0	Incorporative	To 18 months	Reflexes related to sensing and moving	None	None	Sensorimotor	Physiological survival
1	Impulsive	2 to 7	Impulses and perceptions	Reflexes related to sensing and moving	Punishment/obedience	Preoperational	Physiological satisfaction
2	Imperial Balance	Preadolescent (7-10)	Needs, desires and interests	Impulses and perceptions	Instrumental	Concrete operational	Safety orientation
3	Interpersonal Balance	Postadolescent	Social environment	Needs, desires and interests	Interpersonal concordance orientation	Early formal operational	Love, affection and belongingness
4	Institutional	Postadolescent	Personality, identity, values and ideology	Social environment	Social contract	Full formal operational	Esteem and self-esteem
5	Interindividual	After age 40	Interindividuality & interpenetrability of self systems	Unique personality, identity, values, ideology	Principled orientation	Post formal	Self-actualization

Kegan described a first pre-stage called "Incorporative." There is no sense of self because there is no differentiation between subject and object: the baby (up to 18 months) can only see his or her own subjective perspective.

Subject-object relations become possible at Stage 1, "Impulsive." The child (ages 2 to 7) is subject to impulses and perceptions; the object is the reflexes related to sensing and moving.

"The emerging capacity to 'take the role' of another, to see that others have a perspective of their own" signals Stage 2, the "Imperial Balance" (Kegan, 1982, p. 137). Preadolescents are subject to their needs, desires, and interests. The object is one's impulses and perceptions. Self-construct emerges: "Children are aware of others and their needs but have no sense of being responsible to others' needs" (Eriksen, 2006, p. 293). Relationships are extrinsically valuable (what can this person do for me?).

At Stage 3, "Interpersonal Balance," the socialized mind takes its subject as the social environment and the socialization process. The object is one's needs, desires, and interests. Identity is determined by social roles and the motivation at this stage is to fit in and not disappoint others; therefore, the opinions of others are dominant in governing behavior. The individual has fully internalized the values of their society. Relationships become intrinsically valuable:

> This balance is "interpersonal" but it is not "intimate," because what might appear to be intimacy here is the self's *source* rather than its aim. There is no self to share with another; instead the other is required to bring the self into being. (Kegan, 1979, p. 14).

In common with Dąbrowski, Kegan saw this as the stage commonly reached by the average individual.

At Stage 4, "Institutional" (modernism), the self-authoring mind is able to make the transition to a subject encompassing the individual's own unique personality, values, and ideology. The social environment becomes the object and the individual is able to stand back for the first time to critically examine and analyze society. This allows the self-authoring individual to create his or her own identity guided by unique individualized values. Approximately 20% to 30% of the population achieves this stage (Eriksen, 2006).

The final Stage 5 is the "Interindividual" (postmodernism). This rare stage (less than 1% of the population) nominally appears later in life, likely after age 40. The subject is "interindividuality and interpenetrability of self systems." The object is the individual's own unique personality, values, and ideology.

Individuality is a category that all persons are potentially eligible to participate in. Individuality is also a recognition of the connections that exist between people; therefore, for Kegan, the construction of individuality is a process of "interindividuality." Further, "neither one person nor the group is an individuated whole, it is a category of interpenetration" (Kegan, 1982, p. 68). It is helpful to look at Bergson's usage of the term interpenetration. For Bergson, the characteristics of the individual parts of a process are defined by their connections with the whole of the overall process; thus, the parts are interpenetrated. It is impossible to divide the whole and to consider one or another part individually as this inherently falsifies the part (Costelloe, 1912).

At this final stage, "people become the directors and creators of systems, understanding how systems fit together meaningfully" (Eriksen, 2006, p. 291). As Eriksen (2006) explained:

> The interindividual person is able to take the transformational process as object, to hold the tension involved in the transformation concurrently with the product that emerges. The interindividual person equates this process, rather than its resolution, with being awake or alive. Suffering or obstacles or lack of resolution are valued as just as important to relationships as are wholeness and transformation and so resolution of difficulties is not the primary aim. Kegan considers true intimacy to require this meaning-making capacity. (p. 296)

The developmental stages described by Kegan resonate with Dąbrowski's. Kegan did not elaborate how individuals move through the stages (the process of development) nor did he describe a rationale for why one individual would advance through the stages while another would not.

7–5–5. Self-authorship

Baxter Magolda (1998, 2001, 2008; Baxter Magolda & King, 2012) extended Kegan's work by researching his construct of "self-authorship," a fundamental shift from external to internal meaning-making, which mirrors the shift from the influence of second factor to third factor in Dąbrowski's theory. Self-authorship is "the internal capacity to define one's beliefs, identity and social relations" (Baxter Magolda, 2008, p. 269). Baxter Magolda (2001) presented this description of self-authorship from a research subject:

> Making yourself into something, not what other people say or not just kind of floating along in life, but you're in some sense a piece of clay. You've been formed into different things, but that doesn't mean you can't go back on the potter's wheel and instead of somebody else's hands building and molding you, you use your own and in a fundamental sense change your values and beliefs. (p. 119)

Baxter Magolda (2008) described three key aspects to self-authorship. The first is for an individual to be able to trust his or her inner voice and also to have the realization that while one cannot control reality, one can control one's reactions to what happens in life. The second key insight is the necessity to build an internal foundation (similar to Dąbrowski's inner psychic milieu). This internal framework includes a self-generated philosophy of life, beliefs and self-identity. The third key insight is a "crossing over" from understanding one's new world view (meaning-making system) to actually putting these principles into action through one's behavior and lifestyle. The study of self-authorship was advanced by Pizzolato (2007) who developed a questionnaire and an open-ended essay to measure the construct.

Highlights of meaning making and self-authorship (Baxter Magolda & King, 2012):

- Development is continuous and cyclical.
- Development incorporates or, where necessary, transforms the prior structure.
- Prior structures are retained as an element of the new, more

complex system.
- New structures are more complex and more adaptive.
- Meaning-making develops through cycles of differentiation and integration.
- Growth is a gradual process with transitional periods involving internal conflicts (disequilibrium) and periods of consolidation reflecting stability.
- Conflicts trigger cycles of differentiation, integration, and the creation of a new structure.
- Change mechanisms (including the role of internal conflict/disequilibrium) are not yet well understood.
- Kegan defined three forms of meaning making: how one knows (knowledge), who one is (identity), and how one relates with others (relationships).
- Initially, one is subject to, is shaped by, and defines oneself by alignment (fitting in) with one's environment.
- The self-authoring individual can objectify the social environment, allowing a critical evaluation and leading to the creation of an internally based value/belief system, self-identity, and way of relating to others and the world.

In summary, we can identify several qualitatively different meaning-making systems, each with a unique worldview. Each advance is more comprehensive, more differentiated and more effective in dealing with the complexities of life than its predecessors (Cook-Greuter, 2004, p. 276). "World views evolve from simple to complex, from static to dynamic and from egocentric to sociocentric to world-centric" (Cook-Greuter, 2004, p. 277).

Cook-Greuter (2004) further differentiated lateral and vertical development:

> Lateral growth and expansion happens through many channels, such as schooling, training, self-directed and life-long learning as well as simply through exposure to life. Vertical development in adults is much rarer. It refers to how we learn to see the world through new eyes, how we change our interpretations of experience and how we transform our views of reality. (p. 276)

In conclusion of this subsection, many other authors have presented descriptions of the meaning-making developmental levels and transitions seen in personality development (e.g., Arasteh, 1965b, 1974/2008, 1975, 1980/1990; Erikson, 1959, 1968; Graves, 1970, [on Graves see also Beck & Cowan, 1996]; Jung, 1940; Kegan, 1982, 1994; Kohlberg, 1981; Loevinger, 1976; Maslow, 1943d, 1968, 1970, 1971/1976; Piaget, 1954; Wilber, 1996, [on Wilber see also Rowan, 2007]. Although there is no agreement on the specific details, there is a broad consensus in describing personality development, providing rich ground for future researchers to explore.

Consensus items:

- However named, three general developmental categories are described:
  - "Basic" (preconventional)
  - "Medium" (conventional)
  - "Advanced" (postconventional)
- Advanced development is extremely rare.
- Internal conflict or disequilibrium is often associated with growth.
- Advanced development is characterized by decreasing reliance upon environmental cues and by increasing self-determination and self-definition.
- Elimination of ego is associated with advanced development.
- Mechanisms or processes of development are seldom described.
- Factors differentiating non-developers from developers are rarely described.

7–5–6. Contemporary personality theory

Many excellent resources exist introducing personality theory (e.g., Cervone & Mischel, 2002; Cervone & Pervin, 2013; Ellis, Abrams, Abrams, Nussbaum, & Frey, 2009; Funder, 2013; Larsen & Buss, 2013; McCrae & Costa, 2003; E. Taylor, 2009).

Mendaglio (2008b) proclaimed Dąbrowski's theory "a personality theory for the 21st century" based primarily on two considerations (p. 13). First, Dąbrowski assigned emotion a critical role in the development of personality, a feature which reflects a shift in psychology toward a renewed appreciation for the potential roles of emotion, both within personality theory and within psychology as a whole. Second, Mendaglio suggested that Dąbrowski's theory was in a prime position to revitalize the field of personality theory in general.

Mendaglio (2008c) suggested that a careful reading of Dąbrowski's theory could challenge one's taken-for-granted assumptions regarding personality and development. He said this could even trigger an introspective review of one's beliefs. Such a process could act as a template for an individual to go on to further reconsider his or her belief system in general, thus triggering the process of positive disintegration.

McAdams and Emmons (1995) noted a renewed appreciation of levels of personality. Many of these works are reminiscent of Dąbrowski's theory and some adeptly encapsulate his ideas. For instance, Emmons (1995) described a sequence of the development of personality reminiscent of Dąbrowski's three factors:

> In the optimal situation, fully integrated individuals would be able to liberate themselves from genetic commands and cultural constraints to gain control and develop an autonomous and self-determined life, while at the same time benefiting humankind by shaping the direction of future generations. (p. 354)

Other level-based approaches echo Dąbrowski and also involve a progression from lower levels that are more biological and social, to higher, more autonomous levels. For example, McAdams's three levels of personality (introduced above) warrant a closer review. To recap, the first level consists of dispositional traits depicting the most general and observable behavioral patterns of people in general. The second level, characteristic adaptations, describe what an individual is striving to do "over time, situated in place and role, expressing herself or himself in and through strategies, tactics, plans, and goals" (McAdams, 1995, p. 380). As Emmons (1995) summarized, Level I is what a person "has" and level II is what a person "does." These first two levels echo Dąbrowski's first and second factors and both fall within Dąbrowski's first level. Stories form the core of adult personality; "the narration of the events within the life story now becomes part and parcel of personality itself, at Level III. One can now proceed to explain why the individual has created one kind of identity story rather than another" (McAdams, 1995, p. 388). These stories give people "a sense of identity lending a sense of overall meaning and purpose to their lives" (Emmons, 1995, p. 352). In Dąbrowski's terms this would correspond to the process of personality formation described in Levels III, IV and V.

McAdams and Pals (2006) suggested that psychology still lacks a comprehensive understanding of the whole person and they presented five principles required to create an integrative science of the whole person. The five principles of McAdams and Pals (2006) are:

- Human lives are individual variations on a general evolutionary design. These common features describe the underlying essence of what it is to be a human being.

- The dispositional signature reflects one's dispositional traits (for example, extraversion, friendliness, depressiveness) that represent the broad individual differences between people. Traits describe what kind of person this particular person is.

- Characteristic adaptations are the specific motives, goals, values, self-images and so forth that collectively describe what a person does. Characteristic adaptations describe who the person is.

- Life narratives: the challenge for each of us to construct his or her life narrative.

- Culture, society and the day-to-day environment create the proximal contexts within which individuals live. Cultural effects are played out on different levels of personality, creating a complex interplay between culture and individuality. One's culture provides a "menu" of stories from which one chooses his or her individual narrative. (pp. 205-211)

7–6. THE LEGACY OF JOHN HUGHLINGS JACKSON

Hughlings Jackson's hierarchical model of brain organization has had a major influence on neurology (e.g., Franz & Gillett, 2011; Kennard & Swash, 1989; Kolb & Whishaw, 2014). The forebrain, brainstem, and spinal cord are the three major levels in Hughlings Jackson's model. Hughlings Jackson concluded that the newer, higher levels are laid over existing structures and act by controlling lower levels. In his integrative framework, the highly complex conscious mind is the highest and latest layer of evolution—emerging from, but smoothly integrating with, simpler, lower, and older elements. If a higher level becomes disrupted or disinhibited, then lower-level consciousness and lower-level processes are disinhibited and resurface.

A hierarchical approach was fundamental to Paul MacLean's (1913-2007) model of the triune brain, a model describing three-levels of brain function (Cory & Gardner, 2002; MacLean, 1991). The lower level reptilian brain ("R-complex") controls instinctive survival behavior patterns. At the second level, MacLean introduced the term limbic system to describe the brain's source of emotions and higher (mammalian) instincts such as fighting, fleeing, and sexual behavior. The third level, the neocortex, is the highest and newest level and controls higher order thinking, reasoning, and speech. It should be noted that MacLean's model has been severely criticized (e.g., Bear, Conners, & Paradiso, 2007; Reiner, 1990), as has his construct of the limbic system (e.g., LeDoux, 2012).

Dalgleish (2004) explained that MacLean also formulated a neo-Jamesian model, where stimuli lead to bodily changes and messages about these "changes return to the brain where they are integrated with ongoing perception of the outside world. It is this integration that generates emotional experience" (p. 593). Dalgleish concluded by noting that although the general brain regions involved in emotion are becoming better understood, much more research is required to understand how these regions interact with each other and, by extension, with the rest of the brain. The understanding and analysis of the brain and its development continues Hughlings Jackson's tradition of using descriptive levels.

MacLean's theory also formed the basis for an educational approach developed by Elaine de Beauport (1996). One of the major implications of MacLean's theory was that older levels of the nervous system are still functional and doing what they were designed to do. Therefore, it comes as no surprise to see primal patterns of behavior occasionally acted out by humans. By understanding the ancient context of these behaviors, we can come to better understand them and deal with their consequences (de Beauport, 1996). For example, MacLean emphasized the importance of establishing and controlling territory, a tendency that de Beauport felt could help explain modern territorial violence often seen in gang violence. Through her integrated theory of multi-modal intelligence, de Beauport provided us with an important interpretation of the implications of the evolutionary strata seen in the nervous system.

K. G. Bailey (1987) enlarged and refined the triune model in his book, *Human Paleopsychology,* and suggested a continuum between the lower and higher levels. K. G. Bailey suggested that we can move up through the levels—a construct he called "upshifting"—or, under certain conditions of stress, higher levels can falter, leading to "downshifting" to lower levels of function. Our behavior reflects this continuum; at one extreme is our authentic humanity, while at the other lies our animal heritage. There is an ongoing struggle between these higher and lower elements and one's behavior is determined in response to one's inner urges and external circumstances.

In K. G. Bailey's (1987) model, at least a part of upshifting is a conscious, volitional process, a function similar to what Dąbrowski outlined:

> Phylogenetic progression, as defined here, is basically an active process of transcending our basic animality through neocortical inhibition of our generally amoral and acultural natural tendencies on the one hand and cultural reshaping on the other. (p. 95)

K. G. Bailey (1987) continued: "phylogenetic progression may be partly passive up through the lower levels of cultural conformity, but becomes distinctly active on through the higher sublevels of cultural innovation and technocultural advancement" (p. 95).

The failure of higher cortical control can lead to phylogenetic regression in a downward spiral leading to primitive and sometimes animalistic behavior. K. G. Bailey (1987) gave the example of an individual who becomes intoxicated and, in an uncontrollable rage, commits murder. Likewise, Dąbrowski observed that it is relatively common for a person to regress to an animal-like level. An individual may feel a strong need to express lower impulses, either in social situations or as an individual. To illustrate, an individual may regress in situations of mob violence or, in a wartime situation, may be "caught up in the heat of battle" and commit atrocities. On an individual level, socialization (the second factor) sometimes fails to control impulses and the individual runs amok.

7–7. CREATIVITY

Amend (2008) provided a summary of the links between Dąbrowski's approach and creativity—links that are deep and obvious. Dąbrowski's definition of positive disintegration included creativity: "Disintegration is described as positive when it enriches life, enlarges the horizon and brings forth creativity" (Dąbrowski, 1964b, p. 10). "Crises are periods of increased insight into oneself, creativity, and personality development" (Dąbrowski, 1964b, p. 18).

Higher levels of creativity (multilevel creativity) are non-ontogenetic and do not appear in all human beings (Dąbrowski, 1973). Multilevel creativity is an expression "of emotional, imaginational and intellectual overexcitability, with emotional being clearly the strongest" (Dąbrowski, 1996, p. 36).

The creative instinct was also an important construct in Dąbrowski's thinking, although not appearing until at least the level of unilevel disintegration and not substantially until multilevel disintegration. "Creative dynamisms are connected with the process of disintegration in general, and with the process of multilevel disintegration in particular" (Dąbrowski, 1970b, p. 69). Initially, the creative instinct is narrow and strives for artistic expression or the expression of something new, in particular, the search for new forms of reality. Creative abilities represent "a search for new higher ways of understanding reality and of creating or discovering these new ways" (1972b, p. 196) Dąbrowski (1996) made it clear that the benefits in pursuing new forms of reality outweighed the price paid:

It is better to be restless, to suffer depressions and even to be gravely ill, if these afflictions give in return the possibility of finding access to the world of "higher reality," a world of new ideas, new creative stimuli, new intense dreams, rather than remain in the world of everyday reality, full of boredom, full of trivial relations, a reality repulsive in its monotony and uneventfulness. (pp. 61-62)

The creative instinct is a sort of stepping stone; highly creative individuals often become disenchanted with their creations and eventually may destroy them, as was the case with Michelangelo. In these cases, the artist, disenchanted with his or her material creations, begins a new search for "more important matters," for example, existential questions and the problems of transcendence and self-perfection. The narrower creative instinct fades as it is transformed into the broader instinct of self-perfection. The instinct of self-perfection becomes the next step in pushing the search for something new, but now most significantly, something that is not merely new, but higher. Perfection through artistic expression shifts to a concern and even a preoccupation with self-perfection.

Dąbrowski described creativity in unilevel disintegration as impulsive and spontaneous, essentially isolated from personality development as a whole. On the other hand, creativity in spontaneous multilevel disintegration is part of the process of hierarchization seen in personality development and expresses the tragedy and agony of human existence: "Multilevel creativity is a manifestation of the conjunction of emotional, imaginational and intellectual overexcitability, with emotional being clearly the strongest" (Dąbrowski, 1996, p. 36).

Creativity is commonly seen in psychoneurotics and intense creativity may predispose an individual to be seen as mentally ill. Dąbrowski (1964) said:

Are creative people mentally healthy? . . . They are not healthy according to the standard of the average individual, but they are healthy according to their unique personality norms and insofar as they show personality development: the acquiring and strengthening of new qualities in the realization of movement toward their personality ideal. (p. 115)

Dąbrowski was also concerned that psychiatric interventions could dull creativity and cited the case of Janusz Korczak (the pen name of Henryk Goldszmit, 1878-1942). Korczak, a Polish author and pediatrician, is known for his self-sacrifice in protecting a group of orphans caught in the Warsaw ghetto. In describing Korczak, Dąbrowski (1973) said:

On the other hand, having thought about himself, about the qualities of his character and personality, he came to this opinion: "I have too much madness not to be afraid of the thought that somebody—against my will—will try to treat me." It was a symptom such as was exhibited by Kierkegaard, de Unamuno, Kafka—they accustomed themselves to psychoneuroses and to torment. They felt that they (psychoneuroses) played a major role in authentic thinking and experiencing. Here was also the need for autopsychotherapy. Korczak was then a normal person, not in the statistical approach, but in the approach to health on the highest level; health which is approaching to the ideal. (pp. 181-182)

Feist (1998) pointed out that both the study of personality and the study of creativity examine many of the same characteristics of the individual. Feist concluded that in general:

Creative people are more autonomous, introverted, open to new experiences, norm-doubting, self-confident, self-accepting, driven, ambitious, dominant, hostile and impulsive. Out of these, the largest effect sizes are on openness, conscientiousness, self-acceptance, hostility and impulsivity. (p. 299)

Feist (1998) reviewed models incorporating personality and creativity:

Creative people behave consistently over time and situation and in ways that distinguish them from others. It is safe to say that in general a "creative personality" does exist and personality dispositions do regularly and predictably relate to creative achievement in art and science. (p. 304)

Henri-Louis Bergson (1859-1941) was a major influence on Dąbrowski in terms of creativity. Bergson, a French philosopher and polymath, conceived of the ultimate creation as the creation of the self—an ongoing process of maturation. "[F]or a conscious being, to exist is to change, to change is to mature, to mature is to go on creating oneself endlessly" (Bergson, 1922, p. 8). Bergson (1911) saw this self-creation as fundamental to the meaning of life:

> Might we not think that the ultimate reason of human life is a creation which, in distinction from that of the artist or man of science, can be pursued at every moment and by all men alike; I mean the creation of self by self, the continual enrichment of personality, by elements which it does not draw from outside, but causes to spring forth from itself. (pp. 42-43)

Research on creativity and the theory of positive disintegration is plentiful (e.g., Chavez-Eakle, 2004; Chavez-Eakle, Lara, & Cruz-Fuentes, 2006; Daniels & Piechowski, 2010; Gallagher, 1986; He, Wong, & Chan, 2017; Nixon, 2016; Piechowski & Cunningham, 1985).

7–8. OVEREXCITABILITY VERSUS ATTENTION DEFICIT HYPERACTIVITY DISORDER (ADHD)

The issue of attention deficit hyperactivity disorder (ADHD) has exploded over the past few years (e.g., DuPaul & Stoner, 2014; Hinshaw & Scheffler, 2014; Hinshaw et al., 2012; Schwarz, 2016; Ustun et al., 2017).

ADHD in gifted children has been a concern for some time (Webb & Latimer, 1993). In addition, the complexity of diagnosis in gifted children and the common aspect of dual diagnoses in this group has been noted (e.g., Baum & Olenchak, 2002; Lee & Olenchak, 2015; Webb et al., 2004). It has been suggested that the gifted and talented form a subgroup who see the world in a unique way and therefore present unique issues which must be clearly understood by counsellors and educators, especially when psychological or psychiatric diagnosis is required (Levy & Plucker, 2003). Further, the possible presence of characteristics of psychomotor overexcitability further complicates a diagnosis, as they are readily confused with the characteristics of ADHD.

Flint (2001) asked the question: "Is it ADHD or overexcitability?" An article by Hartnett, Nelson and Rinn (2004) on the question of ADHD and overexcitability stimulated a lively debate (e.g., Goerss, Amend, Webb, Webb, & Beljan, 2006; Mika, 2006; Nelson, Rinn, & Hartnett, 2006). Hartnett et al. (2004) made the case that misdiagnosis may lead to "dire consequences" and that that misdiagnosis of ADHD may have a harmful impact on gifted children.

Mika (2006) ably addressed mistakes and misconceptions presented in Hartnett et al. (2004). Mika (2006) stated "there is no evidence that: (a) gifted children are misdiagnosed as ADHD; (b) gifted children misdiagnosed with ADHD are unnecessarily medicated; and (c) gifted children misdiagnosed as ADHD, and medicated as a result, experience negative effects from stimulant medication" (p. 237). As well, Mika clarified that the intensity of overexcitability is not directly related to being gifted and is not an index of development because its expression is dependent upon many other factors, notably other aspects of development potential including the third factor. Mika (2006) also clarified that "Dąbrowski's views on etiology and symptomatology of psychomotor OE almost completely overlap with our current understanding of ADHD" (p. 241).

Despite the succinct analysis provided by Mika (2006), Rinn and Reynolds (2012) again reviewed the literature and supported the potential to confuse overexcitability in gifted children with ADHD. Rinn and Reynolds repeated the misimpression that overexcitabilities, in this case, imaginational, intellectual, and emotional, "are more likely to lead to higher levels of development" (p. 40). As Mika (2006) made clear, overexcitabilities alone can contribute little to development—several other interactive factors are required to lead to a developmental outcome. The results reported by Rinn and Reynolds showed "a significant relationship between the psychomotor overexcitability scores and the DSM-IV" (p. 43)—supporting Mika (2006)—and concluded that:

Individuals with an imaginational overexcitability are most

likely to display symptoms characteristic of ADHD, which would increase the likelihood of an ADHD misdiagnosis, or are more likely to actually have an ADHD diagnosis. The imaginational overexcitability is included as a higher form of overexcitability, though, which is supposed to allow for higher levels of development, as previously mentioned. (pp. 43-44)

Kennedy, Banks and Grandin (2011) provided "a good overview of the problems facing our kids who are gifted and labelled as ADHD, ODD, Asperger's syndrome, or learning disabled" (p. xvi). The work focused on "twice exceptional" (2e) children, those who have "exceptional gifts (creative, academic, intellectual or physical abilities) along with a learning or developmental disability like ADHD or an autism spectrum disorder" (Kennedy et al., 2011, p. xv). Again, echoing the theme of a blurring of OE and ADHD, the authors suggested, "each OE can lead to behaviors identical to those found in children with ADHD, Asperger's or autism, and related conditions. . . . This confusion between traits of giftedness and traits of disability often leads to misdiagnosis, missed diagnosis, and even missed giftedness in 2e children" (Kennedy et al., 2011, pp. 15-16).

Fugate and Gentry (2016) provide the latest review, a consideration of gifted girls with ADHD, although the issue of overexcitabilities was not discussed.

7–9. OVEREXCITABILITY AS HEIGHTENED AWARENESS

Traditionally, overexcitability has been described in terms of increased sensitivity and increased reactivity of the nervous system. I propose that overexcitability may also be viewed in terms of one's awareness. We have already seen several authors suggesting that the average person tends to go through life in a semi-somnambulant state. Experiencing overexcitability is analogous to being fully awake both in terms of self-awareness and in terms of one's awareness of one's environment. In the fully awake state, an individual is acutely in tune with his or her inner psychic milieu—the individual knows exactly and minutely how he or she feels, thinks, and reacts both to intrapsychic stimuli and to stimuli from the environment. Environmental stimuli take on a more complex, deeper, and richer meaning when the perceiver is fully awake. The qualitative nature of external stimuli becomes critically important; that is to say, the meaning of stimuli becomes more important than the strength of the stimuli. When the perceiver is fully awake, even minute stimuli can have a dramatic impact. In turn, the reaction of the individual to stimuli reflects its strong initial impact, and reactions are therefore perceived as higher in comparison to the reactions of the average individual. Two aspects of the reaction are critical from Dąbrowski's perspective: first, reactions tend to be stronger and second, reactions are not immediately rendered; they are carefully considered before they are translated into behavior.

Awareness rather than sensitivity implies a more conscious reaction. An individual can be sensitive without realizing or being aware of the source of his or her sensitivity. There are several psychological descriptions that could be used to examine heightened awareness in relation to overexcitability. For example, the construct of elevation (Haidt, 2003a), Csíkszentmihályi's (1990) construct of flow, or Jamison's (2004) description of exuberance may be useful constructs to compare and contrast.

7–9–1. Curiosity

It has always been strange to me that curiosity has not played more of a role in the discussion of overexcitability. As a child, I had an insatiable curiosity; I wanted to learn everything; I wanted to see everything; I wanted to hear what everyone was saying.

Curiosity was once seen as a dangerous trait associated with substance abuse, experimentation with high-risk behaviors, and with delinquency (Jovanovic & Brdaric, 2012). This viewpoint is also associated with positive well-being among adolescents (Jovanovic & Brdaric, 2012) and is seen as a necessary part of a child's intellectual growth (Engel, 2009). Karwowski (2012) defined curiosity "as a trait—a (relatively) stable disposition to feel curiosity and be curious" (p. 548). This research examined the relationship between curiosity and creative self-efficacy (CSE)—"an individual's set of beliefs that she or he is able to solve problems requiring creative thinking and to function creatively" and creative personal identity (CPI)—"an individual's belief that creativity is an important element of the individual's functioning" (p. 549). Karwowski (2012) concluded that curiosity is an essential component in enhancing one's creative self in both creative self-efficacy and creative personal identity.

Kashdan and Fincham (2002) described curiosity as a motivational mechanism of self-regulation, facilitating "intrinsic goal effort, perseverance, personal growth and, under the right conditions, creativity" (p. 373). The authors presented curiosity as a prerequisite for exploring both the environment and one's own ideas and emotions (the self) and concluded that high curiosity is necessary, though not sufficient, for creativity.

Curiosity has been seen as a basic biological drive shared by both humans and animals and a key component in motivation for learning and discovery (Jepma, Verdonschot, Van Steenbergen, Rombouts, & Nieuwenhuis, 2012). A neurobiological study by Jepma et al. (2012) found support for a classic psychological theory of curiosity, which postulates that curiosity is caused by increased arousal produced by the presentation of ambiguous stimuli, which lead to an aversive condition that an individual will want to terminate. The authors went on to conclude that termination is rewarding to the individual and is associated with enhanced memory and learning. Interestingly, the authors described how people differ in the level of knowledge to which they aspire: "The same actual level of knowledge will evoke curiosity in some people but not in others. . . . People with a higher level of aspired perceptual knowledge experience stronger negative feelings when confronted with an ambiguous perceptual input" (Jepma et al., 2012, p. 7). Some people aspire to know more and this aspiration is correlated to increased curiosity.

Interestingly, research has supported a prediction by Erikson showing that people in crisis experience higher levels of curiosity (Robinson, Demetre, & Litman, 2017). Excellent reviews of curiosity are available (e.g., Leslie, 2014; Levens, 2017; Livio, 2017).

7–10. NEUROPSYCHOLOGICAL VIEWS OF OVEREXCITABILITY

7–10–1. Overexcitability

Dąbrowski was not the only one to suggest that excitability varies among individuals. Eysenck (1967) said:

> Human beings differ with respect to the speed with which
> excitation and inhibition are produced, the strength of the
> excitation and inhibition produced and the speed with which
> inhibition is dissipated. These differences are properties of the
> physical structures involved in making stimulus response
> connections. (p. 79)

Eysenck used Hughlings Jackson's model whereby higher
structures exert a controlling and restraining role over lower
structures. Thus, increased cortical excitation would increase the
inhibition of lower levels and be expressed in behavior as a *decrease*
in excitability (more inhibition). The argument was illustrated by the
example of the effects of alcohol; inhibiting the higher cortical centers
(decreasing cortical excitation) and releasing lower centers from
control produces excited and disinhibited behavior (Eysenck, 1967, p.
76). With this in mind, Eysenck explained:

> Individuals in whom excitatory potential is generated slowly
> and in whom excitatory potentials so generated are relatively
> weak, are thereby predisposed to develop extraverted patterns
> of behavior and to develop hysterical—psychopathic disorders
> in cases of neurotic breakdown. (p. 79)

This was expressed in Eysenck's view of people who score high
on extraversion (extraverts having lower cortical excitation) described
as outgoing, changeable, playful, hot-headed, optimistic, active, and
sociable, compared to low scorers (introverts having higher cortical
excitation) who are described as unsociable, thoughtful, controlled,
serious, passive, quiet, and careful.

Eysenck's explanation of the role of physiological arousal is an
important component of his whole theoretical approach to personality.
Matthews, Deary and Whiteman (2009) said:

> Much empirical work has been directed towards Eysenck's
> arousal theory, which links extraversion to low arousability of
> a reticulo-cortical circuit, neuroticism to arousability of a
> limbic-cortical circuit and psychoticism to a fight-flight

system. The basic assumptions of arousal theory have been criticised and it may be too simplistic to accommodate the multiple activating systems of the brain. Experimental studies provide some modest support for the hypothesis that introverts are more easily aroused than extraverts, but there are various inconsistencies in the data. (p. 202)

The reader interested in arousal and extraversion is directed to Matthews and Gilliland (1999) for a detailed review.

7–10–1–1. Neural networks

Many advances in understanding the nervous system can be attributed to Donald Olding Hebb (1904-1985) and the research he generated (e.g., Brown & Milner, 2003; Fentress, 1999; Hebb, 1949, 1972; Klein, 1999; Posner & Rothbart, 2007b). In trying to understand thought processes, Hebb proposed the idea that when cells are triggered in proximity to each other, their synapses are strengthened (now known as Hebb's law: "neurons that fire together wire together"), forming a network of cells referred to as a cell-assembly. These patterns or networks of cells form an ever-changing algorithm describing the brain's response to stimuli. Hebb (1972, p. 71) suggested that the assembly originally organized in response to a particular sensory event was free to continue its activity after the stimulation had ceased—it is made up of "self-re-exciting closed loops," and various loops (cell-assemblies) may interact with each other. In the early days of neurophysiology, the short interval between the stimulus and a response was attributed simply to "mediating processes," processes that Hebb assumed were made up of one or more cell-assemblies. These early ideas laid the foundation for a network approach to cognition and to the analogy that the brain operates as a computer-like, computational machine.

Posner and Rothbart (2007b) promoted Hebb's orientation as a basis for the integration of psychology as a unified science:

Every psychological event, sensation, expectation, emotion, or thought is represented by the flow of activity in a set of interconnected neurons. Learning occurs by a change in the synaptic strength when a synapse conducts excitation at the same time the postsynaptic neuron discharges. This provided a basis for the modification of synapses and showed how neuron networks might be organized under the influence of specific experiences. (p. 4)

Posner and Rothbart (2007b, p. 7) provided an early description of three basic functions of neural networks:

- alerting, achieving, and maintaining a state of high sensitivity to incoming stimuli (modulated by norepinephrine);
- orienting, the selection of information from sensory inputs (modulated by acetylcholine);
- executive attention—mechanisms for monitoring and resolving conflicts among thoughts, feelings, and responses (modulated by dopamine).

Posner and Rothbart (2007b) examined differences in normal individuals in the efficiency of brain networks performing these three functions and found strong heritability for differences in the executive network, some heritability for the orienting network, and no apparent heritability for the alerting network.

Early progress in identifying the genes involved in the control of neural networks was made by Posner and Rothbart (2007b). A group of subjects who were genotyped to examine polymorphisms in genes related to dopamine revealed an association of the dopamine 4 receptor gene and the monoamine oxidase A gene. Differences in the alleles of these two genes were subsequently found to be associated with differences in measurements of the executive attention network (Posner & Rothbart, 2007b). The authors concluded that the same genes involved in individual differences commonly seen in attention are likely also important in the development and operation of attentional networks (e.g., Fan, Wu, Fossella, & Posner, 2001; Sporns, 2011; Sporns & Betzel, 2016).

Posner and Rothbart (2007b) reviewed differences observed between infants, including:

reactive traits such as emotionality, activity level and orienting to sensory events and regulatory traits like attention focusing and shifting and inhibitory control. We believe that these early developing temperamental differences reflect the maturation of particular neural networks. (p. 11)

The authors suggested that research on attentional networks could be generalized and used to study cognitive and emotional networks as well. Individual differences are a significant feature that likely will be understood on the basis of genetic differences underlying neurotransmitter function and the development and operation of networks in the brain (Posner & Rothbart, 2007b). The authors also explored the implications of their findings for education (Posner & Rothbart, 2007a).

Advances in imaging techniques have opened a new window on understanding the large-scale neural networks that characterize the brain (e.g., Bihan, 2015; Bullmore & Sporns, 2009; Hurley & Taber, 2008; Kolb & Whishaw, 2015; Levine & Craik, 2012; Passingham, 2016; Sporns, 2012; Yoshor & Mizrahi, 2012). Collectively, these neural networks are called the connectome (e.g., Lowe et al., 2016; Sporns, 2011, 2012; Swanson & Lichtman, 2016; Zalesky, Keilholz, & Heuvel, 2017).

It has now become clear that the brain is not an all-purpose computing device with a centralized "processor." Rather, it consists of specialized circuits distributed throughout the brain, each performing specific sub-functions, organized and connected to yield an overall seamless flow of experience (Gazzaniga, 2013). Localization has become a dominating theme in brain science, an organization that combines both focal and distributed themes: the functional arrangement of the cortex is a hybrid, an arrangement commonly referred to as modular (e.g., Sevush, 2016; see also Lowe et al., 2016; Marcus & Freeman, 2015; Richmond, Johnson, Seal, Allen, & Whittle, 2016; Swanson & Lichtman, 2016).

7–10–1–2. Neuronal excitability

In overview, the individual neuron displays both intrinsic levels of excitability and ongoing modulation of excitability over time. Intrinsic levels are controlled by genetics—intraindividual differences are introduced as different individuals have slightly different genetics. As well, differences are introduced by epigenetics—one's unique life experience will modify both the architecture and functional expression of one's neurons and subsequently affect neuronal excitability (Armstrong, 2014). Life experience also dynamically modifies levels of brain/network variability, network flexibility, and network connectivity (Zhang et al., 2016). These factors also impact neuronal excitability (e.g., Chen et al., 2016; Meadows et al., 2016). In summary, it is clear that both the architecture and functional expression of individual neurons and the variability, flexibility, and connectivity of neuronal networks represent controls of excitability.

As neurons operate in microcircuits and as part of larger networks, neuronal control of the balance of excitability and inhibition is a critical factor. There are two reasons for this—first, there are many systems in the brain that require strict homeostatic control; for example, the control of blood pressure and respiration must be held within tight limits and cannot afford variability. On the other hand, much of the brain must be plastic and respond to environmental changes. For example, in order to remember things and to learn things, systems within the brain must be open to constant modification.

Genes control excitability partly through calcium homeostasis in neurons (Smoller, 2013). Some of the genes that control voltage-gated ion channels or calcium transport are among the most consistently found in psychiatrically focused genome-wide association studies (GWAS) (Ament et al., 2015). Mäki-Marttunen et al. (2016) concluded: "alteration in the ability of a single neuron to integrate the inputs and scale its excitability may constitute a fundamental mechanistic contributor to mental disease, alongside with the previously proposed deficits in synaptic communication and network behaviour" (p. 1). Further, Mäki-Marttunen et al. (2016) suggested that at least some of the pathology related to schizophrenia "might be an effect of altered ionic channel properties at the single neuron level, and not only of the modified elements in synaptic circuitry as previously thought" (p. 8). On another front, ion channel abnormalities leading to neuronal hyperexcitability have been implied in pathological pain syndromes (Du, Gao, Jaffe, Zhang, & Gamper, 2018).

In summary, the proof of concept for the neurophysiological

mechanisms and genetic (and epigenetic) control of neuronal excitability have now been established (e.g., Gulledge & Bravo, 2016; Mäki-Marttunen et al., 2016; Meadows et al., 2016; Rannals et al., 2016; Remme & Wadman, 2012). Balancing excitation and inhibition on various levels in the nervous system is critically important and abnormalities in control of excitability are implied in psychiatric disorders.

7–10–1–3. Overexcitability: Evolving research support

Dąbrowski spoke of overexcitability in terms of large-scale phenomena (for example, "mental overexcitability" and "emotional overexcitability") but defined overexcitability at the level of the individual neuron: "Each form of overexcitability points to a higher than average sensitivity of its receptors" (Dąbrowski, 1972b, p. 7). Does contemporary neuroscience inform us in terms of overexcitability on macro scales and in terms of the overexcitability of the individual neuron?

The picture of contemporary neurophysiology that is coalescing allows us to make some general conclusions relevant to Dąbrowski and overexcitability as follows:

- **Brain correlates with behaviors and traits.** Contemporary experts assume that the structure and function of internal brain processes correlate with external, observable behaviors. Behavior and traits (like OE) represent corresponding neurophysiological factors and reseach of underlying brain mechanisms of observable behaviors is justified (e.g., Kolb & Gibb, 2014; Kolb & Whishaw, 2014).
- **A continuum of excitability.** There is a physiological continuum of excitability and it seems reasonable to hypothesize that the continuum differs between individuals:
  - too little excitability (leading to pathology)
  - normal levels of excitability
  - Dąbrowski's overexcitabilities
  - pathological neuronal hyperexcitability/excitotoxicity
    - › In support of this hypothesis, in a review of neuronal hyperexcitability in autism spectrum disorders, Takarae and Sweeney (2017) concluded, "the influence of cortical

excitability on cognition and perception is multifaceted, and its impact may vary across brain regions, in different behavioral conditions, and across different individuals" (p. 2). Further, "alterations in cortical excitability seem to exist to varying degrees in individuals with ASD, and only a subset of affected individuals may have neuronal hyperreactivity" (Takarae & Sweeney, 2017, p. 5).

- **Hughlings Jackson's model.** Hughlings Jackson's general hierarchical model of the nervous system (a phylogenetically arranged hierarchy of reflex arcs) is confirmed by contemporary research. The organization of the nervous system has many levels, organized hierarchically (vertically) and also in parallel (horizontally); organization is also both widely distributed and localized (e.g., Bullmore & Sporns, 2009; Freiwald, Duchaine, & Yovel, 2016; Gazzaniga, 2013; Kolb & Whishaw, 2014; Pribram, 1982; Sevush, 2016; Stanley et al., 2013; Uhlhaas et al., 2009).

- **Dynamic and ongoing balancing of inhibition and excitation.** The nervous system functions on the basis of balancing inhibition and excitation on micro, meso, and macro levels. This dynamic and ongoing balancing of both inhibitory and excitatory networks is critical to the healthy functioning of the nervous system and the many networks it employs (e.g., Chen et al., 2016; Froemke, 2015; Goold & Nicoll, 2010; Grashow, Brookings, & Marder, 2010; Kolb & Whishaw, 2014; Lee, Lee, & Kim, 2016; Pozo & Goda, 2010; Remme & Wadman, 2012; Schulz, 2006; Tatti, Haley, Swanson, Tselha, & Maffei, 2017; Turrigiano, 2011, 2012; Turrigiano & Nelson, 2004; Yin & Yuan, 2015). Control of excitability and inhibition in neurons is complex and extremely sensitive; neurons monitor their own excitability and make adjustments to accommodate what nearby neurons are doing (Turrigiano, 2008; Turrigiano & Nelson, 2004). Research on balanced network theory is developing testable models linking brain circuits to brain activity (Rosenbaum, Smith, Kohn, Rubin, & Doiron, 2017).

- **Examples of neuronal controls of excitability and**

inhibition.

o *Control of neuronal excitability.* One aspect of control of neuronal excitability is genetic. Genes control neuronal excitability and each individual's intrinsic neuronal excitability is predicted to vary just as individuals' genetics vary (e.g., Ament et al., 2015; Chen et al., 2016; Davis & Bezprozvanny, 2001; Erwin et al., 2016; Johns, Marx, Mains, O'Rourke, & Marbán, 1999; Mäki-Marttunen et al., 2016; Meadows et al., 2016; Moore, Throesch & Murphy, 2011; Rannals et al., 2016). A second aspect of control of neuronal excitability involves ionic channels. Neuronal excitability is controlled by a suite of ion channels in the membranes of the cell, as well as by the biochemical properties and kinetics of those channels. The intrinsic excitability of neurons is responsible for the translation of synaptic input to the particular output function of a given neuron (Schulz, 2006).

o *Epigenetic mechanisms.* Excitability and inhibition balancing involves epigenetic mechanisms that respond to the activity of the synapse and that alter the structural architecture of the neuron—adding or deleting dendritic spines and arborizations (the fine branching structures at the end of a nerve fiber), and thereby raising or lowering the number of synapses (McCann & Ross, 2017). In another example, it is well established that depression is associated with the loss of dendritic spines and a subsequent loss of synapses (Nasrallah, 2015). These epigenetic architectural (physical) changes dynamically affect the intrinsic excitability of neurons and subsequently impact meta-scale, ongoing network behaviors.

o *Firing patterns.* In any given neuron, firing impulse patterns take the form of rate of firing, rate of change in firing, onset and offset of firing, and sequential order of firing intervals (Klemm, 2014, p. 30).

o *Graded action potentials.* Some neurons also generate graded action potentials that vary in intensity (Kolb &

Whishaw, 2014).

o *Dendrite modifiability.* Dendrites on the neuron are modifiable—their numbers are increased or decreased on an ongoing basis—thus, the neuron has considerable latitude in controlling its operation. The more dendrites, the more synapses available to interact with neighboring neurons. We are used to seeing standard textbook illustrations of the axon of the neuron connecting with a few synapses to the next neighboring neuron. But when we consider that each neuron can have from 40,000 to 100,000 synaptic connections to each neighboring neuron, the complexity involved becomes huge (e.g., Sevush, 2016; Turrigiano, 2008).

o *Autapses.* Neurons can connect their synapses with themselves—self-looping structures—a phenomenon called autapses. Research supports a role for autaptic connections in influencing network dynamics (Wiles et al., 2017).

o *Excitability and inhibition balancing: An illustration.* Excitability and inhibition balancing may be seen in conscious motor behaviors. For example, to raise one's arm, motor neurons are excited. When the desired height is reached, inhibition stops movement and rebalancing holds the arm in place. Likewise, EI balancing may reflect unconscious brain operations. For example, stress or fear temporarily spike excitability in the autonomic nervous system in preparation for fight or flight. As the threat abates, adjustments in inhibition eventually bring systems back to normal levels and homeostatic balance is restored.

• **Neuronal plasticity**. Synaptic plasticity describes the capability of individual synapses to change their strength of transmission in response to different stimuli or environmental cues. These experience-dependent, moment-to-moment modifications of neural circuits play a critical role in brain function. As behavioral contexts constantly change, different neuromodulatory systems are activated that shift cortical excitatory-inhibitory balance to induce long-term synaptic plasticity (Froemke, 2015, pp. 211-212). These lasting changes involve long-term potentiation (LTP), which increases the efficacy of synaptic transmission and long-term depression (LTD), which decreases it. "LTP and LTD are also thought to play a crucial role in the network hyperexcitability [excitotoxicity] observed in pathological conditions and in the establishment of appropriate synaptic connections" (Gaiarsa & Ben-Ari, 2006, p. 23). Plasticity in inhibitory synapses is controlled by many neuromodulators, especially during learning. "Many modulators transiently alter excitatory-inhibitory balance by decreasing inhibition, and thus disinhibition has emerged as a major mechanism by which neuromodulation might enable long-term synaptic modifications" (Froemke, 2015, p. 195).

- **Homeostasis versus plasticity**. Maintaining homeostasis is critical to the function of many neural networks. Homeostatic plasticity is the capacity of neurons to monitor and regulate their own excitability relative to network activity, a measure of robustness (e.g., Chen et al., 2016; Lyttle, Gill, Shaw, Thomas, & Chiel, 2017; Schulz, 2006; Turrigiano & Nelson, 2004). The term homeostatic plasticity is an oxymoron essentially meaning "staying the same through change." Neural plasticity is now a well understood phenomenon referring to ongoing alterations in the brain that occur throughout an individual's life. Plasticity plays critical roles in processes such as learning, memory, and other activity-dependent forms of neural function. "Neural networks strike a balance between altering individual neurons in the name of plasticity, while maintaining long-term stability in neural system function. The balance of plasticity and stability in neural networks plays a critical role in the normal functioning of the nervous system" (Schulz, 2006, p. 4821; see also Chen et al., 2016; Turrigiano, 2008; Turrigiano & Nelson, 2000).

- **Inhibitory Synaptic Plasticity (ISP).** Through both feedforward and feedback control, inhibitory synaptic plasticity (ISP) plays an important part in the organization of neural circuits. Although much fewer in number compared to excitatory neurons, inhibitory neurons exert powerful control in stabilizing and balancing brain circuits (Hennequin, Agnes, & Vogels, 2017).

- **Balance within microcircuits and networks**. As noted above, as neurons operate in microcircuits and as part of larger networks, broad neuronal control of the balance of excitability and inhibition is a critical factor. This balance is maintained by homeostatic metaplasticity. Mechanisms of metaplasticity reflect the reciprocal relationship between neural architecture and neuronal activity. Individual synapses either strengthen or weaken depending upon the relative timing of action potentials in connected neurons, both in their microcircuits and in larger networks. This phenomenon is referred to as spike timing-dependent plasticity (STDP) (e.g., Ocker, Litwin-Kumar, & Doiron, 2015; Murakami, Müller-Dahlhaus, Lu, & Ziemann, 2012).
  - o *Synaptic Coordination*. "Diverse synaptic plasticity mechanisms often act in concert with one another, and their efficacy is tightly controlled by the activity of other synapses in their proximity" (Hennequin, Agnes, & Vogels, 2017, p. 559). "Changes to specific excitatory synapses must be coordinated within existing networks of numerous other excitatory and inhibitory synapses" (Froemke, 2015, p. 196). As excitatory synapses are modified, inhibitory synapses must correspondingly adjust to maintain homeostasis (Froemke, 2015).
- **Epigenetics**. Epigenetic influences during the lifetime of an individual are constantly remodeling the properties of individual neurons and network excitability via altered gene expression (e.g., Fagiolini, Jensen, & Champagne, 2009; Lilienfeld & Treadway, 2016; Maletic & Raison, 2014; Meadows et al., 2016; Pliszka, 2016).
  - o *Illustration*. To illustrate, a child with a high level of inherited overexcitability being raised in a severely impoverished orphanage with very little contact or stimulation may experience epigenetic muting of excitability and reduced overexcitability later in life; whereas the same child raised in a stimulus rich

environment may display an epigenetic enhancement of his or her inherited overexcitability as seen later in life.

- **Neuronal mosaicism**. Neuronal genomes are dynamic, with single individual neurons displaying considerable genomic plasticity and diversity—a phenomenon known as somatic mosaicism. A number of mechanisms have been linked to this neuronal diversity operating at several levels, including: genomic, epigenomic, transcriptomic, and the posttranscriptomic. As Linker, Bedrosian, and Gage (2017) highlighted:

> Brain cells in particular may be as unique as the people to which they belong. This genetic, molecular, and morphological diversity of the brain leads to functional variation that is likely necessary for the higher-order cognitive processes that are unique to humans. (p. 46)

Somatic mutations occurring in a cell are passed on to all of its daughter cells. These mutations can be introduced in early development or at any point during the lifetime, and the timing of when they occur determines their frequency. Linker et al. (2017) noted that neuronal variations add great complexity to the traditional classification of neuronal cell types,

> Diversification of neurons arising from somatic gene mutations or subtle molecular and environmental differences may help explain the origin of cognitive and behavioral individuality. The findings thus far highlight the importance of moving away from a blanket definition of "cell types" that are assumed to behave in a stereotyped manner toward a more nuanced view of neurons that includes the multidimensional combination of transcriptome, epigenome, and genome when attempting to understand the impact of a given cell state. (p. 42)

Neuronal mosaicism may contribute to functional differences in individual neurons, personality, and behavioral differences among individuals, as well as to various neurological or psychiatric disorders.

- **Modular communication and intelligence**. Hilger, Ekman, Fiebach, and Basten (2017) demonstrated that an important component in general intelligence is the degree of interconnectedness between modules and sub-networks of the brain. It was noted that "intrinsic functional networks are closely related to underlying anatomical connections, constrain brain activity during cognitive demands, and are associated with fundamental differences between persons, e.g., in personality or psychopathology" (Hilger et al., 2017, p. 1). Hilger et al. (2017) concluded,

> Region-specific profiles of intrinsic functional connectivity within and between different brain modules are relevant for individual differences in general cognitive ability. Although our results do not allow for causal inferences, our findings lend support to the idea that the *integration* of processing between functionally specialised brain regions plays an important role for intelligence. (p. 10)

In summary, contemporary research generally supports Dąbrowski's approach to overexcitabilities and presents several plausible explanations to account for differences in levels of excitability between individuals. This would support Dąbrowski's contention that excitability varies in the population, with "average" excitability as the norm and "overexcitable" individuals as the exception. Studies confirm that the control of excitability largely occurs within the individual neuron—each neuron monitors its own firing activity through feedback and can modify its rate of firing to maintain overall network stability. Individual neurons exhibit intrinsic levels of excitability and ongoing modulation of excitability. These features are largely controlled by genetics and epigenetics. It seems reasonable to hypothesize that the degree of interconnectedness between neural networks, the number of connected networks, network flexibility, and the frequency with which these networks interact with one another may also act as an index of overexcitability. Fewer networks, less frequent interaction, or lower inter-network flexibility would be associated with lower levels of excitability.

7–10–2. Other contemporary approaches

Research has demonstrated individual differences in emotional responding in both positive and negative trait affect scores (Ripper, Boyes, Clarke, & Hasking, 2018). Ongoing research continues to elaborate the factors underlying these differences. Three factors are described by Ripper et al. (2018):

- Emotional reactivity or frequency (an increased probability of experiencing affect in response to situations or stimuli);
- Emotional perseveration or duration (a disposition to experiencing prolonged emotional reactions);
- Emotional/Affective intensity (the magnitude of the emotional experience that is triggered).

Ripper et al. (2018) have developed an instrument that "demonstrates that reactivity, intensity, and perseveration account for independent variance in trait affect and are differentially associated with general psychological distress and symptoms of depression, anxiety, and stress" (p. 98). It would certainly be germane to compare the OEQII with the scale developed by Ripper and her associates, and/or the other gold standard measurements in the field (e.g., Watson, Clark, & Tellegen, 1988).

7–11. CHAPTER SUMMARY

This chapter placed the theory of positive disintegration into a contemporary context. Dąbrowski's idea that growth requires disintegration was examined in the context of the role of suffering in development. The theory falls into the category of posttraumatic growth and uses a positive approach. Therefore, posttraumatic growth and recent approaches to this new area of psychological research were reviewed. Historical and contemporary developments in positive psychology were reviewed.

Other works in personality development were considered, including contributions by Jung and Erickson, and the comparable theories presented by Arasteh and Kegan. A brief review of contemporary personality theory followed.

The legacy of Hughlings Jackson was considered and overexcitability was reviewed as it relates to ADHD. Alternate interpretations of overexcitability were presented including heightened awareness and curiosity. Neurophysiological research supporting Dąbrowski's construct of overexcitability was reviewed.

This chapter demonstrates that Dąbrowski's work is compatible with, and supported by, contemporary advances and remains relevant today. Dąbrowski's work represents an important contribution to personality theory and the field of personality development.

8

THE ROLE OF SELF-ACTUALIZATION IN DĄBROWSKI'S APPROACH

8–1. SELF-ACTUALIZATION

8–1–1. Kurt Goldstein

There are several early usages of the construct of actualization in a psychological context, the first being by Kurt Goldstein (1878-1965). Goldstein (1939/1995) provided a holistic or "organismic theory" of the person in his major work in English, *The Organism: A Holistic Approach to Biology Derived from Pathological Data in Man.* For a review of Goldstein's contribution, see Whitehead (2017). Goldstein's emphasis was on the biological and psychological self-actualization of the organism. In this view, the healthy organism living in optimal conditions with all of his or her basic needs being met, reaches an optimal level of tension which "impels the organism to actualize itself in further activities, according to its nature" (Goldstein, 1939/1995, p. 163). The healthy organism is one "in which the tendency towards self-actualization is acting from within and overcomes the disturbance arising from the clash with the world, not out of anxiety but out of the joy of conquest" (Goldstein, 1939/1995, p. 239).

Self-actualization is not a future-oriented goal; rather, as Goldstein (1939/1995) said, it is a moment-by-moment response to the environment:

> [The foreground is determined by] the task the organism has to fulfil at any given moment, namely, by the situation in which the organism happens to find itself and by the demands with which it has to cope. The tasks are determined by the "nature" of the organism, its "essence," which is brought into actualization through the environmental changes that act on it. The expressions of this actualization are the performances of the organism. Through them the organism can deal with the respective environmental demands and actualize itself. The possibility of asserting itself in the world, while preserving its character, hinges on a specific kind of "coming to terms" of the organism with the environment. This has to take place in such a fashion that each change of the organism, caused by environmental stimuli, is equalized after a definite time, so that the organism regains that "average" state that corresponds to its nature, which is "adequate" to it. (p. 101)

8–1–2. Abraham Maslow

The name most often associated with self-actualization is Abraham Maslow. Initially Maslow was drawn to psychology by his interest in the ideas of the behaviorist John B. Watson.[34] Behaviorism did not satisfy Maslow and he went on to study psychology at the University of Wisconsin under Harry Harlow (1905-1981). Harlow became well known for his work on social and cognitive development, using experiments on rhesus monkeys to study maternal-separation and social isolation. Maslow became Harlow's laboratory assistant and later Harlow was Maslow's doctorate adviser. The two went on to study comparative behavior and psychology with various types of primates.

Maslow began informally interviewing female college students about their sexual behavior (Cullen, 1997; see also Cullen & Gotell, 2002). These studies led to the publication of several papers examining self-esteem, motivation, and sexual behavior in college women (Maslow, 1939, 1940, 1942). Maslow's informal research method became important as it set the precedent of using normal subjects to study psychological behavior and also because Maslow's later research used the same techniques (Maslow, 1945). This work was the precursor to Maslow's (1943d) first critically important paper on human motivation and to his approach to the dynamics of personality organization (1943a; 1943b).

8–1–3. Maslow's self-actualization

After meeting Goldstein, Maslow adopted the term self-actualization and first used it in 1943 (Maslow, 1943c, 1943d). Maslow (1943c) began by asserting that the individual is an integrated and organized whole and also included the point:

> It is a truism to say that a white rat is not a human being, but unfortunately it is necessary to say it again since too often the results of animal experiments are considered basic data on which we must base our theorizing of human nature. (p. 89)

In a footnote, Maslow (1943c) listed five sets of goals, purposes or needs and included in the fifth:

> self-actualization, self-fulfilment, self-expression, working out of one's own fundamental personality, the fulfilment of its potentialities, the use of its capacities, the tendency to be the most that one is capable of being. (p. 91)

One of the foundations of Maslow's model reflected Goldstein's earlier approach: As lower needs are met, higher needs will emerge and when they are satisfied, still higher needs emerge and so on.[35] Maslow (1943d) therefore suggested that gratification becomes as important a construct as deprivation. Maslow (1943d) elaborated his idea of self-actualization:

> The need for self-actualization—Even if all these needs are satisfied, we may still often (if not always) expect that a new discontent and restlessness will soon develop, unless the individual is doing what he is fitted for. A musician must make music, an artist must paint, a poet must write, if he is to be ultimately happy. What a man can be, he must be. This

need we may call self-actualization. (p. 382)

Maslow (1943d) went on to explain that his use of the term was more specific than Goldstein's in that it referred to:

> the desire for self-fulfilment, namely, to the tendency for him to become actualized in what he is potentially. This tendency might be phrased as the desire to become more and more what one is, to become everything that one is capable of becoming. (p. 382)

Actualization was also equated with health: "I should then say simply that a healthy man is primarily motivated by his needs to develop and actualize his fullest potentialities and capacities" (Maslow, 1943d, p. 394). Maslow summarized his position by saying that it is reasonable to assume that "practically every human being" demonstrates an "active will toward health, an impulse toward growth, or toward the actualization of human potentialities" (Maslow, 1971/1976, p. 24). This approach created the paradox that only a small proportion of the population reaches full humanness or self-actualization, and it followed that a failure to achieve self-actualization is a pathological state. Reflecting the fact that the vast majority of people usually function below the level of self-actualization, Maslow described the development of the average person by using the phrase, "the psychopathology of normality" (Loevinger, 1976, p. 140).

8–1–4. Maslow's features of self-actualization

Maslow could not find enough subjects in the college population who demonstrated advanced growth ("superior specimens") so he began to generate descriptions of self-actualized individuals through the study of historical figures (see Winston, 2017). In an approach reminiscent of Dąbrowski's, Maslow selected eminent individuals, both dead and alive, and searched for patterns and common characteristics in their lives. Maslow included such individuals as Abraham Lincoln, William James, Jane Addams, Eleanor Roosevelt, Albert Einstein and Albert Schweitzer (for a full list, see: Krems, Kenrick and Neel, 2017).

Maslow's familiar pyramid of needs begins with four layers of basic needs he referred to as "deficiency needs" or "D-needs." D-needs include physiological needs, safety needs, love/belonging needs, and esteem needs. Significantly, these needs are met by the interaction of the individual with the environment; a non-supportive environment is one major source of human diminution and the frustration of higher growth. Deficiency motivation (D-motivation) is generated to meet these needs and maintain balance. If a need goes chronically unmet, then tension, disequilibrium, and possibly neuroses result. A significant shortfall in a given need during development, such as extreme insecurity as a child, may later be experienced through lifelong insecurity issues represented by various neuroses.

Maslow also described a set of higher metaneeds or being needs ("being values"), usually represented as "B-values" and their associated B-motivations—the metamotivations leading to advanced growth. Maslow (1967) said, "self-actualizing individuals (more matured, more fully-human), by definition, already suitably gratified in their basic needs, are now motivated in other higher ways, to be called 'metamotivations'" (p. 93). These higher motivations are largely associated with values external to the individual, such as truth, goodness, and beauty. When metaneeds are unfulfilled, various corresponding metapathologies result—essentially focused on a lack of meaning in life—involving depression, despair, disgust, alienation or cynicism. Maslow (1971/1976) noted that failures to satisfy metaneeds are rooted in pathologies of the self (not in environmental sources) (Geller, 1982). As mentioned above, most people in Western societies achieve their D-needs, but few progress to the level of metaneeds, primarily because they fear and doubt their own potential abilities (Maslow's "Jonah complex"). Other reasons people fail to progress include a lack of will to progress, fear of losing one's existing level of security, and entrenchment in cultural expectations that stifle progress.

Maslow presented several sets of criteria for self-actualization that I have assembled here, as they rarely appear together in publications (for an alternative analysis see Heylighen, 1992). First, Maslow's being values are presented (Maslow, 1968, 1971/1976).

- Truth: honesty; reality; nakedness; simplicity; richness; essentiality; oughtness; beauty; pure, clean and unadulterated; completeness.
- Goodness: rightness; desirability; oughtness; justice; benevolence; honesty (we love it, are attracted to it, approve of it).
- Beauty: rightness; form; aliveness; simplicity; richness; wholeness; perfection; completion; uniqueness; honesty.
- Wholeness: unity; integration; tendency to oneness; interconnectedness; simplicity; organization; structure; order; not dissociated; synergy; homonomous and integrative tendencies.
- Aliveness: process; non-deadness; spontaneity; self-regulation; full-functioning; changing and yet remaining the same; expressing itself.
- Uniqueness: idiosyncrasy; individuality; noncomparability; novelty; quale; suchness; nothing else like it.
- Perfection: nothing superfluous; nothing lacking; everything in its right place; unimprovable; just-rightness; just-so-ness; suitability; justice; completeness; nothing beyond; oughtness.
- Completion: ending; finality; justice; it's finished; no more changing of the Gestalt; fulfillment; finis and telos; nothing missing or lacking; totality; fulfillment of destiny; cessation; climax; consternation closure; death before rebirth; cessation and completion of growth and development.
- Justice: fairness; oughtness; suitability; architectonic quality; necessity; inevitability; disinterestedness; non-partiality.
- Simplicity: honesty; nakedness; essentiality; abstract unmistakability; essential skeletal structure; the heart of the matter; bluntness; only that which is necessary; without ornament; nothing extra or superfluous.
- Richness: differentiation; complexity; intricacy; totality; nothing missing or hidden; all there; "non-importance," i.e., everything is equally important; nothing is unimportant; everything is less the way it is, without improving, simplifying, abstracting, rearranging.
- Effortlessness: ease; lack of strain, striving or difficulty; grace;

perfect and beautiful functioning.
- Playfulness: fun; joy; amusement; gaiety; humor; exuberance; effortlessness.
- Self-sufficiency: autonomy; independence; not-needing-other-than-itself-in-order-to-be-itself; identity; self-determining; environment-transcendence; separateness; living by its own laws.

Maslow (1970, pp. 153-172) also described fifteen salient characteristics of self-actualized people:

- More efficient perception of reality and more comfortable relations with it.

    [T]hey live more in the real world of nature than in the man-made mass of constructs, abstractions, expectations, beliefs and stereotypes that most people confuse with the world. They are therefore far more apt to perceive what is there rather than their own wishes, hopes, fears, anxieties, their own theories and beliefs, or those of their cultural group. (Maslow, 1970, p. 154)
- Acceptance (self, others, nature). Acceptance of self without complaint, guilt or feelings of shame. Stoically accepting the self as-is with whatever its shortcomings and not feeling concern over discrepancies from the ideal image.
- Spontaneity; simplicity; naturalness. Relatively spontaneous behavior and quite spontaneous in one's inner life, thoughts and impulses. Behavior is simple and natural. Alienation from ordinary conventions reflects an autonomous individual value structure. Motivated to develop to self-perfection.
- Problem-centered. Strongly focused upon problems outside of themselves; rarely are they the focus of problems. Usually concerned with a mission in life. Concerned with universal ethical and philosophical issues—concerned with "the big picture."
- The quality of detachment; the need for privacy. Seek and enjoy solitude. Able to concentrate to a high degree, more objective, more problem-centered than average. Make up their minds for themselves and display more free will than average.

- Autonomy; independence of culture and environment; will; active agents. Self-contained. Not dependent upon the real world, culture or others for their satisfaction. Moved by growth motivation not deficiency motivation. Their satisfaction is based upon the ongoing growth and expression of their own potentialities and resources. They do not require need gratifications (love, safety, respect, prestige, belongingness) from others; they have become strong enough and independent enough that they are now inner-individual and they do not need the approval or affection of others.

- Continued freshness of appreciation. They are able to appreciate the experiences of life freshly and naïvely, as if for the first time—"express an acute richness for subjective experience" (Maslow, 1970, p. 163). Special experiences often involve beautiful objects in nature, music or sexual expression.

- The mystic experience: the peak experience. It is common (but not universal) for these subjects to experience strong emotions associated with mystical experiences. Maslow indicated that his attention to peak experiences was first drawn by his subjects' descriptions of their sexual orgasm. These experiences include feelings of limitless horizons, feeling powerful and at the same time helpless, feeling ecstasy and awe, feeling that something extremely important has occurred and that life has been transformed and strengthened (Maslow, 1970, p. 164).[36]

- Gemeinschaftsgefühl (human kinship). Deep feelings of identification, affection and sympathy for mankind. The self-actualizing individual often feels "saddened, exasperated and even enraged by the shortcomings of the average person and while they are to him ordinarily no more than a nuisance, they sometimes become bitter tragedy" (Maslow, 1970, p. 166). In spite of such feelings, there is a deep underlying kinship with others.

- Interpersonal relations$_{SA}$. Self-actualizing people have deeper relationships with others who also tend to be self-actualizers. Due to the rarity of others like themselves, these people usually have deep ties with only a few others—friendships are deep but few. Express qualities of kindness and patience towards others; express love and compassion for all mankind. They may attract others as admirers or even as worshipers.

- The democratic character structure. Self-actualizing people can be friendly and interact with anyone and do not appear aware of differences like class, education, political belief, race, or color. They tend to protest against evil and they tend to be less ambivalent and less confused about their own anger.

- Discrimination between means and ends, between good and evil. Self-actualizing people are confident in their belief in what is right and wrong and they do not display the inconsistencies or confusion that is commonly seen in the average person over ethical concerns. They are fixed on ends rather than means.

- Philosophical, unhostile sense of humor. Self-actualizing people display an unusual sense of humor reflecting a philosophical position, often finding humor in the foolishness of human beings in general or in making fun of one's self but not finding humor at the expense of another's feelings.

- Creativeness$_{SA}$. Creativity is a universal characteristic of all subjects studied. This creativeness is of a special type, akin to the inborn, naïve, and universal creativity seen in children. Whereas most individuals lose this creativity during the process of enculturation, the self-actualizing person retains it.

- Resistance to enculturation; the transcendence of any particular culture. Display a resistance to enculturation and a certain inner detachment from their less than healthy culture. They display an ongoing concern with improving cultural conditions and will fight for causes if necessary, usually fighting from within, rather than rejecting culture altogether. They tend to be "ruled by the laws of their own character rather than by the rules of society" (Maslow, 1970, p. 174). Maslow went on to say that these individuals display a continuum ranging from relative acceptance of the culture to relative detachment from it.[37]

In addition to these 15 specific elements and their developmental processes, Maslow (1971/1976, pp. 44-47) also described eight general ways by which one self-actualizes:

- Concentration and total absorption. To be able to experience life vividly, selflessly and fully with total absorption of one's experience. This creates a vivid experience of the moment— the self-actualizing moment. We are usually either unaware of what is going on around us, or we are focused on self-awareness and self-consciousness at the expense of seeing life clearly.
- Choices toward growth. Every day presents opportunities to choose regression and stasis or to choose moving forward into growth. Fear must be overcome through will and courage to make a choice toward self-actualization.
- Listening to one's self. The ability to seal out external voices and influences in order to examine one's own self to determine one's own preferences, opinions, likes and dislikes, and ultimately one's values. To listen to one's own self.
- Honesty. To be honest about one's self and one's actions and to avoid playing games, posing or presenting false fronts. To be honest with one's self is to take responsibility, an actualizing of the self.
- Judgment in action. The first four points illustrate one's capacity "for better life choices." Here Maslow emphasizes that we need to follow through in learning about one's self; listening to one's own voice and judgment and following through; daring to be different, unpopular or nonconforming. To have confidence in one's judgment based upon one's own self and one's feelings.
- Growth as a process. Self-actualization is the ongoing process of working to continually be as good as one can be at what one chooses to do.
- Peak experiences. Peak experiences are transient moments during which one experiences a more integrated feeling of knowing, of thinking, and of acting. During these exciting and joyous moments, one becomes deeply connected to and absorbed by, one's experience of the world. The sense of self may dissolve into a sense of the greater whole. These moments represent self-actualization.

- Removing defenses. Self-actualization involves risking the identification of defenses and actively giving them up in order to open oneself to opportunities to be more oneself. One must remove neurosis and other defenses in order to facilitate further self-growth.

8–1–5. Other theories of self-actualization

In looking at other approaches to self-actualization, Carl Rogers (1902-2002) must be mentioned. Das (1989) equally credited Maslow and C. Rogers with introducing the construct of self-actualization. C. Rogers used the description "the fully functioning person" to describe his goal of trying to help the individual achieve his or her full potential. C. Rogers (1961) said:

In this process [therapy] it is not necessary for the therapist to "motivate" the client or to supply the energy which brings about the change. Nor, in some sense, is the motivation supplied by the client, at least in any conscious way. Let us say rather that the motivation for learning and change springs from the self-actualizing tendency of life itself, the tendency for the organism to flow into all the differentiated channels of potential development, insofar as these are experienced as enhancing. (p. 285)

C. Rogers (1961) said that, based on his experience, self-actualization is not a goal in itself. The good life cannot be associated with a state of contentment, happiness, fulfilment or actualization. Nor can it be described in terms of drive-reduction, tension management or homeostasis. C. Rogers (1961) suggested that the good life is a process, a direction: "the direction which constitutes the good life is that which is selected by the total organism, where there is psychological freedom to move in any direction" (pp. 186-187).

The above discussion has confined itself to self-actualization, but it should also be remembered that many other similar and equally important views are also available, for example, the optimal personality (Coan, 1974, 1977). Coan's (1977) outstanding survey of the optimal personality is highly recommended. Coan (1977) concluded his survey with a factor analysis of some 300 subjects producing 19 factors and concluding there was no one general factor related to personality integration or self-actualization. Interestingly, Coan's (1977) first factor was "distress proneness."

Sheldon (2004, p. 200) suggested five "meta-prescriptions" for the optimal human based upon seeking certain types of experiences and incentives that will satisfy basic, universal human needs, including: to try to serve some social or cultural goal beyond one's self; to seek a balanced approach to need satisfaction; to be prepared to resist or modify problematic aspects of oneself or one's environment; to take responsibility for one's goals and choices and to listen to one's organismic valuing processes while being prepared to change one's goals if necessary.

Another series of publications examined "eminent" individuals as defined by the number of biographies written about a subject and focused on childhood and developmental factors thought to influence outcome (Goertzel & Goertzel, 1962; Goertzel, Goertzel, & Goertzel, 1978).

8–2. MASLOW AND DĄBROWSKI

Comparing Maslow's construct of self-actualization and Dąbrowski's descriptions of advanced development, the fundamental approaches and constructs of the two authors concerning human development are quite similar. However, there are also several key differences that prevented Dąbrowski from endorsing Maslow's approach to self-actualization. To fully appreciate why Dąbrowski refused to use the term self-actualization requires further explanation of Maslow's use of the construct: Self-actualization as outlined by Maslow is essentially a unilevel construct.

8–2–1. The animal-human continuum

As part of his graduate work with Harry Harlow, Maslow studied primate behavior, principally at the Bronx zoo and the Henry Vilas Park Zoo in Maadison, and came to the conclusion that human behavior is an extension of animal behavior and instincts. For example, Maslow (1942) said, "in general it is fair to say that human sexuality is almost exactly like primate sexuality with the exception that cultural pressures added to the picture" (p. 291). This led Maslow to the conclusion that our lowest animal-like behaviors and our highest human values both come from the same realization of our "biological life" as he called it. Maslow (1971/1976) said:

> The so-called spiritual or value life, or "higher" life is on the same continuum (is the same kind or quality of thing) with the life of the flesh, or of the body, i.e., the animal life, the material life, the "lower" life. That is, the spiritual life is part of our biological life. It is the "highest" part of it, but yet, part of it. (pp. 313-314)

For Dąbrowski, it made no sense to talk about animal instincts, human authenticity, and higher values as being on a continuum. There must be a qualitative break separating animals from humans, analogous to the qualitative demarcation between unilevel and multilevel experience. Dąbrowski found Maslow's approach unacceptable because, for Dąbrowski, it is precisely overcoming this animal nature that differentiates humans from animals. The "higher mental functions of man, particularly those of an autonomous and authentic nature, differ qualitatively from lower mental functions and from mental functions of animals" (Dąbrowski, 1970b, p. 149). There are many other similar examples in Dąbrowski. For example, Dąbrowski (1964b) said: "The individual human being, through his personality, masters his impulses. This process consists in purifying the primitive animal elements which lie in every impulse or group of impulses" (p. 61).

8–2–2. Actualization of the self as-is

Another important distinction involves the goal of actualization. For Dąbrowski the goal of advanced development is the creation and pursuit of an idealization of whom one wants to be. Maslow, on the other hand, advocated that self-actualization should involve the actualization of oneself as it is and as one discovers it. In the following examples, we again see the influence of Maslow's perception of a continuum of lower instincts to higher values.

In an article originally published in 1967 entitled "Neurosis as a Failure of Personal Growth," Maslow (1971/1976) said that an important task of development is to first "become aware of what one *is*, biologically, temperamentally, constitutionally, as a member of a species, of one's capabilities, desires, needs and also one's vocation, what one is fitted for, what one's destiny is" (p. 31). This amounts to getting in touch with one's "instinctoid," one's animality and specieshood. Maslow (1971/1976) explained that he believed it possible "to carry through this paradigm even at the very highest levels of personal development, where one transcends one's own personality" (p. 31), and he went on to suggest that underlying our highest values lies this instinctoidal character. Maslow (1971/1976) considered it a scientific advantage to utilize a single continuum:

> Think of the great theoretical and scientific advantages of placing on one single continuum of degree or amount of humanness, not only all the kinds of sickness the psychiatrists and physicians talk about but also all the additional kinds that existentialists and philosophers and religious thinkers and social reformers have worried about. (p. 31)

Maslow suggested that various levels of potential exist within a person and said that all of these potentials must be actualized, both the lowest and the highest. Therefore, Maslow (1970) saw the expression of lower instincts as a necessary and healthy feature: "The first and most obvious level of acceptance is at the so-called animal level. Those self-actualizing people tend to be good animals, hearty in their appetites and enjoying themselves without regret or shame or apology" (p. 156). Maslow (1970) went on to say:

> They are able to accept themselves not only on these low levels, but at all levels as well; e.g., love, safety, belongingness, honor and self-respect. All of these are accepted without question as worthwhile, simply because these people are inclined to accept the work of nature rather than to argue with her for not having constructed things to a different pattern. (p. 156)

Maslow was clear that self-actualization does not involve a discrimination of features; all features that are present are accepted and actualized equally. Thus, in describing self-actualizing people, Maslow (1970) said:

> Our healthy individuals find it possible to accept themselves
> and their own nature without chagrin or complaint or, for that
> matter, even without thinking about the matter very much.
> They can accept their own human nature in the stoic style,
> with all its shortcomings, with all its discrepancies from the
> ideal image without feeling real concern. (p. 155)

Emphasizing acceptance of oneself as-is, Maslow (1970) said: "the
self-actualized person sees reality more clearly: our subjects see
human nature as it is and not as they would prefer it to be" (p. 156).
These individuals were described as more objective and less
emotional, less likely to allow hopes, dreams, fears or psychological
defenses to distort their observations of reality.

A careful reading of Maslow reveals that there is no sense of "ought"
in Maslow. He advocated the discovery and actualization of individual
(self) potential as it exists; we need to go from "what we are" to "what
we can be"[38] without a sense of the potential for what one could be or
could become (Maslow, 1970, p. 272). Maslow (1971/1976) said "the
best way for a person to discover what he ought to do is to find out who
and what he is" (p. 108) and that to defy one's nature and "trying to be
what one is not" leads to intrinsic guilt (p. 327).

We have repeatedly seen Dąbrowski's fundamental objection to
this idea: "To be authentic does not mean to be natural, to be as you
are, but as you ought to be" (Cienin, 1972, p. 22).

8–2–3. Developmental potential

Both Dąbrowski and Maslow described developmental potential.
Maslow saw individuals as having a unique essential nature ("some
skeleton") of both needs and potentials. In his model, Maslow
suggested that everyone has an intrinsic impulse or instinct toward
self-actualization and that the higher brain circuits that form the
neurophysiological foundation of self-actualization are not created as
one develops; they already exist, lying dormant and waiting to be
activated. In this sense, the evolution of self-actualizers is
predetermined by the biological structure of the human brain (Wilson,
1972). The universality of the instinct toward, and potential for, self-
actualization was emphasized by the fact that Maslow did not draw a
sharp distinction between self-actualizers and ordinary people

(Wilson, 1972). Maslow suggested that self-actualization is not "an all-or-none affair"—it is "a matter of degree and of frequency" (Maslow, 1968, p. 97).

As we have seen, Dąbrowski's perspective was that the features comprising developmental potential are not universal; some people have little potential; many have equivocal potential; and some people have strong potential.

An important difference between Dąbrowski and Maslow in their approaches to developmental potential relates to the importance of environmental conditions. As we have seen, Dąbrowski believed that strong developmental potential could overcome even a strongly negative environment. But Maslow was clear that self-actualization required positive environmental conditions—"Very good conditions are needed to make self-actualizing possible" (Maslow 1970, p. 99). Initially, Maslow suggested that the emergence of self-actualization depended upon the satisfaction of the lower needs described in his hierarchy (physiological, safety, love, and esteem needs). Later, he suggested such a positive environment might be a necessary precondition, but not a sufficient condition: "It is now more clear to me that gratification of the basic needs is not a sufficient condition for metamotivation, although it may be a necessary precondition" (Maslow, 1971/1976, p. 290).

Herman (1995) believed that self-actualization was a by-product of the conditions found in an affluent post-war America and that "Mental health, the product of a psychic economy of plenty, resulted from economic affluence. It could be bought and sold" (p. 271). This comment also underscored another aspect of humanistic psychology—that it was peculiarly a North American phenomenon (Royce & Mos, 1981).

Traditional views hold that anxiety and actualization are mutually exclusive. Using Dąbrowski's framework, de Grâce (1974) examined the hypothesis that a degree of anxiety is a source of actualization. Further, de Grâce (1974) concluded that mental health is best characterized by the flexibility to move between psychological equilibrium and disequilibrium, and disease signified stability.

8–2–4. Similarities between Dąbrowski and Maslow

Maslow's approach to autonomy and motivation was similar to Dąbrowski's idea of the third factor. As Dąbrowski (1972b) pointed out:

> Both Maslow and I underline that the course of development depends on the strength and character of the developmental potential, on the strength and character of environmental influence and on the strength and range of activity of the third factor which stands for the autonomous dynamisms of self-determination. (p. 249)

Both authors also emphasized unique and individualized values; as we have seen above, Maslow distinguished socialized values (second factor) from individualized values (Dąbrowski's hierarchy of values, third factor and the personality ideal). Maslow (1970) said: "the ordinary ethical behavior of the average person is largely conventional behavior rather than truly ethical behavior, e.g., behavior based on fundamentally accepted principles (which are perceived to be true)" (p. 158).

8–3. MULTILEVEL-ACTUALIZATION

I believe that an amalgamation of multilevelness and self-actualization would produce a stronger and more useful model for describing development. A neo-Dąbrowskian, neo-Maslowian synthesis would retain the important contributions of Maslow and incorporate the critical construct of multilevelness. I call this synthesis *multilevel-actualization*.

When we examine Maslow's characteristics associated with self-actualization, we can readily see that many of these attributes can be applied to most advanced development approaches, including Dąbrowski's. What is missing in Maslow is an appreciation of Dąbrowski's multilevel dimension incorporating vertical differentiations between the lower and the higher. Maslow's "as is" needs to be replaced by Dąbrowski's ideal of what "ought to be." Before actualizing the self, this vertical differentiation must be made—ideally, one will develop the mental image of one's personality ideal and a related hierarchy of values, aims and goals. It is this ideal that must be actualized. As part of this process, the features considered "less like myself" need to be repressed, inhibited and eliminated. Those features one considers "more like myself" can then be a goal of actualization.

Maslow's continuum, beginning with animal instinct and ending with the highest authentic human values, must be bifurcated to reflect the qualitative differences between these vital but largely contradictory aspects. Lower, animal, instinctoid aspects need to be qualitatively differentiated from higher, authentically human and creative aspects that distinguish humans and that set humans apart from animals. These lower, instinctive aspects can then be overcome (to use Nietzsche's framework) or transformed, and their energies applied to higher pursuits.

Multilevel-actualization creates a powerful and satisfying level of analysis with which to analyze human development. Many of the specific descriptions and attributes of Maslow's actualization can readily be applied, especially when perceived in a multilevel context. The use of the term multilevel-actualization makes it clear that we are differentiating a new synthesis in our discussion, thus avoiding any misunderstanding as to Maslow's or Dąbrowski's respective approaches and meanings.

In summary, a synthesis creating an updated neo-approach is called for to provide the multilevel foundation to actualization that allows our authentic humanity to rise above our animal heritage and instincts. A future challenge is to refine and further research the qualities that should be associated with actualization in general and specifically with multilevel-actualization. Unfortunately, it is beyond the scope of this work to pursue this new construct.

8–4. CHAPTER SUMMARY

This chapter reviewed Maslow's contributions to self-actualization in detail. The characteristics of the self-actualized individual were summarized. Similarities and differences with Dąbrowski were highlighted. The construct of multilevel-actualization was introduced.

EDUCATION

9–1. DĄBROWSKI'S GENERAL APPROACH TO EDUCATION

Dąbrowski was extremely critical of American education and its methods: methods that he considered to be equivalent to animal "training" techniques (Dąbrowski, n.d.b). Dąbrowski was also critical of the "objective approach" epitomized by intelligence testing and the heavy emphasis on rote learning and test performance with little appreciation for the roles of emotional intelligence or individual development.

Dąbrowski's views on education were expressed in an undated and unpublished manuscript he wrote with the assistance of Marlene Rankel (Dąbrowski, n.d.b). Rankel (2008) provided a comprehensive summary of this important work. Dąbrowski (n.d.b) defined authentic education:

> All that is truly human expresses a hierarchy of values—a clear indication that the teacher recognizes, in himself and others, better and worse ways of educating and that he consciously chooses "the better." This, then, is authentic education. It is aimed at educating children in an environment of mutual compassion, understanding and positive adjustment—adjustment not just to the changing material

conditions of life, but commitment to individual positive developmental changes. "Authentic" for the child, then, is his commitment to his own particular "developmental inner truth." (p. 1)

Education emphasizes objectivity, epitomized in the measurement of learning by testing. For Dąbrowski, a student's objective behavior (what we can measure) means little as it does not reflect the child's internal psychic processes—for instance, imagination, developmental processes, motivation, and emotional state. Dąbrowski was concerned that traditional education deals with only the external milieu of children while neglecting their developmental potential and inner psychic development. Education must take into account the child's unique personality characteristics, including his or her sensitivities, frustrations, strengths, and creativity. Mirroring his emphasis on overexcitabilities, the child's imaginational and emotional sensitivities must be considered and cultivated in parallel with intellectual capabilities.

It is apparent Dąbrowski's ideas are in stark contrast with the status quo. Gardner (1995/2011) elaborated that the role of education is essentially to pass along the traditions and knowledge of one's culture. "A society features all manner of conventions, rituals, tastes, legal schemes, moral precepts, preferred behaviors, and cherished values, and each of these could be the subject of a targeted education" (Gardner, 1995/2011, p. 126). Dąbrowski advocated a holistic education placing the student at the heart of the educational process. The process of education is fundamentally intermingled with a student's self-development.

9–2. SELF-EDUCATION (EDUCATION-OF-ONESELF)

In addition to traditional schooling, Dąbrowski advocated self-education (education-of-oneself). Self-education plays two critical roles: in self-education, the student explores a wide range of academic topics of interest, and the process of self-education itself contributes to the developmental process.

Based upon the first role, a student will ideally become a polymath (as was Dąbrowski): the best preparation possible for success in life. Traditional education emphasizes specialization and maximizing achievement, usually in a student's particular area of strength. Our technological society demands more and earlier specialization. Individuals often excel at such specialization, leading to the accolades associated with productivity and efficiency. Opposing this, Dąbrowski pitted specialization against creativity: "the developing individual cannot submit to narrow specialization except at the cost of a loss in creativity" (Dąbrowski, 1964b, p. 124).

Dąbrowski (1970b) was concerned that one-sided development could result in a retardation of emotional development and a stunting of development in general:

> One-sided development of some mental functions leads to an integration within the narrow sphere of these functions without loosening and dissolution of a wider scope of structures and dynamisms and without the development of key functions. It increases egocentrism, lack of syntony, tendency towards autocratic attitudes with a simultaneous lack of self-consciousness, self-control and without the development of the inner psychic milieu. (p. 149)

This stunting of individual development also has significant implications for society at large. "Such individuals, when they succeed in attaining positions of power, cause grave, sometimes disastrous, effects for social groups and societies" (Dąbrowski, 1970b, p. 149).

As Bateson and Martin (2000) echoed:

> Through an excessive emphasis by some parents on certain forms of achievement, their children end up with narrow lives. The long-term effects on their social, emotional and intellectual development may ironically result in poorer attainment later in life, as well as personal unhappiness. A faster, narrower development is not a surefire recipe for success. (p. 229)

Secondly, Dąbrowski emphasized the critical role played by self-education in personality development. Self-education is "the process of working out the personality in one's inner self" and is critical in establishing "object-subject" and the relationship between what is educated and what educates (Dąbrowski, 1964b, p. 62). As Mowrer (1967) said:

> Self-education is the highest possible process of a psychological and moral character. It begins at the time when the individual undergoes changes which permit him to make himself partially independent of biological factors and of the influence of the social environment. (p. xxii)

Ideally, self-education leads to self-determination, ultimately expressed through personality development and culminating in the apex of the personality ideal. Self-educational opportunities should be encouraged and facilitated by traditional education.

Dąbrowski made a connection between the developmental instinct, education-of-oneself, and personality development. An individual's education should include issues such as values, moral character, personality, and learning about oneself. Education needs to ask students critical insight questions; for instance, "What am I good at and do I enjoy it?" And, "What do I most enjoy and am I good at it?" This line of self-inquiry helps to guide the student in the discovery of individual aptitudes, personality ideal, and how to integrate personality traits with educational goals. In this way aptitude joins with ability to yield competence and, through performance, to create confidence.

Schneider (2012) presented an interesting description of a German approach to self-education. In this framework, *Bildung*, action is taken to create one's self. Using subject-object, one transforms "from being shaped by the environment to assuming individual self-responsibility. This characterizes the development from [Kegan's] interpersonal to the institutional stage" (Schneider, 2012, p. 310). As Schneider (2012) explained:

> Consequently, it no longer suffices to let ourselves be formed by our environment; much more we are called upon to develop an inner authority that enables us to determine for ourselves what is valuable. This means a process of becoming aware that one's own value system is of importance in order to bring

about self-determined transformations of our own value system. (p. 310)

9–3. ISSUES IN GIFTED EDUCATION

The field of gifted education has been the subject of intense internal examination (e.g., Ambrose, Van Tassel-Baska, Coleman, & Cross, 2010; Sternberg, 2018). The authors reviewed theory and stated that there has been relatively little theoretical activity either in the past or going on today, and it was concluded that theory is rarely the foundation of scholarly progress in the field.

Research was the next topic reviewed by Ambrose et al. (2010). There are various stakeholders participating in research, each bringing their own constructions of giftedness, leading to the conclusion that the field is fractured. None of the popular formulations have a solid foundation based on sound research. The authors concluded that the gifted field "is quite fragmented at the research level, divided among several groups, none of which has yet to establish firm intellectual footing" (Ambrose et al., 2010, p. 466).

Finally, educational practice was considered. The authors said, "at the practice level we are still at the stage of medieval thought characterized by camps, fads and imperfect attempts to gain coherence" (Ambrose et al., 2010, p. 466). The conclusion was that at the level of practice, the field is porous and "does not progress; rather, it stagnates in some places [and] regresses in others" (Ambrose et al., 2010, p. 468).

Dai (2011) provided a response to Ambrose et al. (2010). Dai used the 2009 *International Handbook on Giftedness*, edited by Shavinina, as an illustration of the broad scope of the field. A dual affiliation was noted: on one hand, gifted education is connected to gifted studies, and on the other hand, to general education. Dai (2011) concluded that porosity is a positive feature, creating an open and vital atmosphere interacting with both education and human sciences.

Dai (2011) presented three paradigms. First was the gifted child paradigm. The assumption of this paradigm is that children can be categorized as gifted based upon unique mental qualities. This classification also involves various subcategories such as moderate, high, and profound levels. Numerous subgroups may be created, for instance: gifted girls, underachievers, and the creative. A second paradigm is based on talent development. This paradigm assumes a broader definition of gifted and moves beyond an IQ-based or academic achievement basis. The third paradigm is the differentiation practice paradigm. It uses a non-categorical approach (rejecting gifted or not) based upon diagnosis of specific areas of needs requiring interventions. Dai (2011) concluded that these three paradigms could serve as scaffolds for research, yielding evidence-based practices that will continue to evolve.

In summarizing his career working with the gifted, Pfeiffer (2013) presented three main conclusions. The first conclusion related to the identification of high-ability students. Three myths were identified, the first one being that giftedness is a real attribute. Giftedness is "not real;" instead, it is a socially constructed construct (Borland, 2009). There is no scientific justification in dichotomizing students as gifted or non-gifted. IQ scores are quite arbitrary: There is no difference between an individual with an IQ of 129 compared to an individual with an IQ of 131, although based upon a cut-off score of 130, one student may be identified as gifted and one not.

A second myth is that giftedness is equivalent to high IQ. Pfeiffer (2013) said that although most experts no longer see giftedness as high IQ, many educators and parents still believe that high IQ is equivalent to giftedness and that most studies still rely on IQ as an index of giftedness (Carman, 2013). Pfeiffer (2013) stated that only about 25% of the variance in student achievement can be attributed to IQ scores. Pfeiffer's third myth is that once identified as gifted, always gifted. Typically, once students are identified they are not retested and simply maintain their gifted classification throughout their education.

The second main conclusion presented by Pfeiffer (2013) was that the development of talent requires more than ability. There are many non-academic qualities that are critical, including hard work and practice. The ability to delay gratification and to tolerate frustration are also critical components of success.

The third conclusion of Pfeiffer (2013) was that success requires both "head strengths" and strengths of the heart. Pfeiffer (2013) outlined six heart strengths he considered critical, including humility, persistence, kindness, gratitude, enthusiasm, and playfulness.

Mendaglio (2013) pointed out that giftedness has been associated with underachievement; up to half of gifted students are academic underachievers. In Mendaglio's affective cognitive model of giftedness, intelligence and achievement are considered distinct constructs. In this framework, motivation, effort and persistence must be present for achievement. Further, achievement does not depend on intelligence alone: "students with average intelligence may obtain high achievement when they persistently exert effort in their studies" (Mendaglio, 2013, p. 6). Mendaglio (2013) proposed three motivational characteristics: heightened sensitivity, analytical attitude, and self-criticism.

In reviewing the gifted research literature on topics germane to this work, few definitive answers emerge. Results are often contradictory and even trends are difficult to see. It is difficult to draw conclusions from research due to the low quality of individual studies and the challenges of comparing disparate studies (e.g., Borland, 2003; Carman, 2013; Kerr, 2009; Martin, Burns, & Schonlau, 2010; Neihart, 1999; Pfeiffer, 2008; Shavinina & Ferrari, 2004; Sternberg, Jarvin, & Grigorenko, 2011; Walsh, Kemp, Hodge, & Bowes, 2012). While it is not within the purview of this work to fully explore this topic, a few challenges are noted, including studies using unique definitions of giftedness or creativity; employing various methodologies; using small sample sizes; not differentiating levels of giftedness; using different IQ cut-off scores; not using appropriate nongifted comparison groups; assuming non-relatedness of factors studied; assuming normal population distributions; and research with no theoretical framework.

Many authors have noted the lack of consensus in defining giftedness. For example, Carman (2013) reviewed the topic and pointed out that 10.7% of research articles did not report how their subjects were selected, and only 24.3% identified their own subjects as part of their research protocol.[39] Efforts to develop higher standards in gifted education and research (Coleman, Gallagher, & Job, 2012) and incremental improvements in research will be critical in moving forward.

9–4. DĄBROWSKI AND THE GIFTED

The application of Dąbrowski's theory to gifted populations was not a major focus during his lifetime. Dąbrowski conducted one study in English that dealt with gifted youth. This research was reported on in Dąbrowski (1967, pp. 250-262) and again in Dąbrowski (1972b pp. 202-219). "The subjects were 80 children, of whom 30 were generally intellectually gifted (from elementary schools), and 50 were children and young people from art schools (theatre, ballet, and art)" (Dąbrowski 1972b, p. 203).

Dąbrowski found that "all gifted children and young people display symptoms of increased psychic excitability, or psychoneurotic symptoms of greater or lesser intensity (1972b, p. 218) and went on:

> The development of personality among gifted children and young people usually passes through the process of positive disintegration (strictly related to the complexity of the psychoneurosis), and it leads to self-control, education-of-oneself, and autopsychotherapy, in other words, to a conscious inner psychic transformation. (p. 219)

In the unpublished manuscript, *On Authentic Education,* Dąbrowski (n.d.b) said:

> The nervous and psychoneurotic individual is present in an overwhelming percentage of highly gifted children and youths, artists, writers, etc. This tendency to reach beyond the statistical norm and mediocre development presents the privilege and drama of psychoneurotic people. (p. 49)

Further elaborating the psychological issues highlighted in the gifted child, Dąbrowski (n.d.b) said:

> The extremely sensitive child by contact with conflict in everyday life, with death and injustice and the child who experiences greatly feelings of inferiority can elaborate or realize, besides his giftedness, anxiety (psychoneurotic), the fears of darkness and loneliness and aggressiveness. Such anxiety comes most often from unpleasant experience, usually

being the dominant influence of hereditary potential in the form of emotional overexcitability. Such anxiety symptoms are unpleasant for the child, the parents and the larger environment. The sensitive child usually hides, inhibits, or pushes down the symptoms to unconsciousness. (p. 58)

In terms of being gifted, Nixon (2005) reviewed Dąbrowski's works and concluded that IQ was a necessary but not sufficient condition for personality development and, in his reports, Dąbrowski described a very wide range of necessary IQ (of between 70 and 110). In reflecting on this project, Dąbrowski (1972b) concluded:

We think that we shall have reached our goal if this work will focus attention on the positive relation between the development of superior abilities and talents and the development of psychoneuroses in the direction of their higher forms. (p. 219)

9–5. APPLICATIONS OF DĄBROWSKI TO GIFTED POPULATIONS

The impact of Dąbrowski in the field of gifted education has been somewhat uneven. His work is most often associated with the emotional needs of the gifted (see Cross, 2018) and the application of the construct of overexcitability to the gifted. His work is often not mentioned in reviews within the field; for example, recent reviews on the assessment and identification of gifted students do not mention Dąbrowski (Cao, Jung, & Lee, 2017; Sternberg, 2017).

Operationalizing Dąbrowski's constructs has been a challenge. As Mendaglio and Tillier (2006) pointed out, it was "Piechowski and his associates that rose to the challenge of operationalizing overexcitability," (p. 83) and much was accomplished during the first phase of research using overexcitability in gifted education (Silverman, 2008). As well, Dąbrowski's constructs have begun to appear in the context of counseling the gifted (Colangelo & Wood, 2015).

It remains for future researchers to move beyond overexcitabilities and begin to examine Dąbrowski's other constructs and hypotheses.

Fundamentally at issue is Dąbrowski's contention that gifted individuals will be predisposed to, and disproportionately display, issues related to the process of positive disintegration, including psychoneuroses and developmental dynamisms. Anxieties, compulsions, obsessions, inner conflicts, and depressions are predicted to be seen more frequently, in particular, related to issues concerning the self. Dissatisfaction with oneself may be an early and prominent symptom of positive disintegration in this population. Given the possibility, if not the likelihood, that these "symptoms" will be misinterpreted, it seems especially relevant to conduct further research on these issues. If links are demonstrated, then educational personnel and, especially, educational counselors can be alerted to the developmental context of such "symptoms." Once accurately identified, the difficult questions about how to best manage these so-called "symptoms" will need to be carefully discussed both in general and in individual cases.

Dąbrowski's (1972b) goal of focusing attention on the relationship between the development of superior abilities and the development of psychoneuroses has not yet been achieved. I would reframe and enlarge this goal to focus attention on the simultaneous development of one's abilities and talents and of one's personality in general, including an appreciation for the role of emotion in life. In taking this "top-down" approach, much can be achieved if we can emphasize the increased probability of personality and psychological issues arising in the gifted as a group and then advocate for the sensitive and compassionate management of these issues when they arise.

To establish a more sensitive and more responsive school environment seems to be a priority. Many parents report being turned aside when they ask school administrators for compassion and understanding in the management of their children.

In many cases, early and exceptional abilities are exploited, commonly by parents overly anxious for their child to excel or by school systems anxious to take credit for an exceptional student. Alternatively, schools that lack resources may simply ignore gifted students. These children appear to require general support and encouragement to explore their interests, in their own ways and in their own timeframes. A student choosing his or her own path may be more likely to develop the intrinsic motivation and drive necessary to complement his or her particular talents and to go on to a positive life.

9–5–1. Overexcitability and the gifted

Attempts to identify and understand the gifted have sometimes utilized personality-related constructs and tests borrowed from psychology; for example, the Myers-Briggs Type Indicator (Carman, 2011). In this vein, Piechowski introduced the overexcitability construct to the gifted field and the framework became popular (Piechowski, 2008). Piechowski developed the overexcitability questionnaire (OEQ) based on the idea of Dąbrowski's verbal stimuli[40] (Lysy & Piechowski, 1983).

An important early study using the OEQ was conducted by Ackerman (1997), who reported:

> Classificatory analysis performed at the end of the discriminant analysis indicated that a total of 70.9% of all subjects were correctly classified using psychomotor, intellectual, and emotional OE scores; that is, into the groups the schools had placed them. However, 23 subjects were classified incorrectly: 13 of the 37 (35.1%) nongifted subjects were classified as gifted and 10 of the 42 (23.8%) gifted subjects were classified as nongifted. (p. 233)

I present Ackerman's (1997) conclusions in detail because I believe that they had a far-reaching impact on practitioners in the field of gifted education—in assuming that overexcitabilities are synonymous with giftedness:

> Gifted subjects were differentiated from their nongifted peers based on their higher psychomotor, intellectual, and emotional OE scores. While this was an unexpected finding, it clearly illustrates that scores on the OEQ can differentiate between gifted and nongifted students. . . . if teachers were trained to recognize characteristics of overexcitabilities in their students, some students who would normally go unidentified, might be identified in this manner. (p. 235)

Falk, Lind, Miller, Piechowski, and Silverman (1999) developed a revised instrument (the OEQII). The OEQII is a research instrument that "may be used for research with group data but cannot provide diagnostic information about the individual case" (Falk et al., 1999, p. 4). The two questionnaires stimulated many studies that were summarized by Mendaglio and Tillier (2006).

An excellent review of past research conclusions was provided by Pyryt (2008). Research demonstrated that gifted individuals are more likely than those not identified as gifted to show signs of intellectual overexcitability (Pyryt, 2008). It now seems apparent that, based upon the research strategies and testing done to date, the gifted do not consistently demonstrate "the big three": intellectual, imaginational, and emotional overexcitability. This finding does not support Ackerman's suggestion of using overexcitability profiles to identify gifted students who have not been previously identified by conventional means (Ackerman, 1997). As Pyryt (2008) concluded:

> It appears that gifted and average ability individuals have similar amounts of emotional overexcitability. This finding would suggest that many gifted individuals have limited developmental potential in the Dąbrowskian sense and are more likely to behave egocentrically rather than altruistically. (p. 177)

Unfortunately, the conclusions of more recent studies are also contradictory; for instance, Warne (2011b) stated, "It has never been clear what exactly the OEQII measures . . . Further psychometric studies on the instrument should be conducted before the instrument gains widespread acceptance" (p. 688). Warne (2011a) concluded "those who use the OEQII or read studies containing data produced by the instrument [should] use caution in interpreting group or individual differences because such score differences are likely partially psychometric in nature and not psychological" (p. 590). On the other hand, Al-Onizat (2013) found the OEQII to be sound and advocated its use for students to understand themselves and their specific strengths and weaknesses, and to "enable the counselors and the teachers to better understand their students' intelligences" (p. 61) (in contravention of the limitations of using the test only with group data as mentioned above). Carman (2011) concluded that the OEQII is difficult to administer and has questionable reliability; she therefore encouraged further research to develop a more appropriate instrument to measure overexcitabilities. Dai stated, "Some may say that Dąbrowski's notion of overexcitability is misinterpreted in research as it may not reveal itself in psychometric research" (see Henshon, 2013, p. 76).

Winkler and Voight (2016) found high ambiguity, and concluded "Using the presented findings and data, it is possible for scholars and practitioners to believe or disbelieve in the relationship between giftedness and the OEs" (p. 251). It is also important to differentiate the validity and reliability of overexcitability testing and the question of whether or not overexcitability actually exists to a higher degree in gifted populations (see Buntins, Buntins, & Eggert, 2017; Cronbach & Meehl, 1955). To this point, Winkler and Voight (2016) stated:

> Cautious practitioners may want to reserve commitment on the relationship between giftedness and OE and on the OEQ II's viability. One could certainly consider individual students and patients as overexcitable, but the OEQ II might not be the most valid method for confirming or disconfirming such opinions. (p. 253)

As mentioned above, these instruments treat overexcitabilities as five unrelated domains and base their questions on essentially an amalgamation of descriptions of each of the overexcitabilities. The vast differences in the expression and meaning of each overexcitability on each level are not taken into consideration and thus, past research has, by definition, not validly reflected the constructs of the overexcitabilities as described by Dąbrowski. For example, here are the items measuring emotional overexcitability on the OEQ II (Falk et al., 1999)

- I feel other people's feelings
- I worry a lot
- It makes me sad to see a lonely person in a group
- I can be so happy that I want to laugh and cry at the same time
- I have strong feelings of joy, anger, excitement, and despair

- I am deeply concerned about others
- My strong emotions moved me to tears
- I can feel a mixture of different emotions all at once
- I am an unemotional person
- I take everything to heart (pp. 7-8).

It is difficult to see how these items capture the complexity and depth of Dąbrowski's approach to emotional overexcitability.

In an important contribution to the literature, Mendaglio (2012), pointed out that much of the research done on overexcitabilities has made assumptions that are not supported by, or do not reflect, the basic tenets of the theory of positive disintegration. Mendaglio (2012) gave the example that research assumes that overexcitability is a continuous variable, normally distributed in the population, and this violates the basic construct as Dąbrowski presented it. Mendaglio (2012) called for a paradigm shift to encourage researchers to take into account the theoretical context and assumptions of the theory when designing their research.

Finally, although it is beyond the scope of the present work to re-analyse data, it should be noted that publication bias is also a definite possibility in the interpretation of the research findings. "A large literature documents that people are self-serving in their interpretation of ambiguous information and remarkably adept at reaching justifiable conclusions that mesh with their desires" (Simmons, Nelson, & Simonsohn, 2011, pp. 1359-1360). In addition, broader, ongoing concerns about using null hypothesis significance testing (as used in most of this research) continue to beset psychology (Nickerson, 2000; see also García-Pérez, 2017).

In summary, many in the gifted field appear to take for granted that overexcitability has been satisfactorily and significantly linked with gifted children. The meta-analysis of the last 30 years of research calls for a reappraisal of this conclusion, especially as it relates to Dąbrowski's so-called big three: imaginational, intellectual, and emotional overexcitability. As Jane Piirto cautioned, "people in our field should be careful about assuming that the gifted students are more sensitive than other students. This just hasn't been proved" (Sansom, Barnes, Carrizales, and Shaughannesy, 2018, p. 97). Do the gifted disproportionately demonstrate other signs of developmental potential; for example, the third factor? This question awaits future research using instruments specifically designed to measure developmental potential and its other components.

9–5–2. Psychoneuroses, positive disintegration, and the gifted

There are two views on the role of giftedness in terms of psychological well-being, and there is research to support both. As we will see, on one hand, giftedness is seen to enhance resiliency and help individuals cope with life. The other view is that being gifted increases psychological vulnerability (Neihart, 1999).

Do the gifted display a higher incidence of psychoneuroses and positive disintegration? While we don't have a direct answer to this question, perhaps we can approach it by examining three key dimensions of well-being in the gifted: anxiety, depression, and self-harm/suicide.

9–5–2–1. Anxiety and the gifted

Anxiety has been the topic of several reports in the gifted (e.g., Dirkes, 1983; Flescher, 1963; Scholwinski, 1985; Tibbetts, 1979). Flescher (1963) found anxiety unrelated to intellectual ability. Olszewski-Kubilius, Kulieke, and Krasney (1988) found the gifted to be well-adjusted with fewer psychological problems and lower levels of anxiety compared to non-gifted. This study also differentiated achievers from non-achievers, with the achievers showing higher responsibility and self-control. Neihart (1999) reported no significant differences in anxiety levels between high-ability students in gifted programs versus students in the general population. Martin, Burns, and Schonlau (2010) conducted a meta-analysis finding significantly lower levels of anxiety in gifted youth compared to their non-gifted peers.

Harrison and Van Haneghan (2011) used Dąbrowski as a framework in examining insomnia, death anxiety, and fears of the unknown in a sample of 216 students. Overexcitabilities were considered a predictor of anxiety. Levels of insomnia and fear of the unknown were higher in the gifted group (but not death anxiety), as were sensual, intellectual and imaginational overexcitabilities. Emotional overexcitability was the highest in the gifted high school group compared to regular students; however, this was reversed at the middle school level. Gifted groups had higher anxiety even after accounting for overexcitability. Using Harrison and Van Haneghan as a base, Lamont (2012) presented tips for parents and educators in dealing with anxiety and fear in gifted learners.

Supported by his affective cognitive model, Mendaglio (2010, 2011) postulated there are several unique sources of anxiety seen in gifted students including the effect of stigmatization on being gifted and the idea that gifted students think they are perceived as being different by others.

9–5–2–2. Depression and the gifted

A fairly grim picture of the experience of being gifted has been described by various authors. For instance, Grobman (2006) said:

> Despite their growth in intellect and conceptual abilities, these exceptionally gifted adolescents were only dimly aware of the nature and content of their conflicts and anxieties. They were quite aware, however, of the great emotional discomfort that these conflicts and anxieties caused. Because they were unable to tolerate even the smallest bit of emotional discomfort—they could not live with anxiety, struggle with anxiety, or attempt to understand anxiety—they simply tried to eliminate it. (p. 206)

Davidson (2012) found that giftedness is often an unwanted and unappreciated gift:

> It does not make their lives easier nor are they proud to own it . . . it comes with high expectations; and not all gifted children want to be gifted because of the stigma and isolation that can result from it. (p. 263)

Jackson and Peterson (2003) said: "There is indeed clinical evidence that depression can be an insidious and even fatal influence in the lives of some gifted people" (p. 177).

In spite of these viewpoints, both Baker (1995) and Neihart (1999) concluded that the literature does not support the idea that the gifted are more depressed than the non-gifted samples. Missett (2013) summarized research that strongly supported this position, and further concluded that high IQ might serve a protection function against mood disorder. As well, in the meta-analysis conducted by Martin, Burns, and Schonlau (2010), gifted youth had lower rates of depressive symptomatology compared to their nongifted peers.

9–5–2–3. Suicide and the gifted

There does not appear to be firm evidence to support the claim that gifted adolescents have higher suicide rates than other adolescents (Hyatt & Cross, 2009). There are a number of representative reports on the topic (e.g., Bratter, 2003; Cross, 1996, 2013, 2016; Cross, Cook, & Dixon, 1996; Cross, Gust-Brey, & Ball, 2002; Delisle, 1986; Gust-Brey & Cross, 1999; Hayes & Sloat, 1990; Hyatt, 2010; Hyatt & Cross, 2009; Lajoie & Shore, 1981; Sedillo, 2015; Willings & Arseneault, 1986). For an excellent, overall summary see Cross (2013).

Dixon and Scheckel (1996) reported: "the data clearly indicate that the risks of suicide for adolescents have increased dramatically during the past decades" (p. 390). The authors therefore concluded that gifted adolescents are at risk. However, they indicate it is less clear whether or not gifted adolescents have greater suicide risk compared to non-gifted. More research was recommended.

Gust-Brey and Cross (1999) found that there was no significant research to support the claim that the rates of attempted or completed suicide among the gifted differ from rates of non-gifted adolescents. Cassady and Cross (2006) reported that the suicide rate and the amount of suicidal ideation did not differ between gifted students and those from the general population, although all adolescents are committing suicide at increased rates compared to 50 years ago. The authors reported that there may be differences in the structure of suicidal thoughts between the gifted and those from the general population, specifically that the gifted adolescent maintains multifactorial constructions of suicidal ideation and that further research will help link these dimensions of suicidal ideation with established risk factors (Cassady & Cross, 2006).

Grobman (2006) presented his clinical insights that passive and active self-destruction in gifted adolescents is often used to create distractions that undermine achievement, interfering with concentration and dedication. The author concluded that most such students could not accept responsibility for their behavior and were only dimly aware of its implications. Grobman concluded:

> Their most troublesome conflicts and anxieties arose not from fears of ostracism, fears of failure, or lost opportunities, but from fear that giftedness had distorted and twisted them as human beings. Would their developing power, grand ambitions and charisma turn them into self-involved narcissistic destructive people? (p. 209)

Wood and Craigen (2011) presented a review and guidelines for dealing with self-injurious behavior in the gifted. A psychological autopsy of a gifted youth was presented by Hyatt (2010). In one case culminating in suicide, the impressive abilities of the young man appeared to obscure any view of obvious signs of problems, such as boredom and depression (Konigsberg, 2006, 2007). This case was also notable for the after the fact rationalization that occurred on the part of the professionals involved (Konigsberg, 2007, pp. 265-267).

Although statistics and research are not available to determine with certainty that the gifted are at increased risk, suicide is a major concern for all adolescents and therefore represents a significant threat that must always be taken seriously. Our approach ought to be sensitive, compassionate, and watchful for signs of depression and suicide potential in all adolescents.

A review of the research about gay, gifted adolescent suicide and suicidal ideation is available (Sedillo, 2015). Cross (2016), responding to a rash of suicides in several schools, used a community-based perspective and focused on contagion as a factor. Cross (2016) concluded that "although suicide is not specifically a SWGT [students with gifts and talents] phenomenon, there are suicides among this group" (p. 65).

Cross and Cross (2018) reviewed psychological autopsies on several students with gifts and talents who committed suicide and found that:

> All   four   subjects   exhibited   overexcitabilities.   Their

overexcitabilities were expressed in ways or levels beyond the norm even among their gifted peers. The four subjects had minimal prosocial outlets. All four subjects experienced difficulty separating facts from fiction, especially over-identification with negative asocial or aggressive characters or themes in books and movies. They experienced intense emotion, felt conflicted, and wanted to rid themselves of emotions. (p. 64)

Reflecting Dąbrowski's theory, the subjects were found to express behaviors consistent with Levels II or III. Cross and Cross (2018) concluded:

[First lesson] Students with gifts and talents are in many ways the same as their average peers, and what little research has compared their suicide ideation has found no statistically significant difference. This indicates that research from the general population can inform our explorations. Exceptional abilities, however, alter the lived experience for these students and, quite possibly, the way they think about that experience and the possibility of suicide, itself. Risk factors may differ when they are experienced in the context of exceptional abilities. A second lesson represents areas that seemingly are specific to students who are gifted. For example, the descriptions of overexcitabilities in all of the psychological autopsies are believed by many to be unique among students with gifts and talents. Using Dąbrowski's theory may afford suicidologists hints as to the more vulnerable among gifted students. (p. 72)

In terms of the present work, using suicide as an index of positive disintegration, there is not enough evidence to conclude the gifted differ from the general population. I end this subsection with the conclusion Neihart (1999) presented:

What do we know? Intellectually or academically gifted children who are achieving and participate in special educational program for gifted students are at least as well adjusted and are perhaps better adjusted than their nongifted peers. These children do not seem to be any more at-risk for social or emotional problems. (p. 16)

In summary, examination of anxiety, depression, and self-harm in the gifted did not yield clear results that could be generalized to psychoneuroses and positive disintegration. It is also possible that other vulnerabilities exist that were not covered; for example, an association between giftedness and alcohol use has been documented (e.g., Batty et al., 2008; Peairs, Eichen, Putallaz, Costanzo, & Grimes, 2011). As well, one study by Gross, Rinn, and Jamieson (2007) linked overexcitabilities with psychological vulnerability in general. Gross et al. (2007) found correlations between the overexcitabilities and self-concept, concluding that overexcitabilities are not socially valued and therefore may negatively impact the self-construct of gifted adolescents. The findings of Cross and Cross (2018) certainly appear to be the impetus for more research looking at propensity for suicidal ideation and behavior as it may correlate to the characteristics associated with the theory of positive disintegration.

It remains for future research to clarify the incidence of psychoneuroses and positive disintegration in the gifted. This research would be facilitated by the development of instruments specifically designed to measure psychoneuroses and positive disintegration. As indicated, psychoneuroses need to be assessed considering anxiety and depression, but measures of tension, nervousness, and internal conflict are also critical. Overlap would be expected between an instrument that measures psychoneuroses and an instrument measuring positive disintegration. Higher levels of crisis and stress would be predicted during times of disintegration.

9–6. CHAPTER SUMMARY

This chapter began with a review of Dąbrowski's unpublished work presenting his views on education and his constructs of authentic education and self-education. Self-education broadens the traditional approach to education to include an emphasis on developing one's personality. General issues in gifted education introduced Dąbrowski's contribution to the field. Subsequently, research on overexcitabilities in the gifted was reviewed. The unexplored relationship between positive disintegration, psychoneuroses and giftedness was considered by examining research on the gifted in terms of anxiety, depression, and suicide. Based on the ambiguity in the existing research, no conclusions could be drawn.

10

CONCLUSION

Ironically, one of the strengths of Dąbrowski's theory is also one of the obstacles to its broad acceptance—it is extremely rich in interrelated constructs that do not lend themselves to easy comprehension. To fully understand what Dąbrowski is saying requires a broad overview and grasp of his whole approach. Given the depth of the theory, this is a daunting challenge. Most of the work done on the theory since Dąbrowski's passing in 1980 has considered the construct of overexcitability; however, overexcitability was often considered in isolation from its relationship to the other components of developmental potential, or to the broader theory in general.

The theory is dynamic (as are all theories) and requires further research to inform future refinement and theory building. The theory presents major challenges to operationalize, and its complex, interrelated structures will be difficult to assess without the threat of reductionism. Dąbrowski was well aware of these challenges and struggled to find assessment techniques appropriate to measure his constructs. The quality of future theory building will be directly related to the quality of the research that these reformulations are based upon.

Dąbrowski was very supportive of an open approach to future theory building. For over half a century, Dąbrowski was continually updating and revising his theory; he was always observing, looking for ways to make the theory more comprehensive and more descriptive. The seventy-two hypotheses presented in Dąbrowski (1970b) stand as evidence that he felt much more research was required and that this research would inform subsequent theory building. Dąbrowski was purposefully vague and sometimes contradictory in the definitions of his constructs, saying that these framings reflected the vague, contradictory, and complex phenomena he was describing. I look forward to future refinements of the theory. I have no doubt that constructs will be revised; some may be rejected, and some may be added. The process demands a clear differentiation between proposed constructs and the basic tenets of the original theory. This differentiation allows readers to better evaluate revisions and to see the clear pathway from Dąbrowski's contributions to those of subsequent scholars.

One dominant psychological paradigm today is positive psychology. Dąbrowski's work clearly falls under the umbrella of positive psychology. However, I believe Dąbrowski would have major issues with some of the contemporary writings on the topic, writings that appear to be reductionistic and simplistic. In my opinion, Dąbrowski's work makes a significant contribution to positive psychology by adding the subtlety and power of a multilevel framework and by emphasizing the development of one's personality within the context of relating to others (subject-object). Although taking the high road can be arduous, in Dąbrowski's eudaimonic approach, it is the only really meaningful way to confront the realities of life and to make the most of one's potential.

I endorse Mendaglio's (2008b) proclamation that Dąbrowski's is a personality theory suited for the 21st century. The dominant approach to personality today is atheoretical trait analysis involving from three to five factors (depending upon which paradigm one uses). It is important to note that these approaches are not comprehensive descriptions or theories of personality, nor are they accounts of personality development. It is important to keep this in mind when examining factor and trait approaches to see if they can shed light upon Dąbrowski's theory. A comparison between Dąbrowski's theory and trait approaches would be an interesting contribution.

Previous efforts to measure Dąbrowski's theory have been unrealistically reductionistic. Most of these efforts have involved measuring overexcitability, a construct described in terms of the five levels of the theory. This research has not considered the expression of each type of overexcitability on each level and therefore raises validity issues. Any future measure of overexcitability should take into account the major differences in each type of overexcitability on each different level.

Another future challenge is the question of discrete categories versus dimensionality (Haslam, Holland, & Kuppens, 2012). The delineation and demarcation of level boundaries, and different constructs arising from the different levels, appears to be largely dimensional and not discrete. As Buddha suggested, in the sky there is no division between East and West—we create these distinctions and then believe they are true. However, there are major qualitative differences between primary integration and secondary integration and between unilevelness and multilevelness that also must be grappled with. Further thought should be put into these important questions and an open mind kept until further research and theory building can enlighten an appropriate approach.

For the past 30 years, Dąbrowski's theory has found a home in the field of gifted education, in particular the study of overexcitability and its relation to those identified as gifted. We have seen Pyryt's (2008) conclusion that, based on existing research—research using instruments of questionable validity—the gifted generally do not display the types or degrees of overexcitability predicted. It remains to be seen if a useful application of overexcitability can still be found in the gifted population. It also remains to be seen how other aspects of Dąbrowski's theory (for example, third factor, positive disintegration and psychoneuroses) may apply to this population. Clearly, a better understanding of Dąbrowski's theory will contribute to these questions. As well, further, and better, psychological research and study of the theory will benefit its application to gifted education as well as to other areas; for example, to diagnosis and psychotherapy.

I have called for a refined approach to self-actualization that would apply Dąbrowski's construct of multilevelness to Maslow's framework. I refer to this new synthesis as multilevel-actualization.

This work has provided an introduction, overview, and foundation for understanding Dąbrowski's theory. From this portal, the reader is encouraged to further explore the many ideas contained within his work. Many of these ideas could be greatly expanded in their respective fields. For example, dynamisms provide a unique view of emotions, emphasizing not only the awareness of one's emotions, but also the conscious use of emotions in a decision-making and developmental (personality shaping) context. Self-education could be expanded to use as the basis for changes in the traditional curriculum, as well as in contexts such as homeschooling. To give another example, autopsychotherapy could be developed into an important new therapeutic approach, both supplementing and contrasting traditional psychotherapy.

In closing, further elaboration and theory building will provide a sound platform to stimulate more research and to keep honing our theoretical descriptions of the real world. There is much potential to explore in Dąbrowski's unique and rich approach to personality development. Personality theory has gone through many phases over the years, including the development of "grand theories" and today's popular, but reductionistic, trait approaches. I echo Mendaglio in suggesting that Dąbrowski represents a "new" grand theory of personality worthy of careful consideration. As well, there are many sub-themes and secondary applications that justify similar consideration. Dąbrowski's ideas have as much to contribute to contemporary psychology today as they did 50 years ago.

> Sweet are the uses of adversity,
> Which like the toad, ugly and venomous,
> Wears yet a precious jewel in his head;
> (Shakespeare, 1905, p. 222).

APPENDIX 1

A BIOGRAPHY OF KAZIMIERZ DĄBROWSKI

In 2007, I was pleased to provide a biography of Kazimierz Dąbrowski for Sal Mendaglio's book on Dąbrowski (Mendaglio, 2008a). Since then, I discovered a biography of Dąbrowski published in a Polish journal written by Tadeusz Kobierzycki and translated by Anna Przybyłek (Kobierzycki, 2000) and a subsequent update (Kobierzycki, 2010a). Another biography was published by Gawroński (1989). These biographies provided several significant insights and filled in a number of important details. Therefore, I have revised and updated Dąbrowski's biography taking Gawroński's and Kobierzycki's insights into account.

I am proud to provide a biography of Dąbrowski as he had a profound effect on my life. I was just beginning my master's program in Edmonton when one of his colleagues, Marlene Rankel, picked me out of a crowd and said, "I have a book for you to read and someone for you to meet." Reading the book (Dąbrowski, 1972b) gave me a unique perspective and insight into my personality and life history that I had never had before, and I couldn't wait to meet him. I certainly wasn't disappointed, and it was my privilege to be his student and later, to receive his unpublished papers.

Over the years that I knew him, I developed a tremendous appreciation for many aspects of Dr. Dąbrowski, but two particularly stand out. First, in my life experience, he was a unique human being. He had a tremendous energy about him, an animation, a twinkle in his eye, and yet he also had a tremendous sense of calm about him. He was extremely gracious and one of the humblest people I have ever met. Above all, Dąbrowski had a tremendous sense of compassion and an ability to look you in the eye and deeply connect with you—I recall an occasion I was asking him about my anxiety, and he put his hand on my shoulder and said, "Ah yes, but this is not so negative." You couldn't help but feel better after just sitting beside him.

My second appreciation was academic. Dąbrowski, a true Renaissance man, had an astounding command of world cultures, the arts, philosophy, medicine, neurology and, of course, psychiatry and psychology. The list of people Dąbrowski mentored under or worked with is literally a Who's Who of psychiatry and psychology; for example, Błachowski, Mazurkiewicz, Bovet, Piaget, Claparède, Stekel, Janet, Mayer, Mowrer, and Maslow. While many of these people had a major effect on Dąbrowski, his theory stands as a complete and unique system of thought. The more one tries to dissect it, the more its comprehensiveness and integration become obvious. My appreciation for his body of work has grown over the years as I have come to know it more intimately.

Late in his life, Dąbrowski asked me to keep his theory alive after his passing. I have honored his request through my Dąbrowski website (www.positivedisintegration.com/), and by my dissemination of his original writings. There is no question that Dąbrowski left a tremendous legacy, both in terms of his family and in the theory he gave us.

In reflecting back on Dąbrowski, it seems so obvious that he was a human being who lived his theory: he strove to meet his own high standards and acted as an exemplar by action—whatever the peril, you could sense he always chose the higher path in his life.

A-1. DĄBROWSKI'S EARLY LIFE AND EDUCATION

Kazimierz Dąbrowski was born September 1, 1902, in Klarów,

Poland. Dąbrowski's father, Antoni, was an agricultural administrator. Kazimierz was one of four children; he had an older brother and a younger brother and sister. Reflecting on the death of his sister, Dąbrowski (1975) said:

I learned about death very early in my life. Death appeared to me not just something threatening and incomprehensible, but as something that one must experience emotionally and cognitively at a close range. When I was six my little three-year-old sister died of meningitis. (p. 233)

One of the most significant early influences on Dąbrowski was his first-hand experience of World War I. He spoke of being particularly affected by observing the aftermath of a major battle that occurred near his hometown when he was about 12.
Dąbrowski (1975) said:

I remember a battle during the First World War. When the exchange of artillery fire ended, fighting went on with cold steel. When the battle was over, I saw several hundred young soldiers lying dead, their lives cut [short] in a cruel and senseless manner. I witnessed masses of Jewish people being herded toward ghettos. On the way the weak, the invalid, the sick were killed ruthlessly. And then, many times, I myself and my close family and friends have been in the immediate danger of death. The juxtaposition of inhuman forces and inhuman humans with those who were sensitive, capable of sacrifice, courageous, gave a vivid panorama of a scale of values from the lowest to the highest. (p. 233)

As Dąbrowski walked among the dead soldiers lying in his former playfield, he related how he was fascinated by the various positions their bodies took and the different expressions frozen on their faces. Some seemed calm and peaceful while others appeared frightened or horrified (K. Dąbrowski, personal communication, 1977).
Dąbrowski's early education took place at home, where he had a rich family exposure to books and music. His formal education began when he went to the Male College Szkoła Lubelska in Lublin where Catholic priests and pastors schooled him. Among his teachers was

Roman Witold Ingarden (1893-1970) (Kobierzycki, 2000, p. 276). Kobierzycki (2000) said:

In 1921 being still a grammar school student he entered Katolicki Universytet Lubelski, Faculty of Polish Studies as a listener. He also attended philosophy and psychology lectures. Father Jacek Woroniecki (1878-1949) and Henryk Jakubanis (1878-1949) were among his teachers. Before obtaining his secondary school certificate he passed the first and the second-year university exams. (p. 276)

In the autumn of 1923, his education continued in Lublin. He moved to Poznań in 1924 and became a second-year philosophy student at the Adam Mickiewicz University in Poznań. He also attended lectures from Stefan Błachowski (1889-1962), Bogdan Nawroczyński (1882-1974), Stefan Szuman (1889-1972), Florian Znaniecki (1882-1958), Czesław Znamierowski (1888-1967), and Adam Żółtowski (1881-1958) (Gawroński, 1989; Kobierzycki, 2000). During his studies, his best friend and classmate inexplicably committed suicide. At the time, Dąbrowski was uncertain of his future and was contemplating becoming a professional musician. After his friend's suicide, he decided to enter medicine and study human behavior; music became a lifelong and passionate hobby (M. Rankel, personal communication, January, 2007).

After graduating with a degree in philosophy in 1926, Dąbrowski entered Warsaw University, Faculty of Medicine. There, he studied under Edward Loth (1884-1944) and the eminent Polish psychiatrist, Jan Mazurkiewicz (1896-1988). Mazurkiewicz had a profound influence on Dąbrowski's thinking.

In 1928, Dąbrowski was given a grant from the Polish National Culture Foundation to study psychology and education at the Jean-Jacques Rousseau Institute in Geneva, created by the neurologist and child psychologist Édouard Claparède (1873-1940). Claparède recruited philosopher-psychologist Jean Piaget (1896-1980) and the psychologist-educator Pierre Bovet (1878-1965). All three instructed Dąbrowski (Aronson, 1964; Kobierzycki, 2000).

Dąbrowski received his medical degree from the Forensic Medicine Department of the University of Geneva in 1929, completing a doctoral thesis on suicide, entitled *Les Conditions Psycholopique du Suicide* [The Psychological Conditions of Suicide] (Dombrowski, 1929). This work was done under the supervision of Francis Naville (1883-1968).[41] In this thesis, Dąbrowski first used the term "psychic disintegration" (Kobierzycki, 2000).

Dąbrowski's curriculum vitae[42] indicates that in 1929 he also received a Certificat de Pédagogie [Teaching Certificate] from the University of Geneva. After completing his studies at the Jean-Jacques Rousseau Institute in 1931, Dąbrowski was offered an assistant position but decided to return to Poland instead (Kobierzycki, 2000).

Upon his return, Dąbrowski completed a study he had begun under Professor Błachowski and nostrificated a doctorate in psychology from the Adam Mickiewicz University in Poznań, in 1931 (Kobierzycki, 2000). Dąbrowski's thesis, supervised by Błachowski, focused on self-mutilation (Dąbrowski, 1934b) (Kobierzycki, 2000).[43] Dąbrowski also nostrificated a medical diploma from the University of Poznań, 1931 (Kobierzycki, 2000).

From 1931 to 1933, Dąbrowski was a lecturer in Child Psychology and Psychopathology, at the Free Polish University, Warsaw: "In 1931 he organised a clinic for neurotic, mentally disabled and being in moral danger children. In 1932, he established Child Neuropsychiatry Ward in the Public Hospital situated at Złota Street [Warsaw]" (Kobierzycki, 2000, p. 276). Aronson (1964) also indicates that in 1931, Dąbrowski studied child psychiatry in Paris under George Heuyer (1884-1977).

In 1932, Dąbrowski received a two-year research scholarship from the National Culture Fund to study in Vienna and Paris. In Vienna, he studied at the Institute of Active Psychoanalysis under fellow Pole, Wilhelm Stekel (1868-1940), and was given a letter of qualification from Stekel (dated 1934).[44] Kobierzycki (2000) said: "This diploma authorised him to conduct psychoanalysis practice" (p. 276). From 1932 to 1934 Dąbrowski did postgraduate studies in neurology under Otto Mahrburg (1874-1948), developmental psychology studies under Karl Ludwig Bühler (1879-1963) and his wife, Charlotte Bühler (1893-1974); and neurological studies under William Schesinger (Kobierzycki, 2010). During this time, Dąbrowski "met most of the great psychoanalytic personalities, including Sigmund Freud" (K. Dąbrowski, personal communication, 1977).

Kobierzycki (2000) said:

He passed an examination on a thesis on psychopathology of a child presented to qualify himself as assistant professor in 1934 under the guidance of professor E. Claparède and worked with him as privatdozent [a licensed teacher or lecturer] in child psychiatry at the University of Geneva. (p. 276)

Using a grant from the Rockefeller Foundation, in October 1933, Dąbrowski and his first wife went to Harvard University to study at the School of Public Health.[45] From 1933 to 1934, Dąbrowski studied under C. Macfie Campbell (1876-1943), Director of the Boston Psychopathic Hospital and William Healy (1869-1963), first Director of the Judge Baker Foundation (Aronson, 1964). Kobierzycki (2000) said that during this time Dąbrowski also participated in a practice at the clinic of Adolf Mayer (1866-1950) at Johns Hopkins University. Shortly after their return from America, Dąbrowski's wife died of tuberculosis.

In Paris, he took up a practice in clinical psychiatry and psychopathology at the Institute of Mental Prophylaxis and Applied Psychology under the guidance of Jean-Maurice Lahy (1872-1943) and the French neurologist and psychologist Pierre Janet (1859-1947). Dąbrowski noted in his diary:

At that time, I began to clearly crystallize my views on the scope and approaches of multilayered and multi-level mental hygiene, which I began to see as an indispensable science in every department of psychology, psychotherapy, psychiatry and authentic education. I realized more and more that the psychopathological approach is not a simple matter, that it does not express static and statistical abnormality, that high normality meets in this area in the sense of accelerated development, creativity, increased excitability, which is closely related to accelerated development and works. (Gawroński, 1989, p. 3)[46]

Gawroński (1989) indicated Dąbrowski received habilitation in 1934 in the field of child psychopathology and the title of Privatdocent for these studies. In 1934 Dąbrowski published a work on behaviorism (Dąbrowski, 1934a).

Upon Dąbrowski's return to Poland in 1934, he created the Polish League of Mental Hygiene in Warsaw and became its secretary. In 1935, he published *Nervousness of Children and Youth* (Dąbrowski, 1935). With the financial help of the Rockefeller Foundation and the support of the Ministry of Social Welfare, Dąbrowski organised the Institute of Mental Hygiene and became its leader (Kobierzycki, 2000). By 1938, branches of the Institute had been set up in Cieszyn, Gdynia, Kraków, Lublin, Łódź, Stanisławów, Wilno, and Vilnius (Gawroński, 1989; Kobierzycki, 2000). From 1935 to 1948, except for the interruption of the German occupation, Dąbrowski was the director of the Institute (Aronson, 1964). In 1937, Dąbrowski founded the Society of Moral Culture. Also, in 1937, Dąbrowski had his first English publication, "The Psychological Basis of Self-Mutilation," completed with the assistance of C. Macfie Campbell (who also provided a preface) (Dąbrowski, 1937). This monograph was based on his earlier Polish work (Dąbrowski, 1934b). Dąbrowski (1938) followed up with another Polish article, *"Typy wzmozonej pobudliwości psychicznej"* ["Types of increased psychic excitability"]. "In 1939 he bought the Zagórze-Dwór estate in order to create a sanatorium for neurotic children" (Kobierzycki, 2000, p. 277).

In the late 1930's, Dąbrowski was involved with an anthroposophy association in England dedicated to the work of Rudolf Steiner (1861-1925) and run by Alice Bailey (1880-1949) at Cambridge Wells, Kent. Dąbrowski studied Steiner, a polymath best known for developing anthroposophy (a spiritual science), and Waldorf education. Parapsychology and Eastern studies also interested Dąbrowski, and he practiced meditation daily (D. Amend, personal communication, March, 2013).

In 1939 the Germans closed the Institute of Mental Hygiene in Warsaw, and Dąbrowski shifted his operations to the Zagórze estate. A "secret" School of Mental Hygiene and Child Psychiatry was founded at Zagórze, which later was transformed into the College of Mental Hygiene in Warsaw (Kobierzycki, 2010a). "Under conspiratorial conditions, he conducts research and teaching as well as therapeutic and therapeutic activities. Organizes care centers for orphans—war victims" (Gawroński, 1989, p. 3).

A-2. WORLD WAR II

The details of Dąbrowski's life during the war years are sketchy, but there is no doubt that they were very difficult. Dąbrowski said that during his wartime experiences, he saw examples of both the lowest possible inhuman behavior as well as acts of the highest human character (K. Dąbrowski, personal communication, 1979). There were times during the war when Dąbrowski's life hung in the balance, and on at least one occasion his family and friends considered him lost (K. Dąbrowski, personal communication, 1979). Aronson indicated that "of the 400 Polish psychiatrists practicing before the war . . . only thirty-eight survived" (Aronson, 1964, p. x).

Dąbrowski's younger brother was killed in 1941, while his older brother was captured in the Warsaw Insurrection and sent to a concentration camp. In 1942, Dąbrowski founded the College of Mental Hygiene and Applied Psychology, which obtained academic rights granted by Polish underground authorities. Clandestine lectures were given by Sergiusz Hessen (1887-1950), Maria Grzywak-Kaczyńska (1886-1979), Piotr Radło (?-1946) and Adam Kunicki (1903-1989) (Gawroński, 1989). Due to co-operation with Polish underground authorities, Dąbrowski was able to provide a hiding-place to soldiers of Armia Krajowa, refugees from the Warsaw ghetto, as well as doctors and priests "acting in conspiracy." Kobierzycki (2000) said:

> In autumn 1942 Dąbrowski was arrested by Gestapo and put into jail together with Maria Zebrowska in Aleja Szucha and Pawiak in Warsaw at first and later in Montelupich in Kraków. After a few month investigation Dąbrowski was set free and came back to his work to Zagórze. (p. 277)

Dąbrowski was arrested more than once, perhaps as many as three or four times, and his second wife, Eugenia (whom he married in 1940), obtained his release by paying ransom money to prison officials (A. Kawczak, personal communication, 2002).[47] Contrary to Battaglia (2002), Dąbrowski was never held in Auschwitz (J. Dąbrowski, personal communication, 2002). Kobierzycki (2000) indicated that Dąbrowski had planned to use the Institute as a hospital for insurgents in preparation for a Warsaw uprising, but that these plans were never realized. After the war, Dąbrowski returned to Warsaw and resumed his former position of director of the Institute of Mental Hygiene, it now being transformed into the High School of Mental Hygiene, and by 1948 there were 12 branches and 20 dispensaries (Kobierzycki, 2000).

Dąbrowski obtained his specialty as a psychiatrist in June 1948 under Adrian Demianowski (1887-1959) at Wrocław University (Kobierzycki, 2000).[48] Also, in 1948, he founded and became president of the Polish Society of Mental Hygiene. In December 1948, Dąbrowski received a six-month Ford Foundation Fellowship, and he returned to the United States where he studied mental health, neuropsychiatry, and child psychiatry in New York and at Harvard (Kobierzycki, 2000). In 1949/1950, some 500 students attended (Gawroński, 1989).

A-3. IMPRISONMENT UNDER STALIN AND "REHABILITATION"

In April 1949, the Polish Government under Stalin closed the Institute of Mental Hygiene and confiscated the Zagórze-Dwór estate. In May 1950, Dąbrowski was declared a *persona non grata* and transferred to the position of director of a psychiatric hospital in Świecie (Gawroński, 1989). Attempting to flee Poland, Dąbrowski and his wife secretly arranged passage, and on the night before they left, they went to their best friends to say goodbye. Their friends (a couple) turned them in to the authorities in exchange for political immunity. This was a devastating betrayal to Dąbrowski (P. Roland, personal communication, 1990).

The Polish communists imprisoned Dąbrowski in 1950 for some eighteen months (and Eugenia was briefly imprisoned as well). Our only insight into his treatment during this imprisonment was a comment he made after he had his 1979 heart attack, to the effect that, the torture he had sustained in prison had weakened his heart (K. Dąbrowski, personal communication, 1979). When released, Dąbrowski's activities were kept under strict control. He was assigned work as the head of the psychiatric hospital in Kobierzyn (Gawroński, 1989) and later at the Rabka resort, as a tuberculosis physician.

In 1956, Dąbrowski was declared "rehabilitated" and was again allowed to teach, securing an associate professorship at the Catholic Academy of Theology in Warsaw (Kobierzycki, 2000). In January 1958, the Polish Academy of Sciences employed Dąbrowski as a professor. He reorganized the Department of Mental Hygiene and Child Psychiatry and began research on school youth, "especially highly talented youth" (Gawroński, 1989).

A-4. THE 1960S: DĄBROWSKI ESTABLISHES ROOTS IN NORTH AMERICA

Dąbrowski was able to reinvigorate the Polish Society of Mental Hygiene and in 1962 became its chairman, but he was unable to re-establish the Institute of Mental Hygiene and the High School of Mental Hygiene (Kobierzycki, 2000).

In 1962, Dąbrowski was allowed to travel and with the support of the Ford Foundation went to the United States and France, and was able to attend several international psychiatry congresses (for example, in Spain, France and England). On his return to Poland, Dąbrowski gave lectures at the Catholic University in Lublin.[49]

In the early 1960s, Jason Aronson, editor of *The International Journal of Psychiatry*, traveled behind the iron curtain to invite psychiatrists to submit articles for his journal and he met Dąbrowski in Poland. In 1964, Dąbrowski and Aronson spent two months in New York, translating material[50] that became Dąbrowski's first major book in English, *Positive Disintegration* (Dąbrowski, 1964b). Aronson edited and wrote an introduction for the book. Aronson subsequently published the first chapters of the book in his journal (Aronson, 1966; Dąbrowski, 1966).

Dąbrowski also visited Canada in 1964 at the invitation of the Ministry of Health in Québec and accepted a position at a hospital in Montréal. While in Montréal, he met Andrew [Andrzej] Kawczak

(1926-), a Polish lawyer and subsequently a philosopher, who became an important collaborator. Dąbrowski's second major English publication, *Personality Shaping Through Positive Disintegration,* grew out of discussions with Kawczak and some of Kawczak's graduate students (Dąbrowski, 1967). American learning theorist O. Herbert Mowrer (1907-1982) wrote an introduction to the book.

In 1965, Dąbrowski secured a visiting professorship at the University of Alberta and moved his family to Edmonton. He also held a visiting professorship at Université Laval (Laval University), Québec City, and gave lectures at Feminina University[51] in Lima, Peru, where Sister Alvarez Calderon taught Dąbrowski's theory.

Kobierzycki (2000) indicates that in 1966, "Dąbrowski and his family took advantage of Wanda Rohr Foundation de Connecticut and met with Abraham Maslow, who was interested in his theory" (p. 278). Maslow and Dąbrowski had lengthy discussions and became friends and correspondents. In spite of their differences, Maslow endorsed Dąbrowski's 1970 book, *Mental Growth Through Positive Disintegration,* saying:

> I consider this to be one of the most important contributions to psychological and psychiatric theory in this whole decade. There is little question in my mind that this book will be read for another decade or two and very widely. It digs very deep and comes up with extremely important conclusions that will certainly change the course of psychological theorizing and the practice of psychotherapy for some time to come. (Maslow in Dąbrowski, 1972b, back cover)

Kobierzycki (2000) also said that shortly before Maslow's death in 1970, he had arranged an invitation for Dąbrowski to become leader of the Institute of Psychology at the University of Cincinnati.[52]

A core group of students formed in Edmonton, and several went on to become Dąbrowski's co-authors, including Dexter Amend, Michael M. Piechowski, and Marlene Rankel. In 1969, a series of successful applications were made to the Canada Council to support research on the theory.

A-5. THE 1970S: A FINAL FLURRY OF ACTIVITY

In 1970 Dąbrowski organized an International Conference on the theory at the University of Laval (Québec). Several Polish scholars attended, including Zygmunt A. Piotrowski (1904-1985) and Tadeusz Romer (1894-1978), Director of the Polish Institute of Arts and Science in Canada (Gawroński, 1989). In December 1972, Dąbrowski organized a second International Conference at Loyola College in Montréal.

Dąbrowski spent his last years teaching, writing, and dividing his time among Alberta, Québec and Poland. Several Polish and English publications were the result of this last flurry of activity, including *Mental Growth Though Positive Disintegration* (Dąbrowski, 1970b), *Psychoneurosis is Not an Illness* (Dąbrowski, 1972b), *Dynamics of Concepts* (Dąbrowski, 1973), and the two-volume *Multilevelness of Emotional and Instinctive Functions* (Dąbrowski, 1996; Dąbrowski & Piechowski, 1996). Dąbrowski also maintained a hectic schedule, speaking extensively in both Canada and the United States.

Dąbrowski utilized help in translation from Aronson (Dąbrowski, 1964b), Kawczak (Dąbrowski, 1967) and Piechowski (Dąbrowski, 1970b). He was fluent enough in English to translate several volumes himself (Dąbrowski, 1972b, 1973, 1996). However, many of his Polish publications remain untranslated. Several of his twenty or so major Polish books were also published in French and Spanish. There were major Dąbrowski centers in Spain and in Lima, Peru, where in 1970, Dąbrowski attended the "Congress of the World Federation of Psychic [Mental] Health" (Kobierzycki, 2000).

During the 1970s, Dąbrowski regularly visited Poland. He still maintained his involvement in the Polish Society of Mental Hygiene. "In 1975, he purchased the estate in Aleksandrów bordering to Zagórze and erected buildings with a view to create a scientific and dispensary center there" (Kobierzycki, 2000, p. 279).

In the fall of 1976, I went to the University of Alberta and began a master's program. I came to the attention of Marlene Rankel, who was teaching a course in developmental psychology. She introduced me to Dąbrowski, and I became his student.

In 1977, Dąbrowski organized a "Center of Mental Hygiene for

People of Health" in Warsaw (Gawroński, 1989). In 1979, Dąbrowski asked me to perpetuate his theory after he passed on. In 1979, Dąbrowski had a serious heart attack in Edmonton but was able to return to Poland. He died in Warsaw on November 26, 1980. At his request, Dąbrowski was buried beside his friend and fellow physician, Piotr Radło, in the forest near the Institute at Zagórze. His wife, Eugenia and two daughters, Joanna and Anna, survived him.

A-6. DISSEMINATION OF DĄBROWSKI'S LEGACY

A memorial conference was held for Dr. Dąbrowski in Edmonton in November of 1982. By then, I was a psychologist working with the Government of Alberta; however, over the years, a priority of mine was to keep Dąbrowski's theory alive by maintaining an archive containing his original writings and collections of publications related to his theory. With the development of the World Wide Web, in 1995, I established and continue to maintain the Dąbrowski website (see above). With permission, I have made Dąbrowski's original writings available to interested parties and I have participated in and hosted conferences on the theory. Many of Dąbrowski's original writings are held at the Library and Archives Canada, Ottawa.

One area where Dąbrowski's theory is alive and well is in the study of giftedness and gifted education. In 1965, Dąbrowski published a paper on psychoneuroses in gifted youth. He conducted examinations and testing of children who displayed superior abilities and reported his findings (Dąbrowski, 1967, 1972b). He found that every child displayed characteristics suggestive of positive disintegration, including developmental potential and psychoneurosis. Piechowski (1979, 1991) subsequently introduced Dąbrowski's construct of overexcitability, a component of developmental potential, to the field of gifted education and over the past 35+ years, many research projects and papers have addressed the topic (Mendaglio & Tillier, 2006).

A-7. DĄBROWSKI CONFERENCES

Over the years, many Dąbrowski-related workshops have been held, as have a number of major conferences, including Université Laval (Laval University), Québec City, QC (1970); Loyola College, Montréal, QC (1972); Miami, FL (1980); Warsaw, Poland (1987); Keystone, CO (1994); Kananaskis, AB (1996); Kendall College, Evanston, IL (1998); Mont-Tremblant, QC (2000); Fort Lauderdale, FL (2002); Calgary, AB (2004, 2006, and 2016); Canmore, AB (2008, 2014); St. Charles, IL (2010); and Denver, CO (2012).

An important part of continuing Dąbrowski's legacy has been maintaining friendships with former students of Dąbrowski, who have contributed to the dissemination of the theory in their own ways.

A-8. SCIENTIFIC MEMBERSHIPS

Kazimierz Dąbrowski was a member of many scientific societies, among others, the French Société Médico-psychologique (Paris), affiliate of the Royal Medical Society (London), the Executive Council of World Federation of Mental Health (Geneva), the Psychologists Association of Alberta (Edmonton), the Corporation des Psychologues (Québec), and the Polish Psychiatric Association (Warsaw) (Kobierzycki, 2000).

A-9. OTHER ACCOMPLISHMENTS

Dąbrowski was the founder and editor of *The Biuletyn Instytutu Higieny Psychicznej*, Warsaw, 1937-1939, 1946-1949, and 1958-1965. He was also the editor of a scientific and popular series in the field of mental health published by the Institute of Mental Hygienen, Warsaw, 1937-1939, and 1946-1949.

Dąbrowski's publications number in the hundreds in Polish, including some 20 major books. Translations into French, Spanish, German, and English have been made of many of these books.

APPENDIX 2

SELECTED RESOURCES RELATING TO DĄBROWSKI, 2006-2017

[Not otherwise referred to in the text].

• of particular importance

2006

> Bain, Choate, & Bliss, 2006; • Mendaglio & Peterson, 2006; • Piechowski, 2006; Probst, 2006; Treat, 2006; Yakmaci-Guzel & Akarsu, 2006.

2007

> • Tieso, 2007a; • Tieso, 2007b.

2008

> Falk, Yakmaci-Guzel, Chang, Pardo, & Chavez-Eakle, 2008; • Mendaglio, 2008a; • Mendaglio, 2008b; • Mendaglio, 2008c; Piirto, Montgomery, & May, 2008.

2009

• Ackerman, 2009; • Ackerman & Moyle, 2009a; •
Ackerman & Moyle, 2009b; Forstadt, 2009; Forstadt &
Shaine, 2009; Jackson & Moyle, 2009; Jackson, Moyle, &
Piechowski, 2009; Juntune, 2009; • Kane, 2009; Laycraft,
2009; Miller, Falk, & Huang, 2009; Mroz, 2009;
Piechowski, 2009a; Piechowski, 2009b; Silverman, 2009;
Tieso, 2009; Tillier, 2009.

2010

Dąbrowski, 2010a; Dąbrowski, 2010b; Dąbrowski, 2010c;
Dziekanowski, 2010; Hague, 2010; Hyzy, 2010; •
Kobierzycki, 2010b; Nixon, 2010; Piechowski, 2010;
Piirto, 2010a; Piirto, 2010b; Rinn, Mendaglio, Rudasill, &
McQueen, 2010; Romanowska–Lakomy, 2010; Siu, 2010.

2011

C. L. Bailey, 2011; Dai, Swanson, & Cheng, 2011;
Jennaway & Merrotsy, 2011; Laycraft, 2011; Wirthwein,
Becker, & Loehr, 2011; Wirthwein & Rost, 2011.

2012

Burge, 2012; Nixon, 2012; Piirto & Fraas, 2012; Probst &
Piechowski, 2012.

2013

Alias, Rahman, Majid, & Yassin, 2013; Chang & Kuo,
2013; Romey, 2013.

2014

Acevedo et al, 2014; Battaglia, 2014; Battaglia,
Mendaglio, & Piechowski, 2014; He & Wong, 2014; •
Piechowski, 2014a; Piechowski, 2014b; Silverman &

• Piechowski, 2014a; Piechowski, 2014b; Silverman &
Miller, 2014; Van den Broeck, Hofmans, Cooremans, &
Staels, 2014; S. White, 2014; • Winkler, 2014.

2015

• Dąbrowski, 2015; De Bondt & Van Petegem, 2015;
• Kaufman & Gregoire, 2015; Olszewski-Kubilius, 2015;
Parker Peters, 2015; Perrone-McGovern, Simon-Dack,
Beduna, Williams, & Esche, 2015; Piechowski, 2015.

2016

Ataria, 2016; Beduna & Perrone-McGovern, 2016; •
Dąbrowski, 2016; Her & Haron, 2016; Silverman, 2016;
Thomson & Jaque, 2016a; Thomson & Jaque, 2016b;
Tillier, 2016.

2017

Chia, 2017; Chia & Lim, 2017; De Bondt & Van Petegem,
2017; Eiserman, Lai, & Rushton, 2017; Falk, 2017; •
Harper & Clifford, 2017; • Harper, Cornish, Smith, &
Merrotsy, 2017; Lamare, 2017; Leavitt, 2017; Mika, 2017;
Piechowski, 2017: • Tillier, 2017.

Abbey, R. (2004). Introduction: Timely meditations in an untimely mode—the thought of Charles Taylor. In R. Abbey, (Ed.), *Charles Taylor* (pp. 1–28). New York, NY: Cambridge University Press.

Abraído-Lanza, A. F., Guier, C., & Colón, R. M. (2010). Psychological thriving among Latinas with chronic illness. *Journal of Social Issues, 54*(2), 405–424. https://doi.org/10.1111/j.1540-4560.1998.tb01227.x

Acevedo, B. P., Aron, E. N., Aron, A., Sangster, M. D., Collins, N., & Brown, L. L. (2014). The highly sensitive brain: An fMRI study of sensory processing sensitivity and response to others' emotions. *Brain and Behavior, 4*(4), 580–594. https://doi.org/10.1002/brb3.242

Ackerman, C. M. (1997). Identifying gifted adolescents using personality characteristics: Dąbrowski's overexcitabilities. *Roeper Review, 19*(4), 229–236. https://doi.org/10.1080/02783199709553835

Ackerman, C. M. (2009). The essential elements of Dąbrowski's theory of positive disintegration and how they are connected. *Roeper Review, 31*(2), 81–95. https://doi.org/10.1080/02783190902737657

Ackerman, C. M., & Moyle, V. F. (Eds.). (2009a). Introduction [Special issue]. *Roeper Review, 31*(2), 79–80. https://doi.org/10.1080/02783190902737640

Ackerman, C. M. & Moyle, V. F. (Eds.). (2009b). Introduction [Special issue]. *Roeper Review, 31*(3), 140. https://doi.org/10.1080/02783190902993565

Ackley, D. (2016). Emotional intelligence: A practical review of models, measures, and applications. *Consulting Psychology*

Journal: Practice and Research, 68(4), 269–286.
https://doi.org/10.1037/cpb0000070

Adams, T. V. (2016). *The psychopath factory: How capitalism organises empathy.* London, England: Repeater.

Addington, E. L., Tedeschi, R. G., & Calhoun, L. G. (2016). A growth perspective on post-traumatic stress. In A. M. Wood & J. Johnson (Eds.), *The Wiley handbook of positive clinical psychology* (pp. 223–231). Chichester, West Sussex, UK: Wiley/Blackwell.

Adrian, M., Miller, A. B., McCauley, E., & Vander Stoep, A. (2016). Suicidal ideation in early to middle adolescence: Sex-specific trajectories and predictors. *Journal of Child Psychology and Psychiatry, 57*(5), 645–653.
https://doi.org/10.1111/jcpp.12484

Akhtar, R., Ahmetoglu, G., & Chamorro-Premuzic, T. (2013). Greed is good? Assessing the relationship between entrepreneurship and subclinical psychopathy. *Personality and Individual Differences, 54*(3), 420–425.
https://doi.org/10.1016/j.paid.2012.10.013

Al-Onizat, S. H. (2013). The psychometric properties of a Jordanian version of overexcitability questionnaire-two, OEQII. *Creative Education, 4*(1), 49–61. https://doi.org/10.4236/ce.2013.41008

Alias, A., Rahman, S., Majid, R. A., & Yassin, S. F. M. (2013). Dąbrowski's overexcitabilities profile among gifted students. *Asian Social Science, 9*(16), 120–126.
https://doi.org/10.5539/ass.v9n16p120

Allport, G. W. (1969). Personality: Normal and abnormal. In H. Chiang & A. H. Maslow (Eds.), *The healthy personality: Readings* (pp. 1–15). New York, NY: Van Nostrand Reinhold.

Ambrose, D., Van Tassel-Baska, J., Coleman, L. J., & Cross, T. L. (2010). Unified, insular, firmly policed, or fractured, porous, contested, gifted education? *Journal for the Education of the Gifted, 33*(4), 453–478.
https://doi.org/10.1177/016235321003300402

Amend, D. (2008). Creativity in Dąbrowski and the Theory of Positive Disintegration. In S. Mendaglio (Ed.), *Dąbrowski's theory of positive disintegration* (pp. 123–137). Scottsdale AZ: Great Potential Press.

Ament, S. A., Szelinger, S., Glusman, G., Ashworth, J., Hou, L.,
     Akula, N., . . . Roach, J. C. (2015). Rare variants in neuronal
     excitability genes influence risk for bipolar disorder.
     *Proceedings of the National Academy of Sciences of the
     United States of America, 112*(11), 3576–81.
     https://doi.org/10.1073/pnas.1424958112
American Psychiatric Association. (1952). *Diagnostic and statistical
     manual of mental disorders* (1st ed.). Washington, DC:
     Author.
American Psychiatric Association. (1968). *Diagnostic and statistical
     manual of mental disorders* (2nd ed.). Washington, DC:
     Author.
American Psychiatric Association. (1980). *Diagnostic and statistical
     manual of mental disorders* (3rd ed.). Washington, DC:
     Author.
American Psychiatric Association. (2013). *Diagnostic and statistical
     manual of mental disorders* (5th ed.). Washington, DC:
     Author.
Arasteh, A. Reza (1965a). Final integration in the adult personality.
     American Journal of Psychoanalysis, 25(1), 61–73.
     https://doi.org/10.1007/BF01872032
Arasteh, A. Reza (1965b). *Final integration in the adult personality:
     A measure for health, social change and leadership.* Leiden,
     Netherlands: E. J. Brill.
Arasteh, A. Reza (1965c). Normative psychoanalysis: A theory and
     technique for the development of healthy integration. *The
     Journal of General Psychology, 73*(1), 81–91.
     https://doi.org/10.1080/00221309.1965.9711255
Arasteh, A. Reza (1975). *Toward a final personality integration: A
     measure for health, social change and leadership* (2nd ed.).
     New York, NY: Schenkman.
Arasteh, A. Reza (1990). *Growth to selfhood: The Sufi contribution to
     Islam.* London, England, Arkana. (Original work published
     1980)
Arasteh, A. Reza (2008). *Rumi the Persian, The Sufi.* Routledge
     Library Editions: Islam, Vol. 40. Oxon, UK: Routledge.
     (Original work published 1974)

Arikan, G., Stopa, L., Carnelley, K. B., & Karl, A. (2016). The associations between adult attachment, posttraumatic symptoms, and posttraumatic growth. *Anxiety, Stress, & Coping, 29*(1), 1–20. https://doi.org/10.1080/10615806.2015.1009833

Armstrong, L. (2014). *Epigenetics*. New York, NY: Garland.

Aron, E. N. (1996). *The highly sensitive person: How to thrive when the world overwhelms you.* Secaucus, NJ: Birch Lane Press.

Aron, E. N. (2002). *The highly sensitive child: Helping our children thrive when the world overwhelms them.* New York, NY: Harmony.

Aron, E. N. (2006). The clinical implications of Jung's concept of sensitiveness. *Journal of Jungian Theory and Practice, 8*(2). 11–43.

Aron, E. N. (2010). *Psychotherapy and the highly sensitive person: Improving outcomes for that minority of people who are the majority of clients.* New York, NY: Routledge.

Aron, E. N. (2012). Temperament in psychotherapy: Reflections on clinical practice with the trait of sensitivity. In M. Zentner & R. L. Shiner (Eds.), *Handbook of temperament* (pp. 645–672). New York, NY: Guilford Press.

Aron, E. N., & Aron, A. (1997). Sensory-processing sensitivity and its relation to introversion and emotionality. *Journal of Personality and Social Psychology, 73*(2), 345–368. https://doi.org/10.1037/0022-3514.73.2.345

Aron, E. N., Aron, A., & Jagiellowicz, J. (2012). Sensory processing sensitivity. *Personality and Social Psychology Review, 16*(3), 262–282. https://doi.org/10.1177/1088868311434213

Aronson, J. (1964). Introduction. In K. Dąbrowski, *Positive disintegration* (pp. ix–xxviii). Boston, MA: Little, Brown and Company.

Aronson, J. (1966). Discussion of K. Dąbrowski: The theory of positive disintegration. *International Journal of Psychiatry, 2*, 244–247.

Ashcroft, A. (2016). Donald Trump: Narcissist, psychopath or representative of the people? *Psychotherapy and Politics International, 14*(3), 217–222. https://doi.org/10.1002/ppi.1395

Ataria, Y. (2016). Traumatic and mystical experiences: The dark nights of the soul. *Journal of Humanistic Psychology, 56*(4), 331–356. https://doi.org/10.1177/0022167814563143

Babiak, P., & Hare, R. D. (2006). *Snakes in suits: When psychopaths go to work.* New York, NY: HarperCollins.

Babiak, P., Neumann, C. S., & Hare, R. D. (2010). Corporate psychopathy: Talking the walk. *Behavioral Sciences & the Law, 28*(2), 174–193. https://doi.org/10.1002/bsl.925

Bacharach, B. (Composer), & David, H. (Lyricist). (1964). (There's) Always something there to remind me [Recorded by R. B. Greaves] On *R. B. Greaves* [Vinyl record]. New York, NY: ATCO Records. (1969)

Bäckström, M., Larsson, M. R., & Maddux, R. E. (2009). A structural validation of an inventory based on the Abridged Five Factor Circumplex Model (AB5C). *Journal of Personality Assessment, 91*(5), 462–472. https://doi.org/10.1080/00223890903088065

Bacon, A. M., & Corr, P. J. (2017). Motivating emotional intelligence: A reinforcement sensitivity theory (RST) perspective. *Motivation and Emotion, 41*(2), 254–264. https://doi.org/10.1007/s11031-017-9602-1

Bailey, C. L. (2011). An examination of the relationships between ego development, Dąbrowski's Theory of Positive Disintegration, and the behavioral characteristics of gifted adolescents. *Gifted Child Quarterly 55*(3), 208–222. https://doi.org/10.1177/0016986211412180

Bailey, K. G. (1987). *Human paleopsychology: Applications to aggression and pathological processes.* Hillside, NJ: Lawrence Erlbaum.

Bain, S. K., Choate, S. M., & Bliss, S. L. (2006). Perceptions of developmental, social, and emotional issues in giftedness: Are they realistic? *Roeper Review, 29*(1), 41–48. https://doi.org/10.1080/02783190609554383

Baker, J. (1995). Depression and suicidal ideation among academically gifted adolescents. *Gifted Child Quarterly, 39*(4), 218–223. https://doi.org/10.1177/001698629503900405

Barchard, K. A., Brackett, M. A., & Mestre, J. M. (2016). Taking stock and moving forward: 25 years of emotional intelligence

research. *Emotion Review, 8*(4), 289–289.
https://doi.org/10.1177/1754073916650562

Barcia, J. R., & Zeitlin, M. A. (Eds.). (1967). *Unamuno creator and creation.* Berkeley, CA: University of California Press.

Bateson, P., & Martin, P. (2000). *Design for a life: How behaviour and personality develop.* New York, NY: Simon & Schuster.

Battaglia, M. M. K. (2002). *A hermeneutic historical study of Kazimierz Dąbrowski and his Theory of Positive Disintegration.* Unpublished doctoral dissertation. Virginia Polytechnic Institute and State University, Falls Church, Virginia. Retrieved from https://vtechworks.lib.vt.edu/bitstream/handle/10919/26692/Dissertation.pdf?sequence=2

Battaglia, M. M. K. (2014). The life of Kazimierz Dąbrowski (1902-1980). *Advanced Development, 14*, 12–28.

Battaglia, M. M. K., Mendaglio, S., & Piechowski, M. M. (2014). Kazimierz Dąbrowski: A life of positive maladjustment (1902-1980). In A. Robinson & J. L. Jolly, (Eds.), *Century of contributions to gifted education: Illuminating lives* (pp. 181–198). Florence, KY: Taylor and Francis.

Batty, G. D., Deary, I. J., Schoon, I., Emslie, C., Hunt, K., & Gale, C. R. (2008). Childhood mental ability and adult alcohol intake and alcohol problems: The 1970 British cohort study. *American Journal of Public Health, 98*(12), 2237–43. https://doi.org/10.2105/AJPH.2007.109488

Baum, S. M., & Olenchak, F. R. (2002). The alphabet children: GT, ADHD and more. *Exceptionality, 10*(2), 77–91. https://doi.org/10.1207/S15327035EX1002_3

Baumeister, R. F., Vohs, K. D., DeWall, C. N., & Zhang, L. (2007). How emotion shapes behavior: Feedback, anticipation and reflection, rather than direct causation. *Personality and Social Psychology Review, 11*(2), 167–203. https://doi.org/10.1177/1088868307301033

Baxter Magolda, M. B. (1998). Developing self-authorship in graduate school. *New Directions for Higher Education, 1998*(101), 41–54. https://doi.org/10.1002/he.10104

Baxter Magolda, M. B. (2001). *Making their own way: Narratives for transforming higher education to promote self-development.* Sterling, VA: Stylus.

Baxter Magolda, M. B. (2008). Three elements of self-authorship. *Journal of College Student Development, 49*(4), 269–284. https://doi.org/10.1353/csd.0.0016

Baxter Magolda, M. B., & King, P. M. (Eds.). (2012). Assessing meaning making and self-authorship [Special issue]. *ASHE Higher Education Report, 38*(3), 1–138. https://doi.org/10.1002/aehe.20003

Bear, M. F., Conners, B. W., & Paradiso, M. A. (2007). *Neuroscience: Exploring the brain* (3rd ed.). Baltimore, MD: Lippincott Williams & Wilkins.

Beaty, R. E., Kaufman, S. B., Benedek, M., Jung, R. E., Kenett, Y. N., Jauk, E., . . . Silvia, P. J. (2016). Personality and complex brain networks: The role of openness to experience in default network efficiency. *Human Brain Mapping, 37*(2), 773–779. https://doi.org/10.1002/hbm.23065

Beck, D., & Cowan, C. (1996). *Spiral dynamics: Mastering values, leadership and change.* Hoboken, NJ: Blackwell.

Beduna, K., & Perrone-McGovern, K. M. (2016). Relationships among emotional and intellectual overexcitability, emotional IQ, and subjective well-being. *Roeper Review, 38*(1), 24–31. https://doi.org/10.1080/02783193.2015.1112862

Bennet, E. A. (1983). *What Jung really said* (2nd ed.). New York, NY: Schocken. (Original work published 1966)

Berger, R. (2015). *Stress, trauma, and posttraumatic growth: Social context, environment, and identities.* New York, NY: Routledge.

Bergson, H. (1911). Life and consciousness. *Hibbert Journal, X*(1), 24–44.

Bergson, H. (1922) *Creative evolution* (A. Mitchell, Trans.). London, England: Macmillan. (Original work published 1911)

Bernier, M. (2015). *The task of hope in Kierkegaard.* Oxford, UK: Oxford University Press.

Bertalanffy, L. von. (1967). *Robots, men and minds: Psychology in the modern world.* New York, NY: George Braziller.

Bertini, K. (2016). *Suicide prevention.* Santa Barbara, CA: Praeger.

Bihan, D. L. (2015). *Looking inside the brain: The power of neuroimaging*. Princeton, NJ: Princeton University Press.

Binder, E. B. (2016). The importance of understanding the biological mechanisms of trauma. *Acta Psychiatrica Scandinavica, 134*(4), 279–280. https://doi.org/10.1111/acps.12635

Blackie, L. E. R., Jayawickreme, E., Tsukayama, E., Forgeard, M. J. C., Roepke, A. M., & Fleeson, W. (2016). Post-traumatic growth as positive personality change: Developing a measure to assess within-person variability. *Journal of Research in Personality, 69*, 22–32. https://doi.org/10.1016/j.jrp.2016.04.001

Blair, C., & Dennis, T. A. (2010). In S. Calkins & M. Bell (Eds.), *Child development at the intersection of emotion and cognition* (pp. 17–35). Washington, DC: American Psychological Association.

Blair, R. J. R. (2001). Advances in neuropsychiatry: Neurocognitive models of aggression, the antisocial personality disorders, and psychopathy. *Journal of Neurology, Neurosurgery & Psychiatry, 71*(6), 727–731. https://doi.org/10.1136/jnnp.71.6.727

Bloch, M. H. (2016). Editorial: Reducing adolescent suicide. *Journal of Child Psychology and Psychiatry, 57*(7), 773–774. https://doi.org/10.1111/jcpp.12585

Bloom, P. (2017). Empathy and its discontents. *Trends in Cognitive Sciences, 21*(1), 24–31. https://doi.org/10.1016/j.tics.2016.11.004

Boddy, C. (2011). *Corporate psychopaths: Organisational destroyers*. New York, NY: Palgrave Macmillan.

Boddy, C. R. (2014). Corporate psychopaths, conflict, employee affective well-being and counterproductive work behaviour. *Journal of Business Ethics, 121*(1), 107–121. https://doi.org/10.1007/s10551-013-1688-0

Bonanno, G. A. (2004). Loss, trauma, and human resilience: Have we underestimated the human capacity to thrive after extremely aversive events? *American Psychologist, 59*(1), 20–28. https://doi.org/10.1037/0003-066X.59.1.20

Bonanno, G. A., Westphal, M., & Mancini, A. D. (2011). Resilience to loss and potential trauma. *Annual Review of Clinical*

Psychology, 7, 511–535. https://doi.org/10.1146/annurev-clinpsy-032210-104526

Boniwell, I. (2012). *Positive psychology in a nutshell: The science of happiness* (3rd ed.). Berkshire, England: Open University Press.

Borland, J. H. (Ed.). (2003). *Rethinking gifted education.* New York, NY: Teachers College Press.

Borland, J. H. (2009). Myth 2: The gifted constitute 3% to 5% of the population. moreover, giftedness equals high IQ, which is a stable measure of aptitude: Spinal tap psychometrics in gifted education. *Gifted Child Quarterly, 53*(4), 236–238. https://doi.org/10.1177/0016986209346825

Bostwick, J. M., Pabbati, C., Geske, J. R., & McKean, A. J. (2016). Suicide attempt as a risk factor for completed suicide: Even more lethal than we knew. *American Journal of Psychiatry, 173*(11), 1094–1100. https://doi.org/10.1176/appi.ajp.2016.15070854

Boterberg, S., & Warreyn, P. (2016). Making sense of it all: The impact of sensory processing sensitivity on daily functioning of children. *Personality and Individual Differences, 92*, 80–86. https://doi.org/10.1016/j.paid.2015.12.022

Bratter, T. E. (2003). Surviving suicide: Treatment challenges for gifted, angry, drug dependent adolescents. *International Journal of Reality Therapy, 22*, 32–37.

Braun, C., Bschor, T., Franklin, J., & Baethge, C. (2016). Suicides and suicide attempts during long-term treatment with antidepressants: A meta-analysis of 29 placebo-controlled studies including 6,934 patients with major depressive disorder. *Psychotherapy and Psychosomatics, 85*(3), 171–179. https://doi.org/10.1159/000442293

Brent, D. A. (2018). Contraceptive conundrum: Use of hormonal contraceptives is associated with an increased risk of suicide attempt and suicide. *American Journal of Psychiatry, 175*(4), 300–302. https://doi.org/10.1176/appi.ajp.2018.18010039

Brent, D. A., Poling, D., Goldstein, T. R., & Poling, K. D. (2011). *Treating depressed and suicidal adolescents: A clinician's guide.* New York, NY: Guilford.

Bridge, J. A., Horowitz, L. M., & Campo, J. V. (2017). ED-SAFE—Can suicide risk screening and brief intervention initiated in the emergency department save lives? *JAMA Psychiatry, 294*(5), 623–624. https://doi.org/10.1001/jamapsychiatry.2017.0677

Brodsky, B. S. (2016). Early childhood environment and genetic interactions: the diathesis for suicidal behavior. *Current Psychiatry Reports, 18,* 86. https://doi.org/10.1007/s11920-016-0716-z

Brown, L. A., Armey, M. A., Sejourne, C., Miller, I. W., & Weinstock, L. M. (2016). Trauma history is associated with prior suicide attempt history in hospitalized patients with major depressive disorder. *Psychiatry Research, 243,* 191–197. https://doi.org/10.1016/j.psychres.2016.06.046

Brown, R. E., & Milner, P. M. (2003). The legacy of Donald O. Hebb: More than the Hebb synapse. *Nature Reviews Neuroscience, 4,* 1013–1019. https://doi.org/10.1038/nrn1257

Brundin, L., Bryleva, E. Y., & Thirtamara-Rajamani, K. (2017). Role of inflammation in suicide: From mechanisms to treatment. *Neuropsychopharmacology, 42,* 271–283. https://doi.org/10.1038/npp.2016.116

Brundin, L., & Grit, J. (2016). Ascertaining whether suicides are caused by infections. *JAMA Psychiatry, 73*(9), 895–896. https://doi.org/10.1001/jamapsychiatry.2016.1470

Brundin, L., Sellgren, C. M., Lim, C. K., Grit, J., Pålsson, E., Landén, M., . . . Erhardt, S. (2016). An enzyme in the kynurenine pathway that governs vulnerability to suicidal behavior by regulating excitotoxicity and neuroinflammation. *Translational Psychiatry, 6,* e865. https://doi.org/10.1038/tp.2016.133

Bucke, R. M. (Ed.). (1905). *Cosmic consciousness: A study in the evolution of the human mind.* Philadelphia, PA: Innes. (Original work published in 1901)

Bullmore, E., & Sporns, O. (2009). Complex brain networks: Graph theoretical analysis of structural and functional systems. *Nature Reviews Neuroscience, 10*(3), 186–198. https://doi.org/10.1038/nrn2575

Buntins, M., Buntins, K., & Eggert, F. (2017). Clarifying the concept of validity: From measurement to everyday language. *Theory & Psychology, 27*(5), 703–710. https://doi.org/10.1177/0959354317702256

Burge, M. (2012). *The ADD myth: How to cultivate the unique gifts of intense personalities.* San Francisco, CA: Conari Press.

Butcher, J. N., Hass, G. A., Greene, R. L., & Nelson, L. D. (2015). *Using the MMPI–2 in forensic assessment.* Washington, DC: American Psychological Association. https://doi.org/10.1037/14571-000

Butler, J. A. (2016). Self-harm. *Medicine, 44*(12), 715–719. https://doi.org/10.1016/j.mpmed.2016.09.003

Caine, E. D. (2017). Suicide and attempted suicide in the United States during the 21st Century. *JAMA Psychiatry, 10*(5), e0125730. https://doi.org/10.1001/jamapsychiatry.2017.2524

Calhoun, L. G., & Tedeschi, R. G. (1998). Posttraumatic growth: Future directions. In R. G. Tedeschi, C. L. Park & L. G. Calhoun (Eds.), *Posttraumatic growth: Positive changes in the aftermath of crisis* (pp. 215–238). Mahwah, NJ: Lawrence Erlbaum.

Cao, T. H., Jung, J. Y., & Lee, J. (2017). Assessment in gifted education: A review of the literature from 2005 to 2016. *Journal of Advanced Academics, 28*(3), 163–203. https://doi.org/10.1177/1932202X17714572

Caplan, G. (1961). *An approach to community mental health.* New York, NY: Grune & Stratton.

Carman, C. (2011). Adding personality to gifted identification: Relationships among traditional and personality-based concepts. *Journal of Advanced Academics, 22*(3), 412–446. https://doi.org/10.1177/1932202X1102200303

Carman, C. (2013). Comparing apples and oranges: Fifteen years of definitions of giftedness in research. *Journal of Advanced Academics, 24*(1), 52–70. https://doi.org/10.1177/1932202X12472602

Carver, C. S. (2006). Approach, avoidance, and the self-regulation of affect and action. *Motivation and Emotion, 30*(2), 105–110. https://doi.org/10.1007/s11031-006-9044-7

Carver, C. S., Sutton, S. K., & Scheier, M. F. (2000). Action, emotion
and personality: Emerging conceptual integration. *Personality
and Social Psychology Bulletin, 26*(6), 741–751.
https://doi.org/10.1177/0146167200268008

Caspi, A., Hariri, A. R., Holmes, A., Uher, R., & Moffitt, T. E.
(2010). Genetic sensitivity to the environment: The case of the
serotonin transporter. *The American Journal of Psychiatry,
167*(5), 509–527.
https://doi.org/10.1176/appi.ajp.2010.09101452

Caspi, A., Roberts, B. W., & Shiner, R. L. (2005). Personality
development: Stability and change. *Annual Review of
Psychology, 56*, 453–84.
https://doi.org/10.1146/annurev.psych.55.090902.141913

Cassady, J. C., & Cross, T. L. (2006). A factorial representation of
suicidal ideation among academically gifted adolescents.
Journal for the Education of the Gifted, 29(3), 290–304.
https://doi.org/10.1177/016235320602900303

Castellví, P., Miranda-Mendizábal, A., Parés-Badell, O., Almenara, J.,
Alonso, I., Blasco, M. J., . . . Alonso, J. (2017). Exposure to
violence, a risk for suicide in youths and young adults. A
meta-analysis of longitudinal studies. *Acta Psychiatrica
Scandinavica, 135*(3), 195–211.
https://doi.org/10.1111/acps.12679

Cervone, D. (2005). Personality architecture: Within-person structures
and processes. *Annual Review of Psychology, 56*, 423–452.
https://doi.org/10.1146/annurev.psych.56.091103.070133

Cervone, D., & Mischel, W. (Eds.). (2002). *Advances in personality
science*. New York, NY: The Guilford Press.

Cervone, D., & Pervin, L. A. (2013). *Personality: Theory and
research* (12th ed.). Hoboken, NJ: Wiley.

Chaney S. (2017). *Psyche on the skin: A history of self-harm*. London,
England: Reaktion.

Chang, H. J., & Kuo, C. C. (2013). Overexcitabilities: Empirical
studies and application. *Learning and Individual Differences,
23*, 53–63. https://doi.org/10.1016/j.lindif.2012.10.010

Chaves, C., Lopez-Gomez, I., Hervas, G., & Vazquez, C. (2017). A
comparative study on the efficacy of a positive psychology
intervention and a cognitive behavioral therapy for clinical

depression. *Cognitive Therapy and Research, 41*(3), 417–433. https://doi.org/10.1007/s10608-016-9778-9

Chavez-Eakle, R. A. (2004). On the neurobiology of the creative process. *Bulletin of Psychology and the Arts, 5*, 29–35.

Chavez-Eakle, R. A., Lara, M. C., & Cruz-Fuentes, C. (2006). Personality: A possible bridge between creativity and psychopathology? *Creativity Research Journal, 18*(1), 27–38. https://doi.org/10.1207/s15326934crj1801_4

Chehil, S., & Kutcher, S. P. (2012). *Suicide risk management: A manual for health professionals.* (2nd ed.). Chichester, West Sussex: Wiley-Blackwell.

Chen, F., Moran, J. T., Zhang, Y., Ates, K. M., Yu, D., Schrader, L. A., . . . Hall, B. J. (2016). The transcription factor NeuroD2 coordinates synaptic innervation and cell intrinsic properties to control excitability of cortical pyramidal neurons. *The Journal of Physiology, 594*(13), 3729–3744. https://doi.org/10.1113/JP271953

Chia, K. H. (2017). Understanding overexcitabilities of people with exceptional abilities within the framework of cognition-conation-affect-and-sensation. *European Journal of Education Studies, 130*, 649-672. https://doi.org/10.5281/zenodo.803406

Chia, K. H., Lim, B. H. (2017). Understanding overexcitabilities of people with exceptional abilities within the framework of cognition-conation-affect-and-sensation. *European Journal of Education Studies, 3*(6), 667–690. https://doi.org/10.5281/zenodo.803406

Christensen, A. P., Cotter, K. N., & Silvia, P. J. (2018). Reopening openness to experience: A network analysis of four openness to experience inventories. *Journal of Personality Assessment*, 0(March), 1–15. https://doi.org/10.1080/00223891.2018.1467428

Churchland, P. S. (2011). *Braintrust: What neuroscience tells us about morality.* Princeton, NJ: Princeton University Press.

Cienin, P. (Pseudonym) (1972). *Existential thoughts and aphorisms.* London, England: Gryf.

Cipriani, A., Zhou, X., Del Giovane, C., Hetrick, S. E., Qin, B., Whittington, C., . . . Xie, P. (2016). Comparative efficacy and tolerability of antidepressants for major depressive disorder in children and adolescents: a network meta-analysis. *Lancet,* *388*(10047), 881–90. https://doi.org/10.1016/S0140-6736(16)30385-3

Clark, L. A. (2007). Assessment and diagnosis of personality disorder: Perennial issues and an emerging reconceptualization. *Annual Review of Psychology, 58,* 227–257. https://doi.org/10.1146/annurev.psych.57.102904.190200

Cleckley, H. M. (1988). *The mask of sanity: An attempt to clarify some issues about the so-called psychopathic personality* (5th ed.). Augusta, GA: E.S. Cleckley. Retrieved from http://www.cix.co.uk/~klockstone/sanity_1.pdf

Clouston, T. S. (1899). Stages of over-excitability, hypersensitiveness and mental explosiveness in children and their treatment by the bromides. *Scottish Medical and Surgical Journal, IV,* 481–90.

Coan, R. W. (1974). *Optimal personality: An empirical and theoretical analysis.* New York, NY: Columbia University Press.

Coan, R. W. (1977). *Hero, artist, sage, or saint? A survey of views on what is variously called mental health, normality, maturity, self-actualization and human fulfillment.* New York, NY: Columbia University Press.

Cobb, S., & Lindemann, E. (1943). Symposium on the management of the coconut grove burns at the Massachusetts General Hospital: Neuropsychiatric observations. *Annals of Surgery, 117*(6), 814–824. https://doi.org/10.1097/00000658-194311760-00004

Coid, J., Freestone, M., & Ullrich, S. (2012). Subtypes of psychopathy in the British household population: Findings from the national household survey of psychiatric morbidity. *Social Psychiatry and Psychiatric Epidemiology, 47*(6), 879–891. https://doi.org/10.1007/s00127-011-0395-3

Colangelo, N., & Wood, S. M. (2015). Counseling the gifted: Past, present, and future directions. *Journal of Counseling & Development, 93*(2), 133–142. https://doi.org/10.1002/j.1556-6676.2015.00189.x

Coleman, M. R., Gallagher, J. J., & Job, J. (2012). Developing and sustaining professionalism within gifted education. *Gifted*

Child Today, 35(1), 27–36.
https://doi.org/10.1177/1076217511427511

Conway, C. C., Slavich, G. M., & Hammen, C. (2014). Daily stress reactivity and serotonin transporter gene (5-HTTLPR) variation: internalizing responses to everyday stress as a possible transdiagnostic phenotype. *Biology of Mood & Anxiety Disorders, 4*(1), 2. https://doi.org/10.1186/2045-5380-4-2

Cook-Greuter, S. R. (2004). Making the case for a developmental perspective. *Industrial and Commercial Training, 36*(7), 275–281. https://doi.org/10.1108/00197850410563902

Cooper, J., Kapur, N., Webb, R., Lawlor, M., Guthrie, E., Mackway-Jones, K., & Appleby, L. (2005). Suicide after deliberate self-harm: A 4-Year cohort study. *American Journal of Psychiatry, 162*(2), 297–303. https://doi.org/10.1176/appi.ajp.162.2.297

Cornum, R., Matthews, M. D., & Seligman, M. E. P. (2011). Comprehensive soldier fitness: Building resilience in a challenging institutional context. *The American psychologist, 66*(1), 4–9. https://doi.org/10.1037/a0021420

Corr, P. J. (2004). Reinforcement sensitivity theory and personality. *Neuroscience & Biobehavioral Reviews, 28*(3), 317–332. https://doi.org/10.1016/j.neubiorev.2004.01.005

Corr, P. J. (Ed.). (2008). *The reinforcement sensitivity theory of personality.* New York, NY: Cambridge University Press.

Cory, G. A. Jr., & Gardner, R. Jr. (Eds.). (2002). *The evolutionary neuroethology of Paul Maclean: Convergences and frontiers.* Westport, CT: Praeger.

Costelloe, K. (1912). What Bergson means by "interpenetration." *Proceedings of the Aristotelian Society, 13*(1912/1913), 131–155. Retrieved from http://www.jstor.org/stable/4543838

Courtet, P. (Ed.). (2016). *Understanding suicide: From diagnosis to personalized treatment.* Cham, Switzerland: Springer.

Cowen, E. L., & Kilmer, R. P. (2002). Positive psychology: Some plusses and some open issues. *Journal of Community Psychology, 30*(4), 449–460.
https://doi.org/10.1002/jcop.10014

Cox, G., & Hetrick, S. (2017). Psychosocial interventions for self-harm, suicidal ideation and suicide attempt in children and young people: What? How? Who? and Where? *Evidence Based Mental Health, 20*(2), 35–40. https://doi.org/10.1136/eb-2017-102667

Cox, G., Bailey, E., Jorm, A. F., Reavley, N. J., Templer, K., Parker, A., . . . Robinson, J. (2016). Development of suicide postvention guidelines for secondary schools: A Delphi study. *BMC Public Health, 16*, 180. https://doi.org/10.1186/s12889-016-2822-6

Coyne, J.C., & Tennen, H. (2010). Positive psychology in cancer care: Bad science, exaggerated claims and unproven medicine. *Annals of Behavioral Medicine, 39*, 16–26. https://doi.org/10.1007/s12160-009-9154-z

Crago, H. (2017). *The stages of life: Personalities and patterns in human emotional development.* Devon, UK: Routledge.

Critchley, M., & Critchley, E. A. (1998). *John Hughlings Jackson: Father of English neurology.* New York, NY: Oxford University Press.

Cronbach, L. J., & Meehl, P. E. (1955). Construct validity in psychological tests. *Psychological Bulletin, 52*(4), 281–302. https://doi.org/10.1037/h0040957

Cross, T. L. (1996, May/June). Examining claims about gifted children and suicide. *Gifted Child Today, 18*(1), 46–48. https://doi.org/10.1177/107621759601900114

Cross, T. L. (2013). *Suicide among gifted children and adolescents: Understanding the suicidal mind.* Waco, TX: Prufrock Press.

Cross, T. L. (2016). Social and emotional development of gifted students. *Gifted Child Today, 39*(1), 63–66. https://doi.org/10.1177/1076217515597272

Cross, T. L. (2018). *On the social and emotional lives of gifted children: Understanding and guiding their development* (5th ed.). Waco, Texas: Prufrock Press.

Cross, T. L., Cook, R. S., & Dixon, D. N. (1996). Psychological autopsies of three academically talented adolescents who committed suicide. *Journal of Secondary Gifted Education, 7*(3), 403–409. https://doi.org/10.1177/1932202X9600700305

Cross, T. L., & Cross, J. R. (2018). *Suicide among gifted children and adolescents: Understanding the suicidal mind* (2nd ed.). Waco, Texas: Prufrock Press.

Cross, T. L., Gust-Brey, K., & Ball, B. (2002). A psychological autopsy of the suicide of an academically gifted student: Researchers' and parents' perspectives. *Gifted Child Quarterly, 46*(4), 247–264. https://doi.org/10.1177/001698620204600402

Csíkszentmihályi, M. (1990). *Flow: The psychology of optimal experience*. New York, NY: Harper and Row.

Csíkszentmihályi, M., & Csíkszentmihályi, I. S. (Eds.). (2006). *A life worth living: Contributions to positive psychology*. New York, NY: Oxford University Press.

Cullen, D. (1997). Maslow, monkeys and motivation theory. *Organization, 4*(3), 355–373. https://doi.org/10.1177/135050849743004

Cullen, D., & Gotell, L. (2002). From orgasms to organizations: Maslow, women's sexuality and the gendered foundations of the needs hierarchy. *Gender, Work & Organization, 9*(5), 537–555. https://doi.org/10.1111/1468-0432.00174

Curtin, S. C., Warner, M., & Hedegaard, H. (2016, April). Increase in suicide in the United States, 1999–2014. *NC HS Data Brief, 241*. Available at: http://www.cdc.gov/nchs/products/databriefs/db241.htm

Cutcliffe, J. R., Santos, J., & Links, P. S. (Eds.). (2013). *Routledge international handbook of clinical suicide research*. London, UK: Routledge.

Dąbrowski, K. (1929). See Dombrowski, C. (1929).

Dąbrowski, K. (1934a). *Behawioryzm i kierunki pokrewne w psychologii* [Behaviourism and related schools in psychology]. Warsaw, Poland: Lekarz Polski.

Dąbrowski, K. (1934b). *Pódstawy psychologiczne samodreczenia (automutylacji)* [Psychological basis of self-mutilation]. Warsaw, Poland: Przyszłość.

Dąbrowski, K. (1935). *Nerwowosc dzieci i mlodziez* [The nervousness of children and youth]. Warsaw, Poland: Nasza Ksiegarnia.

Dąbrowski, K. (1937). Psychological basis of self-mutilation (W. Thau, Trans.). *Genetic Psychology Monographs, 19*(1), 1–104. Available at: http://positivedisintegration.com/Dabrowski1937.pdf

Dąbrowski, K. (1938). Typy wzmozonej pobudliwości psychicznej [Types of increased psychic excitability]. *Biuletyn Instytutu Higieny Psychicznej, 1*(1), 12–19. Available at: http://positivedisintegration.com/Dabrowski1938.pdf

Dąbrowski, K. (1964a). *0 dezyntegracji pozytywnej* [On positive disintegration]. Warszawa, Poland: Panstwowy Zaklady Wydawnictw Lekarskich.

Dąbrowski, K. (1964b). *Positive disintegration* (J. Aronson, Ed.). Boston, MA: Little, Brown and Company.

Dąbrowski, K. (1966). The theory of positive disintegration. *International Journal of Psychiatry, 2*, 229–244.

Dąbrowski, K. (1967). *Personality-shaping through positive disintegration.* Boston, MA: Little, Brown and Company.

Dąbrowski, K. (1970a, August 26-30). *Immunization against psychosis through neurosis and psychoneurosis.* Paper presented at the First International Conference on the Theory of Positive Disintegration, Laval, Canada. Available at: http://positivedisintegration.com/EDI-62J-16j.pdf

Dąbrowski, K. (with Kawczak, A., & Piechowski, M. M.). (1970b). *Mental growth through positive disintegration.* London, England: Gryf.

Dąbrowski, K. (1970c, August). *Psychic overexcitability and psychoneurosis.* Paper presented at the First International Conference on the theory of Positive Disintegration, Laval, Canada. Available at: http://positivedisintegration.com/EDI-31.pdf

Dąbrowski, K. (1972a). *A more specific picture of the developmental way—neuroses and psychoneuroses, the philosophy of psychoneuroses.* Unpublished manuscript. Available at: http://positivedisintegration.com/EDI-65H.pdf

Dąbrowski, K. (1972b). *Psychoneurosis is not an illness.* London, England: Gryf.

Dąbrowski, K. (with Kawczak, A., & Sochanska, J.). (1973). *The dynamics of concepts.* London, England: Gryf.

Dąbrowski, K. (1975). Foreword. In M. M. Piechowski, A theoretical and empirical approach to the study of development. *Genetic Psychology Monographs, 92*, 233–237. Available at:

http://www.positivedisintegration.com/Dabrowski1975Forewo rd.pdf

Dąbrowski, K. (1976). On the philosophy of development through positive disintegration and secondary integration. *Dialectics and Humanism, 3-4*, 131–144. https://doi.org/10.5840/dialecticshumanism197633/413

Dąbrowski, K. (1996). *Multilevelness of emotional and instinctive functions. Part 1: Theory and description of levels of behavior.* Lublin, Poland: Towarzystwo Naukowe Katolickiego Uniwersytetu Lubelskiego.

Dąbrowski, K. (2010a). Remarks on Wilhelm Stekel's active psychoanalysis (P. Samborowski, & J. Lucas, Trans.).[54] *Heksis, 1* Retrieved from https://heksis.dezintegracja.pl/en/remarks-on-wilhelm-stekels-active-psychoanalysis/

Dąbrowski, K. (2010b). Theme IX-Janusz Korczak (F. Maj, Trans.)[55] *Heksis, 1*, Retrieved from https://heksis.dezintegracja.pl/en/theme-ix-janusz-korczak/

Dąbrowski, K. (2010c). Increased sensual and motor excitability in children (F. Maj, Trans.).[56] *Heksis, 4*, 54–60. (Original work published 1959) Retrieved from http://positivedisintegration.com/Dabrowski2010c.pdf

Dąbrowski, K. (2015). *Personality-shaping through positive disintegration.* Otto, NC: Red Pill Press. (Original work published 1967)

Dąbrowski, K. (2016). *Positive Disintegration.* Anna Maria, FL: Bassett. (Original work published 1964)

Dąbrowski, K. (with Rankel, M.) (n.d.a). *Developmental psychotherapy: Psychotherapy based on the Theory of Positive Disintegration.* Unpublished manuscript, University of Alberta, Departments of Psychology and Educational Psychology, Edmonton, AB.

Dąbrowski, K. (n.d.b). *On authentic education.* Unpublished manuscript, University of Alberta, Departments of Psychology and Educational Psychology, Edmonton, AB.

Dąbrowski, K. (n.d.c). *Philosophy of essence: Developmental philosophy based on the theory of positive disintegration.*

Unpublished manuscript, University of Alberta, Departments of Psychology and Educational Psychology, Edmonton, AB.

Dąbrowski, K., & Joshi, P. (1972). Different contemporary conceptions of mental health. *Journal of Contemporary Psychotherapy, 4*(2), 97–106. https://doi.org/10.1007/BF02111975

Dąbrowski, K., & Kujawska, J. (1965). Psychonerwice u mlodziezy wybitnie uzdolnionej [Psychoneuroses among particularly gifted youth]. *Zdrowie Psychiczne, 6*(1), 24-35.

Dąbrowski, K., & Piechowski, M. M. (with Rankel M., & Amend, D. R.). (1996). *Multilevelness of emotional and instinctive functions. Part 2: Types and levels of development.* Lublin, Poland: Towarzystwo Naukowe Katolickiego Uniwersytetu Lubelskiego.

Dai, D. Y. (2011). Hopeless anarchy or saving pluralism? Reflections on our field in response to Ambrose, VanTassel-Baska, Coleman and Cross. *Journal for the Education of the Gifted, 34*(5), 705–730. https://doi.org/10.1177/0162353211416437

Dai, D. Y. & Sternberg, R. J. (2004). Beyond cognitivism: Toward an integrated understanding of intellectual functioning and development. In D. Y. Dai & R. J. Sternberg (Eds.), *Motivation, emotion, and cognition: Integrative perspectives on intellectual functioning and development* (pp. 3–38). Mahwah, NJ: Lawrence Erlbaum.

Dai, D. Y., Swanson, J. A., & Cheng, H. (2011). State of research on giftedness and gifted education: A survey of empirical studies published during 1998–2010. *Gifted Child Quarterly 55*(2), 126–138. https://doi.org/10.1177/0016986210397831

Dalai Lama. (2017). *The Dalai Lama's little book of mysticism: The essential teachings.* Charlottesville, VA: Hampton Roads.

Dalgleish, T. (2004). The emotional brain. *Nature reviews neuroscience, 5*, 583–589. https://doi.org/10.1038/nrn1432

Damasio, A. R. (1994). *Descartes' error: Emotion, reason and the human brain.* New York, NY: Putnam.

Daniels, M. (1982). The development of the concept of self-actualization in the writings of Abraham Maslow. *Current Psychological Reviews, 2*(1), 61–76. https://doi.org/10.1007/BF02684455

Daniels, S., & Piechowski, M. M. (2009). *Living with intensity: Understanding the sensitivity, excitability and emotional development of gifted children, adolescents and adults.* Scottsdale, AZ: Great Potential Press.

Daniels, S., & Piechowski, M. M. (2010). When intensity goes to school: Overexcitabilities, creativity, and the gifted child. In R. A. Beghetto, & J. C. Kaufman, (Eds.), *Nurturing creativity in the classroom*, (pp. 313–328). New York, NY: Cambridge University Press.

Darwin, C. (1872). *The expression of the emotions in man and animals.* London, England: John Murray. Available from http://darwin-online.org.uk/

Das, A. K. (1989). Beyond self-actualization. *International Journal for the Advancement of Counselling, 12*(1), 13–27. https://doi.org/10.1007/BF00123452

David, S. A., Boniwell, I., & Ayers, A. C. (Eds.). (2013). *The Oxford handbook of happiness.* Oxford, England: Oxford University Press.

Davidson, J. E. (2012). Is giftedness truly a gift? *Gifted Education International, 28*(3), 252–266. https://doi.org/10.1177/0261429411435051

Davies, J. (2012). *The importance of suffering: The value and meaning of emotional discontent.* New York, NY: Routledge.

Davis, G. W., & Bezprozvanny, I. (2001). Maintaining the stability of neural function: A homeostatic hypothesis. *Annual Review of Physiology, 63*(1), 847–869. https://doi.org/10.1146/annurev.physiol.63.1.847

Davis, K. B. (1929). *Factors in the sex life of twenty-two hundred women.* New York, NY: Harper.

Davis, S. K., & Nichols, R. (2016). Does emotional intelligence have a "dark" side? A review of the literature. *Frontiers in Psychology, 7*, 1316. https://doi.org/10.3389/fpsyg.2016.01316

de Beauport, E. (with Diaz, A. S.). (1996). *The three faces of the mind: Developing your mental, emotional and behavioral intelligences.* Wheaton, IL: Quest.

De Bondt, N., & Van Petegem, P. (2015). Psychometric evaluation of the Overexcitability Questionnaire-Two applying Bayesian

Structural Equation Modeling (BSEM) and multiple–group BSEM-based alignment with approximate measurement invariance. *Frontiers in Psychology, 6*, 1963. https://doi.org/10.3389/fpsyg.2015.01963

De Bondt, N., & Van Petegem, P. (2017). Emphasis on emotions in student learning: Analyzing relationships between overexcitabilities and the learning approach using Bayesian MIMIC modeling. *High Ability Studies, 28*(2), 225-248. https://doi.org/10.1080/13598139.2017.1292897

de Grâce, G. (1974). The compatibility of anxiety and actualization. *Journal of Clinical Psychology, 30*(4), 566–568. https://doi.org/10.1002/1097-4679(197410)30:4<566::AID-JCLP2270300430>3.0.CO;2-O

Degrazia, D. (2000). Prozac, enhancement and self-creation. *The Hastings Center Report, 30*, 34–40. https://doi.org/10.2307/3528313

Delisle, J. R. (1986). Death with honors: Suicide among gifted adolescents. *Journal of Counseling and Development, 64*(9), 558–560. https://doi.org/10.1002/j.1556-6676.1986.tb01202.x

Dick, D. M., Agrawal, A., Keller, M. C., Adkins, A., Aliev, F., Monroe, S., . . . Sher, K. J. (2015). Candidate gene-environment interaction research: Reflections and recommendations. *Perspectives on Psychological Science: A Journal of the Association for Psychological Science, 10*(1), 37–59. https://doi.org/10.1177/1745691614556682

Dirkes, M. A. (1983). Anxiety in the gifted: Pluses and minuses. *Roeper Review, 6*(2), 68–70. https://doi.org/10.1080/02783198309552758

Ditum, S. (2017). The merciless mirror: Sylvia Plath's art, suicide, and influence. *The Lancet Psychiatry, 4*(6), 446–449. https://doi.org/10.1016/S2215-0366(17)30195-5

Dixon, D. N., & Scheckel, J. R. (1996). Gifted adolescent suicide: The empirical base. *Journal of Advanced Academics, 7*(3), 386–392. https://doi.org/10.1177/1932202X9600700303

Dombrowski, C. (1929). *Les conditions psycholopique du suicide* [The psychological conditions of suicide] Geneva, Switzerland: lmprimerie du Commerce.[57] http://positivedisintegration.com/Dabrowski1929.pdf

Donaldson, S. I., Dollwet, M., & Rao, M. A. (2015). Happiness, excellence, and optimal human functioning revisited: Examining the peer-reviewed literature linked to positive psychology. *The Journal of Positive Psychology*, *10*(3), 185–195. https://doi.org/10.1080/17439760.2014.943801

Doris, J. M. (2010). *The moral psychology handbook*. New York, NY: Oxford University Press.

Du, X., Gao, H., Jaffe, D., Zhang, H., & Gamper, N. (2018). M-type K + channels in peripheral nociceptive pathways. *British Journal of Pharmacology, 175*(12), 2158–2172. https://doi.org/10.1111/bph.13978

Duffy, D. F. (2009). Self–injury. *Psychiatry*, *8*(7), 237–240. https://doi.org/10.1016/j.mppsy.2009.04.006

DuPaul, G. J., & Stoner, G. (2014). *ADHD in the schools: Assessment and intervention strategies* (3rd ed.). New York, NY: Guilford Publications.

Dutton, K. (2012). *The wisdom of psychopaths*. Toronto, Canada: Doubleday.

Dziekanowski, C. (2010). Self-actualization and the theory of positive disintegration (B. Jablonski, Trans.) *Heksis, 1*. Retrieved from https://heksis.dezintegracja.pl/en/self-actualization-and-the-theory-of-positive-disintegration/

Eggertson, L., & Patrick, K. (2016). Canada needs a national suicide prevention strategy. *Canadian Medical Association Journal*, *188*(13), E309–E310. https://doi.org/10.1503/cmaj.160935

Eiserman, J., Lai, H., & Rushton, C. (2017). Drawing out understanding. *Gifted Education International*, *33*(3), 197–209. https://doi.org/10.1177/0261429415576992

Ekman, P. (2007). *Emotions revealed: Recognizing faces and feelings to improve communication and emotional life*. New York, NY: Holt.

Elderton, A., Berry, A., & Chan, C. (2017). A systematic review of posttraumatic growth in survivors of interpersonal violence in adulthood. *Trauma, Violence, & Abuse, 18*(2), 223–236. https://doi.org/10.1177/1524838015611672

Eliot, C. W. (Ed.). (1909). *Nine Greek dramas* (The Harvard Classics. Vol. 8). New York, NY: Collier.

Eliot, T.S. (1944). *Four Quartets*. London, England: Faber & Faber.

Elkins, D. N. (2009). Why humanistic psychology lost its power and influence in American psychology: Implications for advancing humanistic psychology. *Journal of Humanistic Psychology, 49*(3), 267–291. https://doi.org/10.1177/0022167808323575

Ellenberger, H. F. (1970). *The discovery of the unconscious: The history and evolution of dynamic psychiatry.* New York, NY: Basic.

Elliot, A. J. (1999). Approach and avoidance motivation and achievement goals. *Educational Psychologist, 34*, 169–189. https://doi.org/10.1207/s15326985ep3403_3

Elliot, A. J., & Covington, M. V. (2001). Approach and avoidance motivation. *Educational Psychology Review, 13*(2), 73–92. https://doi.org/10.1023/A:1009009018235

Ellis, A., Abrams, M., Abrams, L. D., Nussbaum, A., & Frey, R. J. (2009). *Personality theories: Critical perspectives.* Thousand Oaks, CA: Sage.

Emmons, R. A. (1995). Levels and domains in personality: An introduction. *Journal of Personality, 63*(3), 341–364. https://doi.org/10.1111/j.1467-6494.1995.tb00499.x

Engel, S. (2009). Is curiosity vanishing? *Journal of the American Academy of Child and Adolescent Psychiatry, 48*(8), 777–9. https://doi.org/10.1097/CHI.0b013e3181aa03b0

Eriksen, K. (2006). The constructive developmental theory of Robert Kegan. *The Family Journal, 14*(3), 290–298. https://doi.org/10.1177/1066480706287799

Erikson, E. H. (1959). Identity and the life cycle. *Psychological Issues, 1*, 1–171.

Erikson, E. H. (1968). *Identity youth and crisis.* New York, NY: Norton.

Erlich, M. D. (2016, September). Addressing the aftermath of suicide: Why we need postvention. *Psychiatric Times, 33*(9). Retrieved from http://www.psychiatrictimes.com/suicide/addressing-aftermath-suicide-why-we-need-postvention

Erwin, J. A., Paquola, A. C. M., Singer, T., Gallina, I., Novotny, M., Quayle, C., . . . Gage, F. H. (2016). L1–associated genomic regions are deleted in somatic cells of the healthy human brain. *Nature Neuroscience, 19*, 1583–1591. https://doi.org/10.1038/nn.4388

Ewalt, J. R. (1957). Goals of the Joint Commission on Mental Illness and Health. *American Journal of Public Health and the Nation's Health, 47*(1), 19–24. Retrieved from http://ajph.aphapublications.org/doi/pdf/10.2105/AJPH.47.1.19

Eysenck, H. J. (1967). *The biological basis of personality.* Springfield, IL: Thomas.

Fagiolini, M., Jensen, C. L., & Champagne, F. A. (2009). Epigenetic influences on brain development and plasticity. *Current Opinion in Neurobiology, 19*(2), 207–212. https://doi.org/10.1016/j.conb.2009.05.009

Fajkowska, M., & DeYoung, C. G. (Eds.). (2015). Introduction to the special issue on integrative theories of personality [Special issue]. *Journal of Research in Personality, 56*, 1–3. https://doi.org/10.1016/j.jrp.2015.04.001

Falk, R. F. (2017). Personality, intellectual ability, and the self-concept of gifted children: An application of PLS-SEM. In H. Latan, R. Noonan (Eds.), *Partial Least Squares Path Modeling* (pp. 299–310). Cham, Switzerland: Springer. https://doi.org/10.1007/978-3-319-64069-3_14

Falk, R. F., Yakmaci-Guzel, B., Chang, A., Pardo, R., & Chavez-Eakle, R. A. (2008). Measuring overexcitability: Replication across five countries. In S. Mendaglio (Ed.), *Dąbrowski's Theory of Positive Disintegration* (pp. 183–199). Scottsdale AZ: Great Potential Press.

Falk, R. F., Lind, S., Miller, N. B., Piechowski, M. M., & Silverman, L. K. (1999). *The Overexcitability Questionnaire–Two (OEQ–II): Manual, scoring system and questionnaire.* Denver, CO: Institute for the Study of Advanced Development.

Fallon, J. H. (2013). *The psychopath inside: A neuroscientist's personal journey into the dark side of the brain.* New York, NY: Penguin.

Fan, J., Wu, Y., Fossella, J. A., & Posner, M. I. (2001). Assessing the heritability of attentional networks. *BMC Neuroscience, 2*, 14. https://doi.org/10.1186/1471-2202-2-14

Feist, G. J. (1998). A meta–analysis of personality in scientific and artistic creativity. *Personality and Social Psychology Review, 2*(4), 290–309. https://doi.org/10.1207/s15327957pspr0204_5

Fennimore, A., & Sementelli, A. (2016). Public entrepreneurship and sub–clinical psychopaths: A conceptual frame and implications. *International Journal of Public Sector Management, 29*(6), 612–634. https://doi.org/10.1108/IJPSM-01-2016-0011

Fentress, J. C. (1999). The organization of behaviour revisited. *Canadian Journal of Experimental Psychology, 53*(1), 8–20. https://doi.org/10.1037/h0087296

Fernández–Berrocal, P., & Checa, P. (Eds.). (2016). Editorial: Emotional intelligence and cognitive abilities [Special issue]. *Frontiers in Psychology, 7, 955.* https://doi.org/10.3389/fpsyg.2016.00955

Ferrari, G. R. F. (Ed.). (2007). *The Cambridge companion to Plato's Republic.* New York, NY: Cambridge University Press.

Flescher, I. (1963). Anxiety and achievement of intellectually gifted and creatively gifted children. *The Journal of Psychology, 56*(2), 251–68. https://doi.org/10.1080/00223980.1963.9916644

Fletcher, D., & Sarkar, M. (2013). Psychological Resilience. *European Psychologist, 18*(1), 12–23. https://doi.org/10.1027/1016–9040/a000124

Flint, L. J. (2001). Challenges of identifying and serving gifted children with ADHD. *Teaching Exceptional Children, 33*(4), 62–70. https://doi.org/10.1177/004005990103300409

Flynn, M. (1995). Conflicting views on the importance of emotion to human development and growth: Piaget and Whitehead. *Interchange, 26*(4), 365–381. https://doi.org/10.1007/BF01434742

Fogelin, R. J. (1971). Three Platonic analogies. *The Philosophical Review, 80*(3), 371–382. https://doi.org/10.2307/2184102

Fonagy, P., Rost, F., Carlyle, J., McPherson, S., Thomas, R., Pasco Fearon, R. M., . . . Taylor, D. (2015). Pragmatic randomized controlled trial of long-term psychoanalytic psychotherapy for treatment-resistant depression: The Tavistock Adult Depression Study (TADS). *World Psychiatry, 14*(3), 312–321. https://doi.org/10.1002/wps.20267

Forget, E. (2003). Evocations of sympathy: Sympathetic imagery in Eighteenth–Century social theory and physiology. *History of*

Political Economy, 35 (Supp 1), 282–308.
https://doi.org/10.1215/00182702-35-Suppl_1-282

Forstadt, L. (2009). [Review of the book *Living with intensity: Understanding the sensitivity, excitability, and the emotional development of gifted children, adolescents, and adults*, by S. Daniels & M. M. Piechowski (Eds.)]. *Roeper Review, 31*(2), 130–131. https://doi.org/10.1080/02783190902737749

Forstadt, L., & Shaine, J. (2009). [Review of the book *Dąbrowski's theory of positive disintegration* by S. Mendaglio (Ed.)]. *Roeper Review, 31*(2), 129–130. https://doi.org/10.1080/02783190902738036

Fox, E., & Beevers, C. G. (2016). Differential sensitivity to the environment: Contribution of cognitive biases and genes to psychological wellbeing. *Molecular Psychiatry, 21*, 1657–1662. https://doi.org/10.1038/mp.2016.114

Frankl, V. E. (1985). *Man's search for meaning* (Revised and Updated). New York, NY: Washington Square (Pocket Books). (Original work published 1959)

Franklin, J. C., Ribeiro, J. D., Fox, K. R., Bentley, K. H., Kleiman, E. M., Huang, X., . . . Nock, M. K. (2016). Risk factors for suicidal thoughts and behaviors: A meta-analysis of 50 years of research. *Psychological Bulletin.* https://doi.org/10.1037/bul0000084

Franz, E. & Gillett, G. (2011). John Hughlings Jackson's evolutionary neurology: A unifying framework for cognitive neuroscience. *Brain, 134*(10), 3114–20. https://doi.org/10.1093/brain/awr218

Freiwald, W., Duchaine, B., & Yovel, G. (2016). Face processing systems: From neurons to real-world social perception. *Annual Review of Neuroscience, 39*(1), 325–346. https://doi.org/10.1146/annurev-neuro-070815-013934

Freud, S. (1920). *A general introduction to psychoanalysis* (G. Stanley Hall, Trans.) New York, NY: Boni and Liveright.

Freud, S. (1961). *Civilization and its discontents.* (J. Strachey, Ed., Trans.). New York, NY: Norton.

Freud, S. (1984). *On Metapsychology-the theory of psychoanalysis: Beyond the pleasure principle, Ego and the Id and other works* (A. Richards, Ed., J. Strachey, Trans.). The Pelican Freud library, Vol. 11. London, England: Penguin Books. (Original work published 1923)

Froemke, R. C. (2015). Plasticity of cortical excitatory-inhibitory balance. *Annual Review of Neuroscience, 38*(1), 195–219. https://doi.org/10.1146/annurev-neuro-071714-034002

Froh, J. J. (2004). Truth be told. *NYS Psychologist, 16*(May/June), 18–20.

Fugate, C. M., & Gentry, M. (2016). Understanding adolescent gifted girls with ADHD: motivated and achieving. *High Ability Studies, 27*(1), 83–109. https://doi.org/10.1080/13598139.2015.1098522

Fullinwider, S. P. (1983). Sigmund Freud, John Hughlings Jackson and speech. *Journal of the History of Ideas, 44*(1), 151–158. https://doi.org/10.2307/2709311

Funder, D. C. (2013). *The personality puzzle* (6th ed.). New York, NY: Norton.

Gable, S. L., & Haidt, J. (2005). What (and why) is positive psychology? *Review of General Psychology, 9*(2), 103–110. https://doi.org/10.1037/1089-2680.9.2.103

Gaiarsa, J. L., & Ben-Ari, Y. (2006). Long-term plasticity at inhibitory synapses: A phenomenon that has been overlooked. In J. T. Kittler and S. J. Moss (Eds.), *The Dynamic Synapse: Molecular Methods in Ionotropic Receptor Biology* (pp. 23–35). Retrieved from http://www.ncbi.nlm.nih.gov/pubmed/21204478

Galang, A. J. R. (2010). The prosocial psychopath: Explaining the paradoxes of the creative personality. *Neuroscience & Biobehavioral Reviews, 34*(8), 1241–1248. https://doi.org/10.1016/j.neubiorev.2010.03.005

Galang, A. J. R., Castelo, V. L. C., Santos, L. C., Perlas, C. M. C., & Angeles, M. A. B. (2016). Investigating the prosocial psychopath model of the creative personality: Evidence from traits and psychophysiology. *Personality and Individual Differences, 100*, 28–36. https://doi.org/10.1016/j.paid.2016.03.081

Galderisi, S., Heinz, A., Kastrup, M., Beezhold, J., & Sartorius, N. (2015). Toward a new definition of mental health. *World*

Psychiatry, 14(2), 231–233.
https://doi.org/10.1002/wps.20231

Gallagher, S. A. (1986). A comparison of the concept of overexcitabilities with measures of creativity and school achievement in 6th grade students. *Roeper Review, 8*(2), 115–119. https://doi.org/10.1080/02783198509552950

Gao, Y., & Raine, A. (2010). Successful and unsuccessful psychopaths: A neurobiological model. *Behavioral Sciences and the Law, 28*(2), 194–210. http://www.ncbi.nlm.nih.gov/pubmed/20422645

Garbarino, J. (2011). *The positive psychology of personal transformation: Leveraging resilience for life change.* New York, NY: Springer.

García-Pérez, M. A. (2017). Thou shalt not bear false witness against null hypothesis significance testing. *Educational and Psychological Measurement, 77*(4), 631–662. https://doi.org/10.1177/0013164416668232

Gardner H. (2011). *The unschooled mind how children think and how schools should teach.* New York, NY: Basic. (Original work published 1995)

Gasper, K., & Clore G. L. (2000). Do you have to pay attention to your feelings to be influenced by them? *Personality and Social Psychology Bulletin, 26*(6), 698–711. https://doi.org/10.1177/0146167200268005

Gawroński, B. (1989). Biographical note prepared for the book "In Search of Mental Health" Retrieved December 30, 2017, from: http://dezintegracja.pl/nota-bio-w-poszukiwaniu-zdrowia-psychicznego/

Gazzaniga, M. S. (2013). Shifting gears: Seeking new approaches for mind/brain mechanisms. *Annual Review of Psychology, 64*(1), 1–20. https://doi.org/10.1146/annurev-psych-113011-143817

Geller, L. (1982). The failure of self-actualization theory: A critique of Carl Rogers and Abraham Maslow. *Journal of Humanistic Psychology, 22*(2), 56–73. https://doi.org/10.1177/0022167882222004

Gendlin, E. T. (1962). *Experiencing and the creation of meaning.* New York, NY: Free Press.

Gibbons, R. D., Hur, K., & Mann, J. J. (2017). Suicide rates and the declining psychiatric hospital bed capacity in the United States. *JAMA Psychiatry, 44*(4), 1385–1405. https://doi.org/10.1001/jamapsychiatry.2017.1227

Gibbs, J. C. (2014). *Moral development and reality: Beyond the theories of Kohlberg, Hoffman, and Haidt.* (3rd ed.). New York, NY: Oxford University Press.

Glenn, A. L., & Raine, A. (2014). *Psychopathy: An introduction to biological findings and their implications.* New York, NY: New York University Press.

Goble, F. (1970). *The third force: The psychology of Abraham Maslow.* New York, NY: Grossman.

Goerss, J., Amend, E. R., Webb, J. T., Webb, N., & Beljan, P. (2006). Comments on Mika's critique of Hartnett, Nelson and Rinn's article, "Gifted or ADHD? The possibilities of misdiagnosis." *Roeper Review, 28*(4), 249–252. https://doi.org/10.1080/02783190609554372

Goertzel, M. G., Goertzel, V., & Goertzel, T. G. (1978). *300 Eminent personalities.* San Francisco, CA: Jossey-Bass.

Goertzel, V, & Goertzel, M. G. (1962), *Cradles of eminence.* Boston, MA: Little, Brown and Company.

Goldblum, P., Espelage, D. L., Chu, J., & Bongar, B. (Eds.). (2015). *Youth suicide and bullying: Challenges and strategies for prevention and intervention.* Oxford, NY: Oxford University Press.

Goldin, P. R., McRae, K., Ramel, W., & Gross, J. J. (2008). The neural bases of emotion regulation: Reappraisal and suppression of negative emotion. *Biological Psychiatry, 63*(6), 577–586. https://doi.org/10.1016/j.biopsych.2007.05.031

Goldney, R. D., & Berman, L. (1996). Postvention in schools: affective or effective? *Crisis, 17*(3), 98–9. https://doi.org/10.1027/0227-5910.17.3.98

Goldsmith, C. (2017). *Understanding suicide: A national epidemic.* Minneapolis, MN: Twenty-First Century.

Goldstein, K. (1995). *The organism: A holistic approach to biology derived from pathological data in man.* New York, NY: Zone. (Original work published 1939)

Goldston, D. B., Erkanli, A., Daniel, S. S., Heilbron, N., Weller, B. E., & Doyle, O. (2016). Developmental trajectories of suicidal thoughts and behaviors from adolescence through adulthood. *Journal of the American Academy of Child & Adolescent Psychiatry, 55*, 400–407.e1. https://doi.org/10.1016/j.jaac.2016.02.010

Goleman, D. (1995). *Emotional intelligence: Why it can matter more than IQ*. New York, NY: Bantam.

Goold, C. P., & Nicoll, R. A. (2010). Single-Cell optogenetic excitation drives homeostatic synaptic depression. *Neuron, 68*(3), 512–528. https://doi.org/10.1016/j.neuron.2010.09.020

Gould, T. (1969, Spring). Four levels of reality in Plato, Spinoza, and Blake. *Arion: A Journal of Humanities and the Classics, 8*, 20–50.

Grashow, R., Brookings, T., & Marder, E. (2010). Compensation for variable intrinsic neuronal excitability by circuit-synaptic interactions. *Journal of Neuroscience, 30*(27), 9145–9156. https://doi.org/10.1523/JNEUROSCI.0980-10.2010

Graves, C. (1970), Levels of existence: An open system theory of values. *Journal of Humanistic Psychology, 10*(2), 131–155. https://doi.org/10.1177/002216787001000205

Gray, J. A., & McNaughton, N. (2003). *The neuropsychology of anxiety: An enquiry into the functions of the septo-hippocampal system* (2nd, paperback, ed.). Oxford, England: Oxford University Press.

Greene, J., & Haidt, J. (2002). How (and where) does moral judgment work? *Trends in Cognitive Sciences, 6*(12), 517–523. https://doi.org/10.1016/S1364-6613(02)02011-9

Grobman, J. (2006). Underachievement in exceptionally gifted adolescents and young adults: A psychiatrist's view. *Journal of Secondary Gifted Education, 27*(4), 199–210. https://doi.org/10.4219/jsge-2006-408

Groff, E. C., Ruzek, J. I., Bongar, B., & Cordova, M. J. (2016, March 7). Social constraints, loss- related factors, depression, and posttraumatic stress in a treatment-seeking suicide bereaved sample. *Psychological Trauma: Theory, Research, Practice, And Policy, 8*(6), 657-660. http://dx.doi.org/10.1037/tra0000128

Grøn, A., Rosfort, R., & Söderquist, K. B. (Eds.). (2017). *Kierkegaard's existential approach.* Berlin, Germany: De Gruyter.

Gross, C. M., Rinn, A. N. & Jamieson, K. M. (2007). Gifted adolescents' overexcitabilities and self–concepts: An analysis of gender and grade level. *Roeper Review, 29*(4), 240–249. https://doi.org/10.1080/02783190709554418

Gulledge, A. T., & Bravo, J. J. (2016). Neuron morphology influences axon initial segment plasticity. *eNeuro, 3,* 1–24. https://doi.org/10.1523/ENEURO.0085-15.2016

Gulliver, S. B., Pennington, M. L., Leto, F., Cammarata, C., Ostiguy, W., Zavodny, C., . . . Kimbrel, N. (2016). In the wake of suicide: Developing guidelines for suicide postvention in fire service. *Death Studies, 40*(2), 121–8. https://doi.org/10.1080/07481187.2015.1077357

Gurdjieff, G. I. (1969). *Meetings with remarkable men (all and everything).* New York, NY: Dutton.

Gurrister, L., & Kane, R. A. (1978). How therapists perceive and treat suicidal patients. *Community Mental Health Journal, 14*(1), 3–13. https://doi.org/10.1007/BF00781306

Gust-Brey, K., & Cross, T. L. (1999). An examination of the literature base on the suicidal behaviors of gifted students. *Roeper Review, 22*(1), 28–35. https://doi.org/10.1080/02783199909553994

Haan, N., Millsap, R., & Hartka, E. (1986). As time goes by: Change and stability in personality over fifty years. *Psychology and Aging, 1*(3), 220–232. https://doi.org/10.1037/0882-7974.1.3.220

Haas, L., & Hunziker, M. (2006). *Building blocks of personality type: A guide to using the eight-process model of personality type.* Huntington Beach, CA: Unite Business Press.

Hacker, P. M. S. (2018). *The passions: A study of human nature.* Hoboken, NJ: John Wiley.

Hague, W. J. (2010). Development through values and intuition in the theory of positive disintegration (A. Danko, Trans.). *Heksis, 1.* Retrieved from https://heksis.dezintegracja.pl/en/development-through-values-and-intuition-in-the-theory-of-positive-disintegration/

Haidt, J. (2003a). Elevation and the positive psychology of morality. In C. L. M. Keyes, & J. Haidt (Eds.), *Flourishing: Positive psychology and the life well-lived* (pp. 275–289). Washington, DC: American Psychological Association.

Haidt, J. (2003b). The moral emotions. In R. J. Davidson, K. R. Scherer, & H. H. Goldsmith (Eds.), *Handbook of affective sciences* (pp. 852–870). Oxford, England: Oxford University Press.

Haidt, J. (2006). *The happiness hypothesis: Finding modern truth and ancient wisdom*. New York, NY: Basic.

Haidt, J. (2007). The new synthesis in moral psychology. *Science, 316*(5827), 998–1002. https://doi.org/10.1126/science.1137651

Haidt, J. (2012). *The righteous mind: Why good people are divided by politics and religion*. New York, NY: Pantheon.

Haidt, J. (2013). Moral psychology for the twenty-first century. *Journal of Moral Education, 42*(3), 281–297. https://doi.org/10.1080/03057240.2013.817327

Hall, D. (1980). Interpreting Plato's cave as an allegory of the human condition. *Apeiron, 14*(2), 74–86. https://doi.org/10.1515/APEIRON.1980.14.2.74

Halldorsdottir, T., & Binder, E. B. (2017). Gene × Environment interactions: From molecular mechanisms to behavior. *Annual Review of Psychology, 68*(1), 215–241. https://doi.org/10.1146/annurev-psych-010416-044053

Hannay, A., & Marino, G. D. (Eds.). (1998). *The Cambridge companion to Kierkegaard*. Cambridge, England: Cambridge University Press.

Hanson, J. (2017). *Kierkegaard and the life of faith: The aesthetic, the ethical, and the religious in Fear and Trembling*. Bloomington: Indiana University Press.

Hanson, L. W., & Baker, D. L. (2017) Corporate psychopaths in public agencies? *Journal of Public Management & Social Policy, 24*(1), Article 3. http://digitalscholarship.tsu.edu/jpmsp/vol24/iss1/3

Hare, R. D. (1999). *Without conscience: The disturbing world of the psychopaths among us*. New York, NY: Guilford Press. (Original work published 1995)

Harper, A. J., & Clifford, C. (2017). Through the Dąbrowski lens: Philosophy, faith, and the personality ideal. *Roeper Review, 39*(4), 262–268. https://doi.org/10.1080/02783193.2017.1363100

Harper, A. J., Cornish, L., Smith, S., & Merrotsy, P. (2017). Through the Dąbrowski lens: A fresh examination of the Theory of Positive Disintegration. *Roeper Review, 39*(1), 37–43. https://doi.org/10.1080/02783193.2016.1247395

Harpur, T. J., Hare, R. D., & Hakstian, A. R. (1989). Two-factor conceptualization of psychopathy: Construct validity and assessment implications. *Psychological Assessment: A Journal of Consulting and Clinical Psychology, 1*(1), 6–17. https://doi.org/10.1037/1040-3590.1.1.6

Harris, M. A., Brett, C. E., Johnson, W., & Deary, I. J. (2016). Personality stability from age 14 to age 77 years. *Psychology and Aging, 31*(8), 862–874. https://doi.org/10.1037/pag0000133

Harrison, G. E., & Van Haneghan, J. P. (2011). The gifted and the shadow of the night: Dąbrowski's overexcitabilities and their correlation to insomnia, death anxiety and fear of the unknown. *Journal for the Education of the Gifted, 34*(4), 669–697. https://doi.org/10.1177/0162353221103400407

Harrison, M. K. (1965). Lindemann's crisis theory and Dąbrowski's positive disintegration theory–A comparative analysis. *Perspectives in Psychiatric Care, 3*(7), 8–13. https://doi.org/10.1111/j.1744-6163.1965.tb01446.x

Hartnett, D. N., Nelson, J. M., & Rinn, A. N. (2004). Gifted or ADHD? The possibilities of misdiagnosis. *Roeper Review, 26*(2), 73–76. https://doi.org/10.1080/02783190409554245

Haslam, N., Holland, E., & Kuppens, P. (2012). Categories versus dimensions in personality and psychopathology: A quantitative review of taxometric research. *Psychological Medicine, 42*(5), 903–920. https://doi.org/10.1017/S0033291711001966

Hatcher, S., Crawford, A., & Coupe, N. (2017). Preventing suicide in indigenous communities. *Current Opinion in Psychiatry, 30*(1), 21–25. https://doi.org/10.1097/YCO.0000000000000295

Hawton, K., Saunders, K. E., & O'Connor, R. C. (2012). Self-harm and suicide in adolescents. *The Lancet, 379*(9834), 2373–2382. https://doi.org/10.1016/S0140-6736(12)60322-5

Hawton, K., Zahl, D., & Weatherall, R. (2003). Suicide following deliberate self-harm: Long-term follow-up of patients who presented to a general hospital. *The British Journal of Psychiatry, 182*(6), 537–542. https://doi.org/10.1192/bjp.182.6.537

Hayes, M. L., & Sloat, R. S. (1990). Suicide and the gifted adolescent. *Journal for the Education of the Gifted, 13*(3), 229–244. https://doi.org/10.1177/016235329001300304

He, W., & Wong, W. (2014). Greater male variability in overexcitabilities: Domain-specific patterns. *Personality and Individual Differences, 66*, 27–32. https://doi.org/10.1016/j.paid.2014.03.002

He, W., Wong, W., & Chan, M. (2017). Overexcitabilities as important psychological attributes of creativity: A Dąbrowskian perspective. *Thinking Skills and Creativity, 25*, 27–35. https://doi.org/10.1016/j.tsc.2017.06.006

Hearn, C. B., & Seeman, J. (1971). Personality integration and perception of interpersonal relationships. *Journal of Personality and Social Psychology, 18*(2), 138–143. https://doi.org/10.1037/h0030849

Heatherton, T. F., & Nichols, P. A. (1994). Personal accounts of successful versus failed attempts at life change. *Personality and Social Psychology Bulletin, 20*(6), 664–675. https://doi.org/10.1177/0146167294206005

Heatherton, T. F., & Weinberger, J. L. (Eds.). (1994). *Can personality change?* Washington, DC: American Psychological Association.

Hebb, D. O. (1949). *The organization of behavior: A neuropsychological theory*. New York, NY: Wiley.

Hebb, D. O. (1972). *Textbook of psychology* (3rd ed.). Toronto, Canada: Saunders.

Hefferon, K., & Boniwell, I. (2011). *Positive psychology: Theory, research and applications*. Maidenhead Berkshire, England: Open University Press.

Hennequin, G., Agnes, E. J., & Vogels, T. P. (2017). Inhibitory plasticity: Balance, control, and codependence. *Annu. Rev. Neurosci, 40,* 557–79. https://doi.org/10.1146/annurev-neuro-072116-031005

Henshon, S. E. (2013). Finding a new vision of gifted education: An interview with David Yun Dai. *Roeper Review, 35*(2), 72–77. https://doi.org/10.1080/02783193.2013.766958

Her, W. L. E., & Haron, F. (2016). The association of giftedness, creativity, and postformal thinking in Malaysian adults. *Advanced Development, 15,* 47–63.

Herman, E. (1995). *The romance of American psychology: Political culture in the age of experts.* Berkeley, CA: University of California. Retrieved from https://publishing.cdlib.org/ucpressebooks/view?docId=ft696n b3n8&brand=ucpress

Hess, U., & Thibault, P. (2009). Darwin and emotion expression. *American Psychologist, 64*(2), 120–128. https://doi.org/10.1037/a0013386

Heylighen, F. (1992). A cognitive-systemic reconstruction of Maslow's theory of self-actualization. *Behavioral Science, 37*(1), 39–57. https://doi.org/10.1002/bs.3830370105

Hilger, K., Ekman, M., Fiebach, C. J., & Basten, U. (2017). Intelligence is associated with the modular structure of intrinsic brain networks. *Scientific Reports, 7*(1), 16088. https://doi.org/10.1038/s41598-017-15795-7

Hinshaw, S. P., Owens, E. B., Zalecki, C., Huggins, S. P., Montenegro-Nevado, A. J., Schrodek, E., & Swanson, E. N. (2012). Prospective follow-up of girls with attention-deficit/hyperactivity disorder into early adulthood: Continuing impairment includes elevated risk for suicide attempts and self-Injury. *Journal of Consulting and Clinical Psychology, 80*(6), 1041–1051. https://doi.org/10.1037/a0029451

Hinshaw, S. P., & Scheffler, R. M. (2014). *The ADHD explosion: Myths, medication, and money, and today's push for performance.* New York, NY: Oxford University Press.

Hoare, C. H. (Ed.). (2002). *Erikson on development in adulthood: New insights from the unpublished papers.* New York, NY: Oxford University.

Hoffman, E. (1988). *The right to be human: A biography of Abraham Maslow.* Los Angeles: Jeremy Tarcher.

Hoffman, E. (1992). The last interview of Abraham Maslow. *Psychology Today, 25*(1), 68–89.

Hoffmann, P. (1996). *The history of the German resistance 1933-1945* (R. Barry, Trans.). Montréal, Canada: McGill-Queens University Press.

Hofstee, W. K. B., de Raad, B., & Goldberg, L. R. (1992). Integration of the big five and circumplex approaches to trait structure. *Journal of Personality and Social Psychology, 63*(1), 146–163. https://doi.org/10.1037/0022-3514.63.1.146

Hogeveen, J., Salvi, C., & Grafman, J. (2016). Emotional intelligence: Lessons from lesions. *Trends in Neurosciences, 39*(10), 694–705. https://doi.org/10.1016/j.tins.2016.08.007

Homberg, J. R., Schubert, D., Asan, E., & Aron, E. N. (2016). Sensory processing sensitivity and serotonin gene variance: Insights into mechanisms shaping environmental sensitivity. *Neuroscience and Biobehavioral Reviews, 71*, 472–483. https://doi.org/10.1016/j.neubiorev.2016.09.029

Horowitz, M. J. (2016). *Adult personality growth in psychotherapy.* New York, NY: Cambridge University Press.

Hosking, J. G., Kastman, E. K., Dorfman, H. M., Samanez-Larkin, G. R., Baskin-Sommers, A., Kiehl, K. A., . . . Buckholtz, J. W. (2017). Disrupted prefrontal regulation of striatal subjective value signals in psychopathy. *Neuron, 95*(1), 221–231.e4. https://doi.org/10.1016/j.neuron.2017.06.030

Hudson, N.W., Fraley, R.C. (2015). Volitional personality trait change: can people choose to change their personality traits? *Journal of Personality and Social Psychology, 109*(3), 490–507.

Hughlings Jackson, J. (1884). Croonian lectures on the evolution and dissolution in the nervous system. Delivered at the Royal College of Physicians. (In three parts). *The Lancet*, Lecture 1: *123*(3161), 555–558. https://doi.org/10.1016/S0140-6736(02)22511-8;
Lecture 2: *123*(3163), 649–652. https://doi.org/10.1016/S0140-6736(02)22554-4;
Lecture 3: *123*(3165), 739–744. https://doi.org/10.1016/S0140-6736(02)23422-4

Hunt, T. K. A., Slack, K. S., & Berger, L. M. (2017). Adverse childhood experiences and behavioral problems in middle childhood. *Child Abuse & Neglect, 67*, 391–402. https://doi.org/10.1016/j.chiabu.2016.11.005

Hurley, R. A., & Taber, K. H. (2008). *Windows to the brain: Insights from neuroimaging.* Washington, DC: American Psychiatric Publishing.

Hyatt, L. (2010). A case study of the suicide of a gifted female adolescent: Implications for prediction and prevention. *Journal for the Education of the Gifted, 33*(4), 514–535. https://doi.org/10.1177/016235321003300404

Hyatt, L. A., & Cross, T. L. (2009). Understanding suicidal behavior of gifted students: Theory, factors and cultural expectations. In L. V. Shavinina (Ed.), *International Handbook on Giftedness* (pp. 537–556). New York: Springer. https://doi.org/10.1007/978-1-4020-6162-2_25

Hyzy, E. (2010). The theory of emotions and care ethics in the context of Kazimierz Dąbrowski's psychology (D. Scislowska, Trans.). *Heksis, 1.* Retrieved from https://heksis.dezintegracja.pl/en/the-theory-of-emotions-and-care-ethics-in-the-context-of-kazimierz-dabrowskis-psychology/

ICD-10 version: 2016. (2016, February 1). Retrieved December 8, 2016, from http://apps.who.int/classifications/icd10/browse/2016/en - /F60-F69

Jackson, P. S., & Moyle, V. F. (2009). With Dąbrowski in mind: Reinstating the outliers in support of full-spectrum development. *Roeper Review, 31*(3), 150–160. https://doi.org/10.1080/02783190902993607

Jackson, P. S., & Peterson, J. (2003). Depressive disorder in highly gifted adolescents. *Journal of Secondary Gifted Education, 14*(3), 175–187. https://doi.org/10.4219/jsge-2003-429

Jackson, P. S., Moyle, V., & Piechowski, M. M. (2009). Emotional life and psychotherapy of the gifted in light of Dąbrowski's theory. In L. Shavinina (Ed.), *International handbook on giftedness* (437–465). New York, NY: Springer. https://doi.org/10.1007/978-1-4020-6162-2_20

Jacobson, G. F. (1980). Crisis theory. *New directions for mental health services, 1980*, 1–10. https://doi.org/10.1002/yd.23319800603

Jahoda, M. (1958). *Current concepts of positive mental health.* Joint Commission on Mental Illness and Health, Monograph Series No. 1., New York, NY: Basic.

James, W. (1884). II.–What is an emotion? *Mind, os-IX*(34), 188–205. https://doi.org/10.1093/mind/os-IX.34.188

James, W. (1899). *On some of life's ideals.* New York, NY: Holt. Available at: http://positivedisintegration.com/James1899.pdf

James, W. (1907). The energies of men. *The Philosophical Review, 16*(1), 1–20. https://doi.org/10.2307/2177575

James, W. (1929). *Varieties of religious experience: A study in human nature.* New York, NY: Modern Library. (Original work published 1902)

James, W. (1950). *The principles of psychology.* (Vol. 1). New York, NY: Dover. (Original work published 1890)

Jamison, K. R. (2004). *Exuberance: The passion for life.* New York, NY: Knopf.

Jayawickreme, E., & Blackie, L. E. R. (2014). Post-traumatic growth as positive personality change: Evidence, controversies and future directions. *European Journal of Personality, 28*(4), 312–331. https://doi.org/10.1002/per.1963

Jayawickreme, E. & Blackie, L. E. R. (2016). *Exploring the psychological benefits of hardship: A critical reassessment of posttraumatic growth.* New York, NY: Springer.

Jennaway, A., & Merrotsy, P. (2011). Dąbrowski's theory of positive disintegration and its use with gifted children. *TalentEd, 27*, 61–67.

Jensen, P. (2009). *Ignite the third factor: Lessons from a lifetime of working with Olympic athletes, coaches and business leaders* (2nd ed.). Toronto, Canada: Performance Coaching.

Jepma, M., Verdonschot, R. G., Van Steenbergen, H., Rombouts, S. R. B., & Nieuwenhuis, S. (2012). Neural mechanisms underlying the induction and relief of perceptual curiosity. *Frontiers in behavioral neuroscience, 6*, 5. https://doi.org/10.3389/fnbeh.2012.00005

Jobes, D. A. (2016). *Managing suicidal risk: A collaborative approach* (2nd ed.). New York, NY: The Guilford Press.

John B. Watson. (2016, February 17). In Wikipedia, The Free Encyclopedia. Retrieved March 10, 2016, from https://en.wikipedia.org/wiki/John_B._Watson

John, O. P., & Scrivastava, S. (1999). The big five trait taxonomy: History, measurement and theoretical perspectives. In L. A. Pervin, & O. P. John (Eds.), *Handbook of personality: Theory and research* (2nd ed., pp. 102–138). New York, NY: Guilford.

Johns, D. C., Marx, R., Mains, R. E., O'Rourke, B., & Marbán, E. (1999). Inducible genetic suppression of neuronal excitability. *The Journal of Neuroscience, 19*(5), 1691–7. Retrieved from http://www.ncbi.nlm.nih.gov/pubmed/10024355/nhttp://www.ncbi.nlm.nih.gov/pubmed/10024355?dopt=Abstract&holding=npg

Johnson, J., & Wood, A. M. (2017). Integrating positive and clinical psychology: Viewing human functioning as continua from positive to negative can benefit clinical assessment, interventions and understandings of resilience. *Cognitive Therapy and Research, 41*(3), 335–349. https://doi.org/10.1007/s10608-015-9728-y

Johnson, S. F., & Boals, A. (2015). Refining our ability to measure posttraumatic growth. *Psychological Trauma: Theory, Research, Practice, and Policy, 7*(5), 422–429. https://doi.org/10.1037/tra0000013

Jokela, M., Virtanen, M., Batty, G. D., & Kivimäki, M. (2016). Inflammation and specific symptoms of depression. *JAMA Psychiatry, 73*(1), 87–88. https://doi.org/10.1001/jamapsychiatry.2015.1977

Joseph, D. L., & Newman, D. (2010). Emotional intelligence: An integrative meta-analysis and cascading model. *Journal of Applied Psychology, 95*(1), 54–78. https://doi.org/10.1037/a0017286

Joseph, S. (2011). *What doesn't kill us: The new psychology of posttraumatic growth.* New York, NY: Basic.

Joseph, S., & Linley, P. A. (Eds.). (2008). *Trauma, recovery and growth: Positive psychological perspectives on posttraumatic stress.* Hoboken, NJ: John Wiley.

Joseph, S., Murphy, D., & Regel, S. (2012). An affective-cognitive processing model of post-traumatic growth. *Clinical Psychology & Psychotherapy, 19*(4), 316–25. https://doi.org/10.1002/cpp.1798

Jovanovic, V., & Brdaric, D. (2012). Did curiosity kill the cat? Evidence from subjective well-being in adolescents. *Personality and Individual Differences, 52*(3), 380–384. https://doi.org/10.1016/j.paid.2011.10.043

Jung, C. G. (1926). *Psychological types or the psychology of individuation* (H. G. Baynes, Trans.). London, England: Kegan Paul, Trench, Trubner.

Jung, C. G. (1933). *Modern man in search of a soul* (C. F. Baynes, Trans.). London, England: Kegan Paul, Trench, Trubner.

Jung, C. G. (1940). The integration of the personality (S. M. Dell, Trans.). London, England: Kegan Paul, Trench, Trubner.

Juntune, J. E. (2009). Positive disintegration. In B. Kerr (Ed.), *Encyclopedia of giftedness, creativity and talent* Volume 2 (pp. 689–691). Thousand Oaks CA: Sage.

Kagan. J. (1984). *The nature of the child.* New York, NY: Basic.

Kalisch, R., Müller, M. B., & Tüscher, O. (2014). A conceptual framework for the neurobiological study of resilience. *Behavioral and Brain Sciences, 38*, 1–49. https://doi.org/10.1017/S0140525X1400082X

Kane, M. (2009). Contemporary voices on Dąbrowski's theory of positive disintegration. *Roeper Review, 31*(2), 72–76. https://doi.org/10.1080/02783190902737624

Kantor, M. (2006). *The psychopathy of everyday life: How antisocial personality disorder affects all of us.* Westport, CT: Praeger.

Karpinski, R. I., Kinase Kolb, A. M., Tetreault, N. A., & Borowski, T. B. (2017). High intelligence: A risk factor for psychological and physiological overexcitabilities. *Intelligence, 66*, 8–23. https://doi.org/10.1016/j.intell.2017.09.001

Karwowski, M. (2012). Did curiosity kill the cat? Relationship between trait curiosity, creative self-efficacy and creative personal identity. *Europe's Journal of Psychology, 8*(4). https://doi.org/10.5964/ejop.v8i4.513

Kashdan, T. B., & Fincham, F. D. (2002). Facilitating creativity by regulating curiosity: Comment. *American Psychologist, 57*(5), 373–374. https://doi.org/10.1037//0003-066X.57.5.373

Kast, V. (1990). *The creative leap: Psychological transformation through crisis* (D. Witcher, Trans.). Wilmette, IL: Chiron. (Original work published 1987)

Kaufman, S. B., & Gregoire, C. (2015). *Wired to create: Unraveling the mysteries of the creative mind.* New York, NY: Perigee.

Kaufmann, W. (1956). *Existentialism from Dostoevsky to Sartre.* New York, NY: Meridian.

Kegan, R. (1979). The evolving self: A process conception for ego psychology. *The Counseling Psychologist, 8*(2), 5–34. https://doi.org/10.1177/001100007900800203

Kegan, R. (1982). *The evolving self: Problem and process in human development.* Cambridge, MA: Harvard University Press.

Kegan, R. (1994). *In over our heads: The mental demands of modern life.* Cambridge, MA: Harvard University Press.

Kendler, K. S., & Prescott, C. A. (2006). *Genes, environment, and psychopathology: Understanding the causes of psychiatric and substance use disorders.* New York, NY: Guilford Press.

Kendler, K. S., Kessler, R. C., Walters, E. E., MacLean, C., Neale, M. C., Heath, A. C., & Eaves, L. J. (1995). Stressful life events, genetic liability, and onset of an episode of major depression in women. *The American Journal of Psychiatry, 152*(6), 833–842. https://doi.org/10.1176/ajp.152.6.833

Kennard, C., & Swash, M. (Eds.). (1989). *Hierarchies in neurology: A reappraisal of a Jacksonian concept.* London, UK: Springer.

Kennedy, D. M., Banks, R. S., & Grandin, T. (2011). *Bright not broken: Gifted kids, ADHD, and autism.* San Francisco, CA: Wiley.

Kerr, B. (Ed.). (2009). *Encyclopedia of giftedness, creativity and talent.* Thousand Oaks, CA: Sage.

Kierkegaard, S. (1941). *The sickness unto death.* (W. Lowrie, Trans.). Princeton, NJ: Princeton University Press.

Kierkegaard, S. (1962). The point of view of my work as an author: A report to history, and related writings (W. Lowrie, Trans.). New York, NY: Harper Torchbook.

Kierkegaard, S. (1980). *The concept of anxiety: A simple psychologically orienting deliberation on the dogmatic issue of hereditary sin.* (R. Thomte, Ed. & Trans.). Princeton, NJ: Princeton University Press.

Kierkegaard, S. (1987). *Either/or part II* (H. V. Hong & E. H. Hong, Eds. & Trans.). Princeton, NJ: Princeton University Press.

Kierkegaard, S. (2017). *Kierkegaard's journals and notebooks. Volume 9: Journals NB26-NB30.* (N. J. Cappelørn, A. Hannay, B. H. Kirmmse, D. D. Possen, J. D. S. Rasmussen, & V. Rumble, Eds.). Princeton NJ: Princeton University Press.

King, C., Foster, C. E., Rogalski, M. and Rogalski, K. M. (2013). *Teen suicide risk: A practitioner guide to screening, assessment, and management.* New York, NY: Guilford.

King, L. A. (2001). The hard road to the good life: The happy, mature person. *Journal of Humanistic Psychology, 41*(1), 51–73. https://doi.org/10.1177/0022167801411005

Klein, R. M. (1999). The Hebb legacy. *Canadian Journal of Experimental Psychology, 53*(1), 1–3. https://doi.org/10.1037/h0087295

Klemera, E., Brooks, F. M., Chester, K. L., Magnusson, J., & Spencer, N. (2017). Self-harm in adolescence: Protective health assets in the family, school and community. International *Journal of Public Health, 62*(6), 631–638. https://doi.org/10.1007/s00038-016-0900-2

Klemm, W. R. (2014). *Mental biology: The new science of how the brain and mind relate.* New York, NY: Prometheus.

Klonsky, E. D., May, A. M., & Saffer, B. Y. (2016). Suicide, suicide attempts, and suicidal ideation. *Annual Review of Clinical Psychology, 12*, 307–330. https://doi.org/10.1146/annurev-clinpsy-021815-093204

Knabb, J., & Welsh, R. (2009). Reconsidering A. Reza Arasteh: Sufism and psychotherapy. *Journal of Transpersonal Psychology, 41*(1), 44–61. Retrieved from http://www.atpweb.org/jtparchive/trps-41-09-01-044.pdf

Knight E. (1960). *The objective society.* New York, NY: George Braziller.

Knoff, W. F. (1970). A history of the concept of neurosis, with a memoir of William Cullen. *American Journal of Psychiatry, 127*, 80–84. https://doi.org/10.1176/ajp.127.1.80

Kobierzycki, T. (2000). Summaries: Profesor dr. Kazimierz Dąbrowski (1902-1980) (A. Przybyłek, Trans.). *Heksis: Scientific-didactic quarterly devoted to problems of person, health, creativity and spirituality, 1-3*(22–24), 276–279. Retrieved from http://positivedisintegration.com/Kobierzycki2000.pdf

Kobierzycki, T. (2010a). Biography of Kazimierz Dąbrowski (A. Danko, Trans.). *Heksis, 1. Heksis, 1.* Retrieved from http://positivedisintegration.com/Kobierzycki2010.pdf

Kobierzycki, T. (2010b). From creativity to the personality: A psychological study on the theory of positive disintegration (A. Danko & F. Maj, Trans.). *Heksis, 1.* Retrieved from https://heksis.dezintegracja.pl/en/from-creativity-to-the-personality/

Kohlberg, L. (1981). *Essays on moral development, Vol. I: The philosophy of moral development.* San Francisco, CA: Harper & Row.

Kokoszka, A. (2007). *States of consciousness: Models for psychology and psychotherapy.* New York, NY: Springer.

Kolb, B. & Whishaw, I. (2014). *Introduction to brain and behavior* (4th ed.). New York, NY: Worth.

Kolb, B. & Whishaw, I. (2015). *Fundamentals of human neuropsychology* (7th ed.). New York, NY: Worth.

Kolb, B., & Gibb, R. (2014). Searching for the principles of brain plasticity and behavior. *Cortex: A Journal Devoted to the Study of the Nervous System and Behavior, 58,* 251–60. https://doi.org/10.1016/j.cortex.2013.11.012

Kong, B., Li-Kong, H., & Lee, A. (Producers), & Lee, A. (Director). (2000). *Crouching Tiger, Hidden Dragon* [Motion picture]. China: Asia Union Film & Entertainment.

Konigsberg, E. (2006, January 16). Prairie fire. *New Yorker, 81*(44), 44–57. Retrieved from http://go.galegroup.com/ps/i.do?id=GALE|A140970605&v=2.1&u=ucalgary&it=r&p=AONE&sw=w&asid=7d1c4c00b3f97861c825da05f9ee7ecb

Konigsberg, E. (2007). Prairie fire. In *The best American magazine writing 2007, Compiled by the American Society of Magazine Editors* (pp. 235–270). New York, NY: Columbia University Press.

Krebs, D. L., & Denton, K. (2005). Toward a more pragmatic approach to morality: A critical evaluation of Kohlberg's model. *Psychological Review, 112*(3), 629–649. https://doi.org/10.1037/0033-295X.112.3.629

Krems, J. A., Kenrick, D. T., & Neel, R. (2017). Individual perceptions of self-actualization: What functional motives are linked to fulfilling one's full potential? *Personality and Social Psychology Bulletin, 43*(9), 1337–1352. https://doi.org/10.1177/0146167217713191

Kudinova, A. Y., Deak, T., Deak, M. M., & Gibb, B. E. (2017). Circulating levels of brain-derived neurotrophic factor and history of suicide attempts in women. *Suicide and Life-Threatening Behavior.* https://doi.org/10.1111/sltb.12403

Kunst, M. J. J. (2011). Affective personality type, post-traumatic stress disorder symptom severity and post-traumatic growth in victims of violence. *Stress and Health, 27*(1), 42–51. https://doi.org/10.1002/smi.1318

Kutchins, H., & Kirk, S. A. (1997). *Making us crazy: DSM–The psychiatric bible and the creation of mental disorders.* New York, NY: Free Press.

Lachman, G. (2016). *Beyond the robot: The life and work of Colin Wilson.* New York, NY: Penguin.

Lajoie, S. P. & Shore, B. M. (1981). Three myths? The over-representation of the gifted among dropouts, delinquents and suicides. *Gifted Child Quarterly, 25*(3), 138–143. https://doi.org/10.1177/001698628102500312

Lamare, P. (2017). *La theorie de la desintegration positive de Dąbrowski: Un autre regard sur la surdouance, la sante mentale et les crises existentielles.* (French Edition) CreateSpace Independent Publishing Platform.

Lambert, M. J., Hansen, N. B., & Finch, A. E. (2001). Patient-focused research: Using patient outcome data to enhance treatment effects. *Journal of Consulting and Clinical Psychology, 69*(2), 159–172. https://doi.org/10.1037/0022-006X.69.2.159

Lamont, R. T. (2012). The fears and anxieties of gifted learners: Tips for parents and educators. *Gifted Child Today, 35*(4), 271–276. https://doi.org/10.1177/1076217512455479

Large, M., Kaneson, M., Myles, N., Myles, H., Gunaratne, P., & Ryan, C. (2016). Meta-analysis of longitudinal cohort studies of suicide risk assessment among psychiatric patients: Heterogeneity in results and lack of improvement over time. *PLOS ONE, 11*(6), e0156322. https://doi.org/10.1371/journal.pone.0156322

Larsen, R. J. (Ed.). (2000). Emotion and personality: Introduction to the special symposium. *Personality and Social Psychology Bulletin, 26*(6), 651–654. https://doi.org/10.1177/0146167200268001

Larsen, R. J., & Buss, D. M. (2013). *Personality psychology: Domains of knowledge about human nature* (5th ed.). New York, NY: McGraw-Hill.

Laycraft, K. (2009). Positive maladjustment as a transition from chaos to order. *Roeper Review, 31*(2), 113–122. https://doi.org/10.1080/02783190902737681

Laycraft, K. (2011). Theory of Positive Disintegration as a model of adolescent development. *Nonlinear Dynamics Psychol Life Sci, 129–52.*

Leary, T. (1957). *Interpersonal diagnosis of personality: A functional theory and methodology for personality evaluation.* Eugene, OR: Wipf & Stock.

Leavitt, M. (2017). Acclimating to change: Orienting to intensity. In M. Leavitt, *Your passport to gifted education* (pp. 109–118). Cham, Switzerland: Springer. https://doi.org/10.1007/978-3-319-47638-4_9

LeBreton, J. M., Binning, J. F., & Adorno, A. J. (2006). Subclinical psychopaths. In J. C. Thomas & D. Segal (Eds.), *Comprehensive handbook of personality and psychopathology* (Vol. 1), *Personality and everyday functioning* (pp. 388–411). New York, NY: Wiley.

LeDoux, J. (1996). *The emotional brain: The mysterious underpinnings of emotional life.* New York, NY: Simon & Schuster.

LeDoux, J. (2012). A neuroscientist's perspective on debates about the nature of emotion. *Emotion Review, 4*(4), 375–379. https://doi.org/10.1177/1754073912445822

Lee, E., Lee, J., & Kim, E. (2016). Excitation/Inhibition imbalance in animal models of autism spectrum disorders. *Biological Psychiatry, 81*(10), 838–847. https://doi.org/10.1016/j.biopsych.2016.05.011

Lee, K. M., & Olenchak, F. R. (2015). Individuals with a gifted/attention deficit/hyperactivity disorder diagnosis. *Gifted Education International, 31*(3), 185–199. https://doi.org/10.1177/0261429414530712

Leighton, C., Botto, A., Silva, J. R., Jiménez, J. P., & Luyten, P. (2017). Vulnerability or sensitivity to the environment? Methodological issues, trends, and recommendations in gene-environment interactions research in human behavior. *Frontiers in Psychiatry, 8, 106*, 1–14. https://doi.org/10.3389/fpsyt.2017.00106

Lennon, M. (2013). *Norman Mailer: A double life.* New York, NY: Simon & Schuster.

Leslie, I. (2014). *Curious: The desire to know and why your future depends on it.* London, England: Quercus.

Levens, L. R. (2017). Curiosity doesn't kill cats: Passion and pragmatism for adventurous life-long learning. *Review & Expositor, 114*(3), 336–340. https://doi.org/10.1177/0034637317716987

Levine, B. & Craik, F. I. M. (2012). *Mind and the frontal lobes: Cognition, behavior, and brain imaging.* New York, NY: Oxford University Press.

Levine, D. S., & Jani, N. G. (2002). Toward a neural network theory of the triune brain. In G. A. Cory & R. Gardner (Eds.), *The evolutionary neuroethology of Paul Maclean: Convergences and frontiers* (pp. 383–394). Westport, CT: Praeger.

Levy, J. J., & Plucker, J. A. (2003). Assessing the psychological presentation of gifted and talented clients: A multicultural perspective. *Counselling Psychology Quarterly, 16*(3), 229–247. https://doi.org/10.1080/09515070310001610100

Lilienfeld, S. O., & Treadway, M. T. (2016). Clashing diagnostic approaches: DSM-ICD Versus RDoC. *Annual Review of*

Clinical Psychology, 12(1), 435–463.
https://doi.org/10.1146/annurev-clinpsy-021815-093122

Lilienfeld, S. O., Waldman, I. D., Landfield, K., Watts, A. L., Rubenzer, S., & Faschingbauer, T. R. (2012). Fearless dominance and the U.S. presidency: Implications of psychopathic personality traits for successful and unsuccessful political leadership. *Journal of Personality and Social Psychology, 103*(3), 489–505.
https://doi.org/10.1037/a0029392

Linde, K., Treml, J., Steinig, J., Nagl, M., & Kersting, A. (2017). Grief interventions for people bereaved by suicide: A systematic review. *PLOS ONE, 12*(6), e0179496.
https://doi.org/10.1371/journal.pone.0179496

Lindemann, E. (1944). Symptomatology and management of acute grief. *American Journal of Psychiatry, 101*(2), 141–148.
https://doi.org/10.1176/ajp.101.2.141

Lindner, R. (1956). *Must you conform?* New York, NY: Grove Press.

Linker, S. B., Bedrosian, T. A., & Gage, F. H. (2017). The kaleidoscopic brain: No two neurons are alike. What does that mean for brain function? *The Scientist*, November, 41–46.

Linley, P. A., Joseph, S., Harrington, S., Wood, A. M. (2006). Positive psychology: Past, present and (possible) future. *The Journal of Positive Psychology, 1*(1), 3–16.
https://doi.org/10.1080/17439760500372796

Livio, M. (2017). *Why? What makes us curious.* New York, NY: Simon & Schuster.

Lockwood, J., Daley, D., Townsend, E., & Sayal, K. (2017). Impulsivity and self-harm in adolescence: A systematic review. *European Child & Adolescent Psychiatry, 26*(4), 387–402. https://doi.org/10.1007/s00787-016-0915-5

Loevinger, J. (with Blasi, A.) (1976). *Ego development: Conceptions and theories.* San Francisco, CA: Jossey-Bass.

Lopez, S. J. (Ed.). (2009). *The encyclopedia of positive psychology.* Malden, MA: Wiley-Blackwell.

Lowe, M. J., Sakaie, K. E., Beall, E. B., Calhoun, V. D., Bridwell, D. A., Rubinov, M., & Rao, S. M. (2016). Modern methods for interrogating the human connectome. *Journal of the*

International Neuropsychological Society, 22(2), 105–119. https://doi.org/10.1017/S1355617716000060

Lowry, R. (1982). *The evolution of psychological theory: A critical history of concepts and presuppositions* (2nd ed.). New York, NY: Aldine de Gruyter.

Lund-Sørensen, H., Benros, M. E., Madsen, T., Sørensen, H. J., Eaton, W. W., Postolache, T. T., . . . Erlangsen, A. (2016). A nationwide cohort study of the association between hospitalization with infection and risk of death by suicide. *JAMA Psychiatry, 73*(9), 912-919. https://doi.org/10.1001/jamapsychiatry.2016.1594

Lykken, D. T. (1995). *The antisocial personalities*. Hillsdale, NJ: Erlbaum.

Lysy, K. Z., & Piechowski M. M. (1983). Personal growth: An empirical study using Jungian and Dąbrowskian measures. *Genetic Psychology Monographs, 108*, 267–320.

Lyttle, D. N., Gill, J. P., Shaw, K. M., Thomas, P. J., & Chiel, H. J. (2017). Robustness, flexibility, and sensitivity in a multifunctional motor control model. *Biological Cybernetics, 111*(1), 25–47. https://doi.org/10.1007/s00422-016-0704-8

MacLean, P. D. (1991). *The triune brain in evolution: Role in paleocerebral functions.* New York, NY: Plenum.

Macur, J. (2014). *Cycle of lies: The fall of Lance Armstrong.* New York, NY: Harper.

Magai, C., & Haviland-Jones, J. (2002). *The hidden genius of emotion: Lifespan transformations of personality.* Cambridge, England: Cambridge University Press.

Mahmut, M. K., Homewood, J., Stevenson, R. J. (2008). The characteristics of non-criminals with high psychopathy traits: Are they similar to criminal psychopaths? *Journal of Research in Personality, 42*(3), 679–692. https://doi.org/10.1016/j.jrp.2007.09.002

Mailer, N. (1957). The white negro. *Dissent, 4*(3), 276–293.

Mäki-Marttunen, T., Halnes, G., Devor, A., Witoelar, A., Bettella, F., Djurovic, S., . . . Dale, A. M. (2016). Functional effects of schizophrenia-linked genetic variants on intrinsic single-neuron excitability: A modeling study. *Biological Psychiatry:*

Cognitive Neuroscience and Neuroimaging, 1(1), 49–59. https://doi.org/10.1016/j.bpsc.2015.09.002

Maletic, V., & Raison, C. (2014). Integrated neurobiology of bipolar disorder. *Frontiers in Psychiatry, 5*(August), 98. https://doi.org/10.3389/fpsyt.2014.00098

Marcus, G., & Freeman, J. (Eds.). (2015). *The future of the brain: Essays by the world's leading neuroscientists.* Princeton, NJ: Princeton University Press.

Marie Jahoda. (2001, May, 2). [Obituary]. *The Guardian.* Retrieved 7 February 2017, from https://www.theguardian.com/news/2001/may/02/guardianobit uaries.highereducation

Martin, L. T., Burns, R. M., & Schonlau, M. (2009). Mental disorders among gifted and nongifted youth: A selected review of the epidemiologic literature. *Gifted Child Quarterly, 54*(1), 31–41. https://doi.org/10.1177/0016986209352684

Mascolo, M. F., & Griffin, S. (Eds.). (2013). *What develops in emotional development?* North Charleston, SC: Springer-Verlag.

Maslow, A. H. (1939). Dominance, personality and social behavior in women. *Journal of Social Psychology, 10*(1), 3–39. https://doi.org/10.1080/00224545.1939.9713343

Maslow, A. H. (1940). A test for dominance-feeling (self-esteem) in college women. *Journal of Social Psychology, 12*(2), 255–270. https://doi.org/10.1080/00224545.1940.9921471

Maslow, A. H. (1942). Self-esteem (dominance-feeling) and sexuality in women. *Journal of Social Psychology, 16*(2), 259–294. https://doi.org/10.1080/00224545.1942.9714120

Maslow, A. H. (1943a). Dynamics of personality organization. I. *Psychological Review, 50*(5), 514–539. https://doi.org/10.1037/h0062222

Maslow, A. H. (1943b). Dynamics of personality organization. II. *Psychological Review, 50*(6), 541–558. https://doi.org/10.1037/h0062037

Maslow, A. H. (1943c). Preface to motivation theory. *Psychosomatic Medicine, 5*(1), 85–92. https://doi.org/10.1097/00006842-194301000-00012

Maslow, A. H. (1943d). A theory of human motivation. *Psychological Review, 50*(4), 370–396. https://doi.org/10.1037/h0054346

Maslow, A. H. (1945). Experimentalizing the clinical method. *Journal of Clinical Psychology, 1*(3), 241–243. https://doi.org/10.1002/1097-4679(194507)1:3<241::AID-JCLP2270010317>3.0.CO;2-L

Maslow, A. H. (1954a). The instinctoid nature of basic needs. *Journal of Personality, 22*(3), 326-347. https://doi.org/10.1111/j.1467-6494.1954.tb01136.x

Maslow, A. H. (1954b). *Motivation and personality.* New York, NY: Harper.

Maslow, A. H. (1962). *Toward a psychology of being.* Princeton, NJ: Van Nostrand.

Maslow, A. H. (1964). *Religions, values and peak experiences.* New York, NY: Penguin.

Maslow, A. H. (1966). *The psychology of science: A reconnaissance.* Chicago, IL: Regnery.

Maslow, A. H. (1967). A theory of metamotivation: The biological rooting of the value-life. *Journal of Humanistic Psychology, 7*(2), 93–127. https://doi.org/10.1177/002216786700700201

Maslow, A. H. (1968). *Toward a psychology of being* (2nd ed.). New York, NY: Van Nostrand.

Maslow, A. H. (1970). *Motivation and personality* (2nd ed.). New York, NY: Harper and Row.

Maslow, A. H. (1976). *The farther reaches of human nature.* New York, NY: Penguin. (Original work published 1971)

Matthews, G., Deary, I. J., & Whiteman, M. C. (2009). *Personality traits* (3rd ed.). Cambridge, England: Cambridge University Press.

Matthews, G., & Gilliland, K. (1999). The personality theories of H. J. Eysenck and J. A. Gray: A comparative review. *Personality and Individual Differences, 26*(4), 583–626. https://doi.org/10.1016/S0191-8869(98)00158-5

Maturana, H. R., & Varela, F. J. (1987). *The tree of knowledge: The biological roots of human understanding.* Boston, MA: Shambhala.

Mayer, J. D., Caruso, D. R., & Salovey, P. (2016). The ability model of emotional intelligence: Principles and updates. *Emotion

Review, 8(4), 290–300.
https://doi.org/10.1177/1754073916639667

Mayer, J. D., DiPaolo, M. T., & Salovey, P. (1990). Perceiving affective content in ambiguous visual stimuli: A component of emotional intelligence. *Journal of Personality Assessment, 54*, 772–781. https://doi.org/10.1080/00223891.1990.9674037

Mayer, J. D., Roberts, R. D., & Barsade, S. G. (2008). Human abilities: Emotional intelligence. *Annual Review of Psychology, 59*, 507–36. https://doi.org/10.1146/annurev.psych.59.103006.093646

McAdams, D. P. (1995). What do we know when we know a person? *Journal of Personality, 63*(3), 365–396. https://doi.org/10.1111/j.1467-6494.1995.tb00500.x

McAdams, D. P. (2001). The psychology of life stories. *Review of General Psychology, 5*(2), 100–122. https://doi.org/10.1037/1089-2680.5.2.100

McAdams, D. P. (2006). The role of narrative in personality psychology today. *Narrative Inquiry, 16*(1), 11–18. https://doi.org/10.1075/ni.16.1.04mca

McAdams, D. P. (2015). *The art and science of personality development*. New York, NY: Guilford.

McAdams, D. P., & Emmons, R. A. (Eds.). (1995). Levels and domains in personality [Special issue]. *Journal of Personality, 63*(3), 341-727.

McAdams, D. P., & Pals, J. L. (2006). A new big five: Fundamental principles for an integrative science of personality. *American Psychologist, 61*(3), 204–217. https://doi.org/10.1037/0003-066X.61.3.204

McCabe, M. M. (1992). Myth, allegory and argument in Plato. *Apeiron, 25*(4), 47. https://doi.org/10.1515/APEIRON.1992.25.4.47

McCann, R. F., & Ross, D. A. (2017). Clinical commentary a fragile balance: Dendritic spines, learning, and memory. *Biological Psychiatry, 82*(2), e11–e13. https://doi.org/10.1016/j.biopsych.2017.05.020

McCrae, R. R., & Costa, P. T., Jr. (1996). Toward a new generation of personality theories: Theoretical contexts for the five-factor model. In J. S. Wiggins (Ed.), *The five-factor model of personality: Theoretical perspectives* (pp. 51–87). New York, NY: Guilford.

McCrae, R. R., & Costa, P. T. Jr. (2003). *Personality in adulthood: A Five-Factor theory perspective* (2nd ed.). New York, NY: Guilford.

McDonald, W. (2014). Søren Kierkegaard. In E. N. Zalta (Ed.), *The Stanford encyclopedia of philosophy*. Retrieved from http://plato.stanford.edu/archives/win2014/entries/kierkegaard

McGraw, J. G. (1986). Personality and its ideal in K. Dąbrowski's theory of positive disintegration: A philosophical interpretation. *Dialectics and Humanism, 13*, 211–237.

McGuirk, L., Kuppens, P., Kingston, R., & Bastian, B. (2017). Does a culture of happiness increase rumination over failure? *Emotion.* https://doi.org/10.1037/emo0000322

McLeod, S. A. (2016). *Id, ego and superego.* http://www.simplypsychology.org/psyche.html

McMillen, J. C., & Fisher, R. H. (1998). The Perceived Benefits Scales: Measuring perceived positive life changes after negative events. *Social Work Research, 22*(3), 173–187. https://doi.org/10.1093/swr/22.3.173

Meadows, J. P., Guzman-Karlsson, M. C., Phillips, S., Brown, J. A., Strange, S. K., Sweatt, J. D., & Hablitz, J. J. (2016). Dynamic DNA methylation regulates neuronal intrinsic membrane excitability. *Science Signaling, 9*(442), ra83–ra83. https://doi.org/10.1126/scisignal.aaf5642

Meares, R. (1999). The contribution of Hughlings Jackson to an understanding of dissociation. *American Journal of Psychiatry, 156*, 1850–1855. PMID:10588396

Medlock, G. (2012). The evolving ethic of authenticity: From humanistic to positive psychology. *The Humanistic Psychologist, 40*(1), 38–57. https://doi.org/10.1080/08873267.2012.643687

Mendaglio, S. (Ed.). (2008a). *Dąbrowski's Theory of Positive Disintegration.* Scottsdale, AZ: Great Potential Press.

Mendaglio, S. (2008b). Dąbrowski's theory of positive disintegration: A personality theory for the 21st century. In S. Mendaglio (Ed.), *Dąbrowski's theory of positive disintegration* (pp. 13–40). Scottsdale, AZ: Great Potential Press.

Mendaglio, S. (2008c). The theory of positive disintegration (TPD) and other approaches to personality. In S. Mendaglio (Ed.), *Dąbrowski's theory of positive disintegration* (pp. 249–274). Scottsdale, AZ: Great Potential Press.

Mendaglio, S. (2010). Anxiety in gifted students. In J. C. Cassady (Ed.), *Anxiety in schools: The causes, consequences and solutions for academic anxieties* (pp. 153–176). New York, NY: Peter Lang.

Mendaglio, S. (2011). Emotions and giftedness. In T. L. Cross, *On the social and emotional lives of gifted children: Understanding and guiding their development* (4th ed., pp. 55–61). Waco, TX: Prufrock Press.

Mendaglio, S. (2012). Overexcitabilities and giftedness research: A call for a paradigm shift. *Journal for the Education of the Gifted, 35*(3), 207–219. https://doi.org/10.1177/0162353212451704

Mendaglio, S. (2013). Gifted students' transition to university. *Gifted Education International, 29*(1), 3–12. https://doi.org/10.1177/0261429412440646

Mendaglio, S. (2017). Dąbrowski's dynamisms: Shapers of development and psychological constructs. *Advanced Development, 16*, 1–17.

Mendaglio, S., & Peterson, J. S. (2006). *Models of Counseling Gifted Children, Adolescents, And Young Adults.* Waco, TX: Prufrock Press.

Mendaglio, S., & Tillier, W. (2006) Dąbrowski's theory of positive disintegration and giftedness: Overexcitability research findings. *Journal for the Education of the Gifted, 30*(1), 68–87. http://dx.doi.org/10.1177/016235320603000104

Mendaglio, S., & Tillier, W. (2015). Has the time come to emulate Jung? A response to Piechowski's most recent rethinking of the Theory of Positive Disintegration: I. The case against primary integration. *Roeper Review, 37*(4), 219–228. https://doi.org/10.1080/02783193.2015.1077495

Michel, K. & Jobes, D. A. (2011). *Building a therapeutic relationship with the suicidal patient.* Washington, DC: American Psychological Association.

Mika, E. (2006). Giftedness, ADHD and overexcitabilities: The possibilities of misinformation. *Roeper Review, 28*(4), 237–242. https://doi.org/10.1080/02783190609554370

Mika, E. (2015, October 31). On primary integration, psychopathy, and the average person. [Web blog post]. Retrieved November 17, 2017 from https://www.linkedin.com/pulse/primary-integration-psychopathy-average-person-elizabeth-mika/

Mika, E. (2017). Who goes trump? Tyranny as a triumph of narcissism. In B. X. Lee (Ed.), *The dangerous case of Donald Trump: 27 psychiatrists and mental health experts assess a president* (pp. 298-318). New York, NY: Thomas Dunne.

Mikolajczak, M., Petrides, K. V, & Hurry, J. (2009). Adolescents choosing self-harm as an emotion regulation strategy: The protective role of trait emotional intelligence. *The British Journal of Clinical Psychology, 48*(Pt 2), 181–193. Retrieved from http://www.ncbi.nlm.nih.gov/pubmed/19054434

Miller, I. W., Camargo, C. A., Arias, S. A., Sullivan, A. F., Allen, M. H., Goldstein, A. B., . . . Boudreaux, E. D. (2017). Suicide prevention in an emergency department population. *JAMA Psychiatry, 2906*, 1–8. https://doi.org/10.1001/jamapsychiatry.2017.0678

Miller, N. B., Falk, R. F. & Huang, Y. (2009). Gender identity and the overexcitability profiles of gifted college students. *Roeper Review, 31*(3), 161–169. https://doi.org/10.1080/02783190902993920

Millon, T., Simonsen, E., & Birket-Smith, M. (1998). Historical Conceptions of psychopathy in the United States and Europe. In T. Millon, E. Simonsen, M. Birket-Smith, & R. D. Davis (Eds.), *Psychopathy: Antisocial, criminal and violent behavior* (pp. 3–31). New York, NY: Guilford.

Miloseva, L., Milosev, V., & Rihter, K. (2016). Cognition and suicide: Effectiveness of cognitive behaviour therapy. *International Journal of Cognitive Research in Science, Engineering and Education, 4*(1), 79–83. https://doi.org/10.5937/IJCRSEE1601079M

Mishara, B. L., & Kerkhof, Ad J F M (2013). *Suicide prevention and new technologies: Evidence based practice*. Basingstoke, UK: Palgrave Macmillan.

Missett, T. C. (2013). Exploring the relationship between mood disorders and gifted individuals. *Roeper Review, 35*(1), 47–57. https://doi.org/10.1080/02783193.2013.740602

Miu, A. C., Bîlc, M. I., Bunea, I., & Szentágotai-Tătar, A. (2017). Childhood trauma and sensitivity to reward and punishment: Implications for depressive and anxiety symptoms. *Personality and Individual Differences, 119*, 134–140. https://doi.org/10.1016/j.paid.2017.07.015

Mofield, E. L., & Parker Peters, M. (2015). The relationship between perfectionism and overexcitabilities in gifted adolescents. *Journal for the Education of the Gifted, 38*(4), 405–427. https://doi.org/10.1177/0162353215607324

Moore, S. J., Throesch, B. T., & Murphy, G. G. (2011). Of mice and intrinsic excitability: Genetic background affects the size of the postburst afterhyperpolarization in CA1 pyramidal neurons. *Journal of Neurophysiology, 106*(3), 1570–1580. https://doi.org/10.1152/jn.00257.2011

Morgan, J. K., & Desmarais, S. L. (2017). Associations between time since event and posttraumatic growth among military veterans. *Military Psychology, 29*(5), 456–463. https://doi.org/10.1037/mil0000170

Morris, D. B. (1991). *The culture of pain.* Berkeley, CA: University of California.

Morrison, K. H., Bradley, R., & Westen, D. (2003). The external validity of controlled clinical trials of psychotherapy for depression and anxiety: A naturalistic study. *Psychology and Psychotherapy: Theory, Research and Practice, 76*(2), 109–132. https://doi.org/10.1348/147608303765951168

Mos, L. P. (1994). We ought to be fighting over the meaning of authenticity. *Theory & Psychology, 4*(3), 447–454. https://doi.org/10.1177/0959354394043009

Mos, L. P., & Kuiken, D. (1998). Theoretical psychology at the University of Alberta 1965-1998. *History and Philosophy of Psychology Bulletin, 10*(1), 3–12.

Moss, D. (2001). The roots and genealogy of humanistic psychology. In K. J. Schneider, J. F. T. Bugental, & J. F. Pierson (Eds.), *The handbook of humanistic psychology: Leading edges in theory, research and practice* (pp. 5–20). Thousand Oaks, CA: Sage.

Mowrer, O. H. (1967). Introduction. In K. Dąbrowski, *Personality-shaping through positive disintegration* (pp. xi–xxxiv). Boston, MA: Little, Brown and Company.

Mroz, A. (2009). Theory of positive disintegration as a basis for research on assisting development. *Roeper Review, 31*(2), 96–102. https://doi.org/10.1080/02783190902737665

Mulligan, K., & Scherer, K. R. (2012). Toward a working definition of emotion. *Emotion Review, 4*(4), 345–357. https://doi.org/10.1177/1754073912445818

Murakami, T., Müller-Dahlhaus, F., Lu, M. K., & Ziemann, U. (2012). Homeostatic metaplasticity of corticospinal excitatory and intracortical inhibitory neural circuits in human motor cortex. *Journal of Physiology, 590*(22), 5765–5781. https://doi.org/10.1113/jphysiol.2012.238519

Murphy, A. (2017). *Out of this world: Suicide examined.* London, England: Karnac.

Myers, K., & Comer, J. S. (2016). The case for telemental health for improving the accessibility and quality of children's mental health services. *Journal of Child and Adolescent Psychopharmacology, 26*(3), 186–191. https://doi.org/10.1089/cap.2015.0055

Nadelhoffer, T., Nahmias, E. A., & Nichols, S. (Eds.). (2010). *Moral psychology: Historical and contemporary readings.* Malden, MA: Wiley-Blackwell.

Nasrallah, H. A. (2015). 10 Recent paradigm shifts in the neurobiology and treatment of depression. *Current Psychiatry, 14*(2), 10–13.

Neihart, M. (1999). The impact of giftedness on psychological well-being: What does the empirical literature say? *Roeper Review, 22*(1), 10–17. https://doi.org/10.1080/02783199909553991

Neimeyer, R. A., Fortner, B., & Melby, D. (2001). Personal and Professional factors and suicide intervention skills. *Suicide and Life-Threatening Behavior, 31*(1), 71–82. https://doi.org/10.1521/suli.31.1.71.21307

Nelson, J. M., Rinn, A. N., & Hartnett, D. N. (2006). The possibility of misdiagnosis of giftedness and ADHD still exists: A

response to Mika. *Roeper Review 28*(4), 243–249.
https://doi.org/10.1080/02783190609554371

Neve, M. (2004). Neurosis. *The Lancet, 363*(9415), 1170.
https://doi.org/10.1016/S0140-6736(04)15924-2

Newman, R. (2002, October). The road to resilience. *Monitor on psychology* (American Psychological Association), *33*(9).
Retrieved from http://www.apa.org/monitor/oct02/pp.aspx

Ngwena, J., Hosany, Z., & Sibindi, I. (2017). Suicide: A concept analysis. *Journal of Public Health, 25*(2), 123–134.
https://doi.org/10.1007/s10389-016-0768-x

Nickerson, R. S. (2000). Null hypothesis significance testing: A review of an old and continuing controversy. *Psychological Methods, 5*(2), 241–301. https://doi.org/10.1037/1082-989X.5.2.241

Nielsen, K. (2017). Kierkegaard and the modern search for self. *Theory & Psychology.*
https://doi.org/10.1177/0959354317742741

Nietzsche, F. (1966). *Thus spoke Zarathustra: A book for all and none* (W. Kaufmann, Trans.). New York, NY: Viking Press.

Nietzsche, F. (1968). *The will to power* (W. Kaufmann, Ed., W. Kaufmann & R. J. Hollingdale, Trans.). New York, NY: Vintage.

Nietzsche, F. (1989). *Beyond good and evil* (W. Kaufmann, Trans.). New York, NY: Vintage.

Nietzsche, F. (2001). *The gay science* (B. A., Williams, Ed., J. Nauckhoff, Trans.). Cambridge, UK: Cambridge University Press.

Nietzsche, F. W. (2007). *Ecce homo: How to become what you are* (D. Large, Trans.). New York, NY: Oxford University Press.

Nixon, L. F. (2005, Winter). Potential for positive disintegration and IQ. *The Dąbrowski Newsletter, 10*, 1–5. Available at:
http://positivedisintegration.com/nixon05.pdf

Nixon, L. F. (2010). Individual identity and union with the Absolute: An analysis of Dąbrowski's critique of Asian religions, *Advanced Development, 12*, 49–67.

Nixon, L. F. (2012). The function of mystical experiences in personality development. *Advanced Development, 13*, 42–67.

Nixon, L. F. (2016). Creativity and positive disintegration. *Advanced Development, 15*, 12–32.

Nock, M. K. (Ed.). (2014). *The Oxford handbook of suicide and self-injury*. New York, NY: Oxford University Press.

Nock, M. K. (2016). Recent and needed advances in the understanding, prediction, and prevention of suicidal behavior. *Depression and Anxiety, 33*, 460–463. https://doi.org/10.1002/da.22528

Norlander, T., Bood, S. A., & Archer, T. (2002). Performance during stress by different occupational groups: Affective personality, age and regularity of physical exercise. *Social Behavior and Personality, 30*(5), 495–508. https://doi.org/10.2224/sbp.2002.30.5.495

Norlander, T., Schedvin, H. Von, & Archer, T. (2005). Thriving as a function of affective personality: Relation to personality factors, coping strategies and stress. *Anxiety, Stress & Coping, 18*(2), 105–116. https://doi.org/10.1080/10615800500093777

Obsieger, B. (2017). Anxiety as the origin of freedom and responsibility. In A. Grøn, R. Rosfort, & K. B. Söderquist (Eds.), *Kierkegaard's Existential Approach* (pp. 171–191). Berlin, Germany: De Gruyter. https://doi.org/10.1515/9783110493016-009

Ocker, G. K., Litwin-Kumar, A., & Doiron, B. (2015). Self-organization of microcircuits in networks of spiking neurons with plastic synapses. *PLoS Computational Biology, 11*(8), 1–40. https://doi.org/10.1371/journal.pcbi.1004458

O'Connor, R. C. & Pirkis, J. (Eds.). (2016). *The international handbook of suicide prevention: Research, policy and practice* (2nd ed.). Hoboken, NJ: Wiley.

O'Connor, R. C., Ferguson, E., Scott, F., Smyth, R., McDaid, D., Park, A. L., . . . Armitage, C. J. (2017). A brief psychological intervention to reduce repetition of self-harm in patients admitted to hospital following a suicide attempt: A randomised controlled trial. *The Lancet Psychiatry, 4*(6), 451–460. https://doi.org/10.1016/S2215-0366(17)30129-3

O'Donovan, A., Rush, G., Hoatam, G., Hughes, B. M., McCrohan, A., Kelleher, C., . . . Malone, K. M. (2013). Suicidal ideation is associated with elevated inflammation in patients with major depressive disorder. *Depression and Anxiety, 30*(4), 307–14. https://doi.org/10.1002/da.22087

O'Leary, V. E., & Ickovics, I. R. (1995). Resilience and thriving in response to challenge: An opportunity for a paradigm shift in women's health. *Women's Health: Research on Gender, Behavior and Policy, 1*, 121–142.

Olfson, M., Blanco, C., Wall, M., Liu, S. M., Saha, T. D., Pickering, R. P., & Grant, B. F. (2017). National trends in suicide attempts among adults in the United States. *JAMA Psychiatry, 74*(11), 1095–1103. https://doi.org/10.1001/jamapsychiatry.2017.2582

Olfson, M., Wall, M., Wang, S., Crystal, S., Gerhard, T., & Blanco, C. (2017). Suicide following deliberate self-harm. *American Journal of Psychiatry, 174*(8), 765–774. https://doi.org/10.1176/appi.ajp.2017.16111288

Olszewski-Kubilius, P. M. (2015). Overexcitabilities: Interview with Daniel Winkler. Available from https://www.ctd.northwestern.edu/summer-2015-talent-newsletter

Olszewski-Kubilius, P. M., Kulieke, M. J., & Krasney, N. (1988). Personality dimensions of gifted adolescents: A review of the empirical literature. *Gifted Child Quarterly, 32*(4), 347–352. https://doi.org/10.1177/001698628803200403

Ormsby, E. (2006, November 29). T. S. Eliot's subway metaphysics readings. *The New York Sun.* Retrieved March 7, 2016 from http://www.nysun.com/article/44277

Ouspensky, P. D. (1971). *The fourth way.* New York, NY: Vintage.

Ouspensky, P. D. (1973). *The psychology of man's possible evolution.* New York, NY: Vintage. (Original work published 1945)

Owens, D., Horrocks, J., & House, A. (2002). Fatal and non-fatal repetition of self-harm: Systematic review. *The British Journal of Psychiatry, 181*(3), 193–199. https://doi.org/10.1192/bjp.181.3.193

Palma-Gudiel, H., & Fañanás, L. (2017). An integrative review of methylation at the serotonin transporter gene and its dialogue with environmental risk factors, psychopathology and 5-HTTLPR. *Neuroscience & Biobehavioral Reviews, 72*, 190–209. https://doi.org/10.1016/j.neubiorev.2016.11.011

Parappully, J., Rosenbaum, R., van den Daele, L., & Nzewi, E. (2002). Thriving after trauma: The experience of parents of murdered children. *Journal of Humanistic Psychology, 42*(1), 33–70. https://doi.org/10.1177/0022167802421003

Park, C. L., Cohen, L. H., & Murch, R. L. (1996). Assessment and prediction of stress-related growth. *Journal of Personality, 64*(1), 71–105. https://doi.org/10.1111/j.1467-6494.1996.tb00815.x

Parkes, G. (1994) *Composing the soul: Reaches of Nietzsche's psychology.* Chicago, IL: University of Chicago Press.

Passingham, R. E. (2016). *Cognitive Neuroscience: A very short introduction.* Oxford, UK: Oxford University Press.

Patrick, J. H., & Henrie, J. (2016). Up from the ashes: Age and gender effects on post-traumatic growth in bereavement. *Women & Therapy, 39*(3/4), 296–314. https://doi.org/10.1080/02703149.2016.1116863

Pawelski, J. O. (2016a). Defining the 'positive' in positive psychology: Part I. A descriptive analysis, *The Journal of Positive Psychology, 11*(4), 339–356, https://doi.org/10.1080/17439760.2015.1137627

Pawelski, J. O. (2016b). Defining the 'positive' in positive psychology: Part II. A normative analysis, *The Journal of Positive Psychology, 11*(4), 357–365. https://doi.org/10.1080/17439760.2015.1137628

Peairs, K. F., Eichen, D., Putallaz, M., Costanzo, P. R., & Grimes, C. L. (2011). Academic giftedness and alcohol use in early adolescence. *The Gifted Child Quarterly, 55*(2), 95–110. https://doi.org/10.1177/0016986210392220

Pérez-Álvarez, M. (2016). The science of happiness: As felicitous as it is fallacious. *Journal of Theoretical and Philosophical Psychology, 36*(1), 1–19. https://doi.org/10.1037/teo0000030

Perrone-McGovern, K. M., Simon-Dack, S. L., Beduna, K. N., Williams, C. C., & Esche, A. M. (2015). Emotions, cognitions, and well-being: The role of perfectionism, emotional overexcitability, and emotion regulation. *Journal for the Education of the Gifted, 38*(4), 343–357. https://doi.org/10.1177/0162353215607326

Peterson, C., Park, N., & Seligman, M. E. P. (2006). Greater strengths of character and recovery from illness. *The Journal of Positive Psychology, 1*(1), 17–26. https://doi.org/10.1080/17439760500372739

Petrides, K. V., Mikolajczak, M., Mavroveli, S., Sanchez-Ruiz, M. J., Furnham, A., & Pérez-González, J. C. (2016). Developments in trait emotional intelligence research. *Emotion Review, 8*(4), 335–341. https://doi.org/10.1177/1754073916650493

Pfeiffer, S. I. (2013). Lessons learned from working with high-ability students. *Gifted Education International, 29*(1), 86–97. https://doi.org/10.1177/0261429412440653

Pfeiffer, S. I. (Ed.). (2008). *Handbook of giftedness in children: Psychoeducational theory, research and best practices.* New York, NY: Springer.

Phelps, E. A. (2006). Emotion and cognition: insights from studies of the human amygdala. *Annual Review of Psychology, 57*, 27–53. https://doi.org/10.1146/annurev.psych.56.091103.070234

Piaget. J. (1954). *The construction of reality in the child.* New York, NY: Basic Books.

Piechowski, M. M. (1979). Developmental potential. In N. Colangelo and R. T. Zaffrann (Eds.), *New voices in counseling the gifted* (pp. 25–57). Dubuque, IA: Kendall Hunt.

Piechowski, M. M. (1991). Emotional development and emotional giftedness. In N. Colangelo & G. Davis (Eds.), *A Handbook of gifted education* (pp. 285–306). Boston, MA: Allyn & Bacon.

Piechowski, M. M. (2006). *"Mellow out," They say. If only I could: Intensities and sensitivities of the young and bright.* Madison, WI: Yunasa.

Piechowski, M. M. (2008). Discovering Dąbrowski's theory. In S. Mendaglio (Ed.), *Dąbrowski's theory of positive disintegration* (pp. 41–77). Scottsdale, AZ: Great Potential Press.

Piechowski, M. M. (2009a). The innerworld of the young and bright. In D. Ambrose & T. Cross (Eds.), *Morality, ethics, and gifted minds* (pp. 177–194). New York: Springer.

Piechowski, M. M. (2009b). Peace Pilgrim, exemplar of level V. *Roeper Review, 31*(2), 103–112. https://doi.org/10.1080/02783190902737673

Piechowski, M. M. (2010). Comment on Jane Piirto's: 21 Years with the Dąbrowski's Theory. *Advanced Development, 12*, 93–94.

Piechowski, M. M. (2014a). Rethinking Dąbrowski's Theory: I. The case against primary integration. *Roeper Review, 36*(1), 11–17. https://doi.org/10.1080/02783193.2013.856829

Piechowski, M. M. (2014b). The roots of Dąbrowski's Theory. *Advanced Development, 14*, 28–42.

Piechowski, M. M. (2015). A reply to Mendaglio and Tillier. *Roeper Review, 37*(4), 229–233. https://doi.org/10.1080/02783193.2015.1077496

Piechowski, M. M. (2017). Rethinking Dąbrowski's theory II: It's not all flat here. *Roeper Review, 39*(2), 87-95. https://doi.org/10.1080/02783193.2017.1289487

Piechowski, M. M., & Cunningham, K. (1985). Patterns of overexcitability in a group of artists. *Journal of Creative Behavior, 19*(3), 153–174. https://doi.org/10.1002/j.2162-6057.1985.tb00655.x

Piirto, J. (2010a). 21 Years with the Dąbrowski Theory: An autoethnography. *Advanced Development, 12*, 68–90.

Piirto, J. (2010b). Rejoinder. *Advanced Development, 12*, 95–96.

Piirto, J., & Fraas, J. (2012). A mixed-methods comparison of vocational and identified-gifted high school students on the Overexcitability Questionnaire. *Journal for the Education of the Gifted, 35*(1), 3–34. https://doi.org/10.1177/0162353211433792

Piirto, J., Montgomery, D., & May, J. (2008). A comparison of Dąbrowski's overexcitabilities by gender for American and Korean high school gifted students. *High Ability Studies, 19*(2), 141–153. https://doi.org/10.1080/13598130802504080

Pizarro, D. (2000). Nothing more than feelings? The role of emotions in moral judgment. *Journal for the theory of social behavior, 30*(4), 355–375. https://doi.org/10.1111/1468-5914.00135

Pizzolato, J. E. (2007). Assessing self-authorship. *New Directions for Teaching and Learning, 2007*(109), 31–42. https://doi.org/10.1002/tl.263

Plato. (1991). *The Republic of Plato* (2nd ed., A. D. Bloom, Trans.). New York, NY: Basic.

Plato. (2004). *Republic*. (C. D. C. Reeve, Trans.). Indianapolis, IN: Hackett.

Pliszka, S. R. (2016). *Neuroscience for the mental health clinician* (2nd ed.). New York, NY: Guilford.

Pluess, M., Assary, E., Lionetti, F., Lester, K. J., Krapohl, E., Aron, E. N., & Aron, A. (2017). Environmental sensitivity in children: Development of the highly sensitive child scale and identification of sensitivity groups. *Developmental Psychology. 54*(1), 51–70. https://doi.org/10.1037/dev0000406

Plutchik, R., & Conte, H. R. (Eds.). (1996). *Circumplex models of personality and emotions.* Washington, DC: American Psychological Association.

Pompili, M. (Ed.). (2018) *Phenomenology of suicide: Unlocking the suicidal mind.* New York, NY: Springer Berlin Heidelberg.

Posner, M. I., & Rothbart, M. K. (2007a). *Educating the human brain.* Washington, DC: American Psychological Association.

Posner, M. I., & Rothbart, M. K. (2007b). Research on attention networks as a model for the integration of psychological science. *Annual Review of Psychology, 58*, 1–23. https://doi.org/10.1146/annurev.psych.58.110405.085516

Power, M. J. (2016). *Understanding happiness: A critical review of positive psychology.* New York, NY: Routledge.

Power, M. J., & Dalgleish, T. (2008). *Cognition and emotion: From order to disorder* (2nd ed.). New York, NY: Psychology Press.

Pozo, K., & Goda, Y. (2010). Unraveling mechanisms of homeostatic synaptic plasticity. *Neuron, 66*(3), 337–351. https://doi.org/10.1016/j.neuron.2010.04.028

Pribram, K. H. (1982). Localization and distribution of function in the brain. In J. Orbach (Ed.), *Neuropsychology after Lashley* (pp. 273–296). New York, NY: Erlbaum.

Prince, M. (1929). Why we have traits—normal and abnormal: The theory of the integration of dispositions. *Journal of Abnormal Psychology, 23*(4), 422–433. https://doi.org/10.1037/h0063814

Priya, P. K., Rajappa, M., Kattimani, S., Mohanraj, P. S., & Revathy, G. (2016). Association of neurotrophins, inflammation and stress with suicide risk in young adults. *Clinica Chimica Acta;*

International Journal of Clinical Chemistry, 457, 41–5.
https://doi.org/10.1016/j.cca.2016.03.019

Probst, B. (2006). Issues in school placement for "twice exceptional" children: Meeting a dual agenda. *Journal of Therapeutic Schools and Programs, 1*(2), 174–188.
https://doi.org/10.19157/JTSP.issue.01.02.10

Probst, B., & Piechowski, M. (2012). Overexcitabilities and temperament. In T. L. Cross, & J. R. Cross (Eds.), *Handbook for counselors serving students with gifts and talents* (pp. 53-74). Waco, TX: Prufrock Press.

Putney, S., & Putney, G. J. (1964). *The adjusted American.* New York, NY: Harper and Row.

Pyryt, M. C. (2008). The Dąbrowskian lens: Implications for understanding gifted individuals. In S. Mendaglio (Ed.), *Dąbrowski's theory of positive disintegration* (pp. 175–182). Scottsdale, AZ: Great Potential Press.

Quinlivan, L., Cooper, J., Davies, L., Hawton, K., Gunnell, D., & Kapur, N. (2016). Which are the most useful scales for predicting repeat self-harm? A systematic review evaluating risk scales using measures of diagnostic accuracy. *BMJ Open, 6*, e009297. https://doi.org/10.1136/bmjopen-2015-009297

Quinlivan, L., Cooper, J., Meehan, D., Longson, D., Potokar, J., Hulme, T., . . . Kapur, N. (2017). Predictive accuracy of risk scales following self-harm: Multicentre, prospective cohort study. *The British Journal of Psychiatry, 210*(6), 429–436.
https://doi.org/10.1192/bjp.bp.116.189993

Raine, A. (2018). Antisocial personality as a neurodevelopmental disorder, (January), 1–31.
https://doi.org/10.1146/ANNUREV-CLINPSY-050817-084819

Ramos, C., & Leal, I. (2013). Posttraumatic Growth in the Aftermath of Trauma: A Literature Review About Related Factors and Application Contexts. *Psychology, Community & Health, 2*(1), 43–54. https://doi.org/10.5964/pch.v2i1.39

Rankel, M. D. (2008). Dąbrowski on authentic education. In S. Mendaglio (Ed.), *Dąbrowski's theory of positive disintegration* (pp. 79–100). Scottsdale, AZ: Great Potential Press.

Rannals, M. D., Hamersky, G. R., Page, S. C., Campbell, M. N., Briley, A., Gallo, R. A., . . . Maher, B. J. (2016). Psychiatric risk gene transcription factor 4 regulates intrinsic excitability of prefrontal neurons via repression of SCN10a and KCNQ1. *Neuron, 90*(1), 43–55. https://doi.org/10.1016/j.neuron.2016.02.021

Rathunde, K. (2001). Toward a psychology of optimal human functioning: What positive psychology can learn from the "experiential turns" of James, Dewey, and Maslow. *Journal of Humanistic Psychology, 41*(1), 135–153. http://doi.org/10.1177/0022167801411008

Reiner, A. (1990). An explanation of behavior? [Review of the book *The Triune Brain in Evolution. Role in Paleocerebral Functions*. By P. D. MacLean]. *Science, 250*(4978), 303–305. https://doi.org/10.1126/science.250.4978.303-a

Reiss, S. (2008). *The normal personality: A new way of thinking about people*. New York, NY: Cambridge University Press.

Remme, M. W. H., & Wadman, W. J. (2012). Homeostatic Scaling of Excitability in Recurrent Neural Networks. *PLoS Computational Biology, 8*(5), e1002494. https://doi.org/10.1371/journal.pcbi.1002494

Rendon, J. (2015). *Upside: The new science of post-traumatic growth*. New York, NY: Simon & Schuster.

Rich, G. J. (2001). Positive psychology: An introduction. *Journal of Humanistic Psychology, 41*(1), 8–12. https://doi.org/10.1177/0022167801411002

Rich, G. J. (2017a). Positive psychology and humanistic psychology. *Journal of Humanistic Psychology*, (January). https://doi.org/10.1177/0022167817698820

Rich, G. J. (2017b). The promise of qualitative inquiry for positive psychology: Diversifying methods. *The Journal of Positive Psychology, 12*(3), 220–231. https://doi.org/10.1080/17439760.2016.1225119

Rich, G. J. (2018). Positive psychology and humanistic psychology: Evil twins, sibling rivals, distant cousins, or something else? *Journal of Humanistic Psychology, 58*(3), 262–283. https://doi.org/10.1177/0022167817698820

Richards, D. A., Ekers, D., McMillan, D., Taylor, R. S., Byford, S., Warren, F. C., . . . Finning, K. (2016). Cost and outcome of behavioural activation versus cognitive behavioural therapy for depression (COBRA): A randomised, controlled, non-inferiority trial. *The Lancet, 388*(10047), 871-880. https://doi.org/10.1016/S0140-6736(16)31140-0

Richmond, S., Johnson, K. A., Seal, M. L., Allen, N. B., & Whittle, S. (2016). Development of brain networks and relevance of environmental and genetic factors: A systematic review. *Neuroscience and Biobehavioral Reviews, 71,* 215–239. https://doi.org/10.1016/j.neubiorev.2016.08.024

Rinn, A. N. & Reynolds, M. J. (2012). Overexcitabilities and ADHD in the gifted: An examination. *Roeper Review, 34*(1), 38–45 https://doi.org/10.1080/02783193.2012.627551

Rinn, A. N., Mendaglio, S., Rudasill, K. M., & McQueen, K.S. (2010). Examining the relationship between the overexcitabilities and self-concepts of gifted adolescents via multivariate cluster analysis. *Gifted Child Quarterly, 54*(1), 3–17. https://doi.org/10.1177/0016986209352682

Ripper, C. A., Boyes, M. E., Clarke, P. J. F., & Hasking, P. A. (2018). Emotional reactivity, intensity, and perseveration: Independent dimensions of trait affect and associations with depression, anxiety, and stress symptoms. *Personality and Individual Differences, 121,* 93–99. https://doi.org/10.1016/j.paid.2017.09.032

Risk factors and warning signs (n.d.). In *American foundation for suicide prevention*. Retrieved from https://afsp.org/about-suicide/risk-factors-and-warning-signs/

Rizzo, M. J. (1999). The coming slavery: The determinism of Herbert Spencer. *Review of Austrian Economics, 12*(2), 115–130. https://doi.org/10.1023/A:1007802424614

Roberts, B. W., Luo, J., Briley, D. A., Chow, P. I., Su, R., & Hill, P. L. (2017). A systematic review of personality trait change through intervention. *Psychological Bulletin, 143*(2), 117–141. http://doi.org/10.1037/bul0000088

Robinson, O. C., Demetre, J. D., & Litman, J. A. (2017). Adult life stage and crisis as predictors of curiosity and authenticity.

International Journal of Behavioral Development, 41(3), 426–431. https://doi.org/10.1177/0165025416645201

Robinson, R. G. (2006). *The clinical neuropsychiatry of stroke: Cognitive, behavioral and emotional disorders following vascular brain injury* (2nd ed.). Cambridge, England: Cambridge University.

Rodway, C., Tham, S. G., Ibrahim, S., Turnbull, P., Windfuhr, K., Shaw, J., . . . Appleby, L. (2016). Suicide in children and young people in England: A consecutive case series. The *Lancet Psychiatry, 3*(8), 751–759. https://doi.org/10.1016/S2215-0366(16)30094-3

Roepke, A. M. (2014). Psychosocial interventions and posttraumatic growth: A meta-analysis. *Journal of Consulting and Clinical Psychology, 83*(1), 129–142. https://doi.org/10.1037/a0036872

Roepke, A. M., & Seligman, M. E. P. (2015). Doors opening: A mechanism for growth after adversity. *The Journal of Positive Psychology, 10*(2), 107–115. https://doi.org/10.1080/17439760.2014.913669

Rogers, B. (2008, February). Charles Taylor. *Prospect Magazine, 143*. Retrieved February 16, 2016, from http://www.prospectmagazine.co.uk/features/charles-taylor-profile-secular-age

Rogers, C. (1961). *On becoming a person: A therapist's view of psychotherapy*. Boston, MA: Houghton Mifflin.

Romanowska-Lakomy, H. (2010). The problem of the meaning of life in Kazimierz Dąbrowski's psychotherapy (M. Uminski, Trans.). *Heksis, 1*. Retrieved from https://heksis.dezintegracja.pl/en/the-problem-of-the-meaning-of-life-in-kazimierz-dabrowskis-psychotherapy/

Romey, E. A. (2013). How Tony Stark can save the world: Overexcitability and positive disintegration in popular culture. In E. A. Romey (Ed.), *Finding John Galt: People, politics, and practice in gifted education* (pp. 255–269). Charlotte, NC: Information Age.

Rosenbaum, R., Smith, M. A., Kohn, A., Rubin, J. E., & Doiron, B. (2017). The spatial structure of correlated neuronal variability. *Nature Neuroscience, 20*(1), 107–114. https://doi.org/10.1038/nn.4433

Roskies, A. L. (2012). Don't panic: Self-authorship without obscure metaphysics. *Philosophical Perspectives, 26*(1), 323–342. https://doi.org/10.1111/phpe.12016

Rowan, J. (2007). On leaving flatland and honoring Maslow. *Humanistic Psychologist, 35*(1), 73–79. https://doi.org/10.1207/s15473333thp3501_6

Roy, B., & Dwivedi, Y. (2017). Understanding epigenetic architecture of suicide neurobiology: A critical perspective. *Neuroscience & Biobehavioral Reviews, 72*, 10–27. https://doi.org/10.1016/j.neubiorev.2016.10.031

Royce, J. R. (1983). Personality integration: A synthesis of the parts of the wholes of individuality theory. *Journal of Personality, 51*(4), 683–706. https://doi.org/10.1111/j.1467-6494.1983.tb00874.x

Royce, J. R., & Mos, L. (1981) Introduction. In J. Royce & L. Mos (Eds.), *Humanistic psychology: Concepts and criticisms* (pp. xiii–xx). New York, NY: Plenum.

Rubens, R. L. (1992). *Psychoanalysis and the tragic sense of life. New Ideas in Psychology, 10*(3), 347–362. https://doi.org/10.1016/0732-118X(92)90010-W

Rubin, J. (2000). William James and the pathologizing of human experience. *Journal of Humanistic Psychology, 40*(2), 176–226. https://doi.org/10.1177/0022167800402006

Rudd, M. D., Bryan, C. J., Wertenberger, E. G., Peterson, A. L., Young-McCaughan, S., Mintz, J., … Bruce, T. O. (2015). Brief cognitive-behavioral therapy effects on post-treatment suicide attempts in a military sample: Results of a randomized clinical trial with 2-year follow-up. *American Journal of Psychiatry, 172*(5), 441–449. https://doi.org/10.1176/appi.ajp.2014.14070843

Ryan, R. M., & Deci, E. L. (2001). On happiness and human potentials: A review of research on hedonic and eudaimonic well-being. *Annual Review of Psychology, 52*, 141–166. https://doi.org/10.1146/annurev.psych.52.1.141

Rycroft, C. (1995). *A critical dictionary of psychoanalysis* (2nd ed.). London, England: Penguin. (Original work published 1968)

Saint-Exupéry, A. de. (1939). *Wind, sand and stars* (L. Galantiere, Trans.). New York, NY: Reynal & Hitchcock.

Salovey, P., & Mayer, J. D. (1990). Emotional intelligence. *Imagination, Cognition and Personality, 9*(3), 185–211. https://doi.org/10.2190/DUGG-P24E-52WK-6CDG

Samanez-Larkin, G. R., Hollon, N. G., Carstensen, L. L., & Knutson, B. (2008) Individual differences in insular sensitivity during loss anticipation predict avoidance learning. *Psychological Science, 19*(4), 320–323. https://doi.org/10.1111/j.1467-9280.2008.02087.x

Sansom, S., Barnes, B., Carrizales, J., & Shaughnessy, M. F. (2018). A reflective conversation with Jane Piirto. Gifted Education International, 34(1), 96–111. https://doi.org/10.1177/0261429416650950

Santas, G. (Ed.). (2006). *The Blackwell guide to Plato's Republic.* Cornwall, England: Blackwell.

Sapolsky, R. M. (2017). *Behave: The biology of humans at our best and worst.* New York, NY: Penguin Press.

Saunders, K. E. A. (2016). Risk factors for suicide in children and young people: Common yet complex. *The Lancet. Psychiatry, 3*(8), 699–700. https://doi.org/10.1016/S2215-0366(16)30102-X

Schilling, E. A., Aseltine, R. H., & James, A. (2016). The SOS suicide prevention program: Further evidence of efficacy and effectiveness. *Prevention Science, 17*(2), 157–166. https://doi.org/10.1007/s11121-015-0594-3

Schneider, K. (2012). The subject-object transformations and "bildung." *Educational Philosophy and Theory, 44*(3), 302–311. https://doi.org/10.1111/j.1469-5812.2010.00696.x

Scholwinski, E. (1985). Dimensions of anxiety among high IQ children. *Gifted Child Quarterly, 29*(3), 125–130. https://doi.org/10.1177/001698628502900305

Schulte, M. J., Ree, M. J., & Carretta, T. R. (2004). Emotional intelligence: Not much more than g and personality. *Personality and Individual Differences, 37*(5), 1059–1068. https://doi.org/10.1016/j.paid.2003.11.014

Schulz, D. J. (2006). Plasticity and stability in neuronal output via changes in intrinsic excitability: It's what's inside that counts. *Journal of Experimental Biology, 209*(24), 4821–4827. https://doi.org/10.1242/jeb.02567

Schwarz, A. (2016). *ADHD nation: Children, doctors, big Pharma, and the making of an American epidemic.* New York, NY: Scribner.

Secker, J. (1998). Current conceptualizations of mental health and mental health promotion. *Health Education Research, 13*(1), 57–66. https://doi.org/10.1093/her/13.1.57

Sedillo, P. J. (2015). Gay gifted adolescent suicide and suicidal ideation literature. *Gifted Child Today, 38*(2), 114–120. https://doi.org/10.1177/1076217514568557

Seeman, J. (1959). Toward a concept of personality integration. *American Psychologist, 14*(10), 633–637. https://doi.org/10.1037/h0042986

Seeman, J. (1966). Personality integration in college women. *Journal of Personality and Social Psychology, 4*(1), 91–93. http://dx.doi.org/10.1037/h0023521

Seeman, J. (1983). Personality integration in children and adults: Some developmental continuities. *Peabody Journal of Education, 60*(3), 29–44. https://doi.org/10.1080/01619568309538405

Seeman, J. (1989). Toward a model of positive health. *American Psychologist, 44*(8), 1099–1109. https://doi.org/10.1037/0003-066X.44.8.1099

Seeman, J., Barry, E., & Ellinwood, C. (1963). Personality integration as a criterion of therapy outcome. *Psychotherapy: Theory, Research & Practice, 1*(1), 14–16. https://doi.org/10.1037/h0088566

Seligman, M. E. P. (1999). The president's address. *American Psychologist, 54*, 559–562.

Seligman, M. E. P. (2002). *Authentic happiness: Using the new positive psychology to realize your potential for lasting fulfillment.* New York, NY: Free Press/Simon and Schuster.

Seligman, M. E. P., & Csíkszentmihályi, M. (2000). Positive psychology: An introduction. *American Psychologist, 55*(1), 5–14. https://doi.org/10.1037/0003-066X.55.1.5

Seligman, M. E. P., & Fowler, R. D. (2011). Comprehensive soldier fitness and the future of psychology. *The American psychologist, 66*(1), 82–6. https://doi.org/10.1037/a0021898.

Seligman, M. E. P., Ernst, R., Gillham, J., Reivich, K., & Linkins, M. (2009). Positive education: Positive psychology and classroom interventions. *Oxford Review of Education, 35*(3), 293–311. https://doi.org/10.1080/03054980902934563

Sevush, S. (2016). *The single-neuron theory: Closing in on the neural correlate of consciousness.* Cham, Switzerland: Springer.

Shaffer, D. R. (2009). *Social and personality development* (6th ed.). Belmont, CA: Wadsworth/Cengage Learning.

Shakespeare, W. (1905). *Shakespeare Complete Works.* (W. J. Craig, Ed.). London, England: The Oxford University Press. (As You Like It, Act II. Scene I)

Shavinina, L. V., & Ferrari, M. (Eds.). (2004). *Beyond knowledge: Extracognitive aspects of developing high ability.* Mahwah, NJ: Lawrence Erlbaum.

Shedler, J. (2012). The efficacy of psychodynamic psychotherapy. *Psychodynamic Psychotherapy Research, 65,* 9–25. https://doi.org/10.1007/978-1-60761-792-1_2

Sheftall, A. H., Asti, L., Horowitz, L. M., Felts, A., Fontanella, C. A., Campo, J. V., & Bridge, J. A. (2016). Suicide in elementary school-aged children and early adolescents. *Pediatrics, 138,* e20160436. https://doi.org/10.1542/peds.2016-0436

Sheldon, K. M. (2004). *Optimal human being: An integrated multi-level perspective.* Mahwah, NJ: Lawrence Erlbaum.

Sheldon, K. M., Kashdan, T. B., & Steget, M. F. (Eds.). (2011). *Designing positive psychology: Taking stock and moving forward.* Oxford Scholarship Online https://doi.org/10.1093/acprof:oso/9780195373585.001.0001

Sherrington C. (1948). *The integrated action of the nervous system: With a new forward by the author and a bibliography of his writings.* Cambridge, England: Cambridge University Press. (Original work published 1906)

Shuwiekh, H., Kira, I. A., & Ashby, J. S. (2017). What are the personality and trauma dynamics that contribute to posttraumatic growth? *International Journal of Stress Management.* https://doi.org/10.1037/str0000054

Silverman, L. K. (2008). The theory of positive disintegration in the field of gifted education. In S. Mendaglio (Ed.), *Dąbrowski's*

Theory of Positive Disintegration (pp. 157–173). Scottsdale, AZ: Great Potential Press.

Silverman, L. K. (2009). My love affair with Dąbrowski's theory: A personal odyssey. *Roeper Review, 31*(3),141–149. https://doi.org/10.1080/02783190902993912

Silverman, L. K. (2016). Empathy: The heart of Dąbrowski's Theory. *Advanced Development, 15*, 32–47.

Silverman, L. K., & Miller, N. B. (2014). Dąbrowski's Theory and Advanced Development: How it began and where we are today. *Advanced Development, 14*, 73–88.

Simanowitz, V., & Pearce, P. (2003). *Personality development.* Maidenhead, UK: Open University Press.

Simmons, J. P., Nelson, L. D., & Simonsohn, U. (2011). False-positive psychology: Undisclosed flexibility in data collection and analysis allows presenting anything as significant. *Psychological Science, 22*(11), 1359–1366. https://doi.org/10.1177/0956797611417632

Sinnott-Armstrong, W. (Ed.) (2008-2014). *Moral Psychology* (Vols. 1-4). Cambridge, MA: MIT Press.

Siu, Angela F. Y. (2010). Comparing overexcitabilities of gifted and non-gifted school children in Hong Kong: Does culture make a difference? *Asia Pacific Journal of Education, 30*(1), 71–83. https://doi.org/10.1080/02188790903503601

Skovlund, C. W., Mørch, L. S., Kessing, L. V., Lange, T., & Lidegaard, Ø. (2017). Association of hormonal contraception with suicide attempts and suicides. *American Journal of Psychiatry, 73*(11), https://doi.org/10.1176/appi.ajp.2017.17060616

Slaney, K. L. (2017). *Validating psychological constructs: Historical, philosophical, and practical dimensions.* London, UK: Palgrave.

Slaney, K. L., & Racine, T. P. (2013). What's in a name? Psychology's ever evasive construct. *New Ideas in Psychology, 31*(1), 4–12. https://doi.org/10.1016/j.newideapsych.2011.02.003

Smith, T. W. (1979). Happiness: Time trends, seasonal variations, intersurvey differences and other mysteries. *Social Psychology Quarterly, 42*(1), 18–30. https://doi.org/10.2307/3033870

Smoller, J. W. (2013). Identification of risk loci with shared effects on five major psychiatric disorders: a genome-wide analysis. *The Lancet, 381*(9875), 1371–1379. https://doi.org/10.1016/S0140-6736(12)62129-1

Snyder, C. R., & Lopez, S. J. (Eds.). (2002). *Handbook of positive psychology*. New York, NY: Oxford University Press.

Snyder, C. R., Lopez, S. J., & Pedrotti, J. T. (2010). *Positive psychology: The scientific and practical explorations of human strengths* (2nd ed.). Thousand Oaks, CA: Sage.

Sokolov, E. N. (1963). Higher nervous functions: The orienting reflex. *Annual Review of Physiology, 25*(1), 545–580. https://doi.org/10.1146/annurev.ph.25.030163.002553

Solomon, R. C. (1999). *The joy of philosophy: Thinking thin versus the passionate life*. New York, NY: Oxford University Press.

Souza, L. D. L., Lopez Molina, M., Azevedo da Silva, R., & Jansen, K. (2016). History of childhood trauma as risk factors to suicide risk in major depression. *Psychiatry Research*, 246, 612-616. https://doi.org/10.1016/j.psychres.2016.11.002

Spencer, H. (1900). *First principles* (4th ed.). Akron, OH: Werner.

Sporns, O. (2011). *Networks of the brain.* Cambridge, MA: Massachusetts Institute of Technology.

Sporns, O. (2012). *Discovering the human connectome*. Cambridge, MA: Massachusetts Institute of Technology.

Sporns, O., & Betzel, R. F. (2016). Modular Brain Networks. *Annual Review of Psychology, 67*(1), 613–640. https://doi.org/10.1146/annurev-psych-122414-033634

Srivastava, S., Oliver, P. J., Gosling, S. D., & Potter, J. (2003). Development of personality in early and middle adulthood: Set like plaster or persistent change? *Journal of Personality and Social Psychology, 84*(5), 1041–1053. https://doi.org/10.1037/0022-3514.84.5.1041

Stanley, M. L., Moussa, M. N., Paolini, B. M., Lyday, R. G., Burdette, J. H., & Laurienti, P. J. (2013). Defining nodes in complex brain networks. *Frontiers in Computational Neuroscience, 7*(November), 169. https://doi.org/10.3389/fncom.2013.00169

Stasiak, K., Fleming, T., Lucassen, M. F. G., Shepherd, M. J., Whittaker, R., & Merry, S. N. (2016). Computer-Based and online therapy for depression and anxiety in children and adolescents. *Journal of Child and Adolescent Psychopharmacology, 26*(3), 235–45. https://doi.org/10.1089/cap.2015.0029

Sternberg, R. J. (2017). ACCEL: A new model for identifying the gifted. *Roeper Review, 39*(3), 152–169. https://doi.org/10.1080/02783193.2017.1318658

Sternberg, R. J. (2018). 21 Ideas: A 42-year search to understand the nature of giftedness. *Roeper Review, 40*(1), 7–20. https://doi.org/10.1080/02783193.2018.1393609

Sternberg, R. J., Jarvin, L., & Grigorenko, E. L. (2011). *Explorations in giftedness*. Cambridge NY: Cambridge University Press.

Stokes, P. (2015). *The naked self: Kierkegaard and personal identity*. Oxford, UK: Oxford University Press.

Storr, A. (1983). Introduction. In E. A. Bennet, *What Jung really said* (2nd ed., pp. vii–xiii). New York, NY: Schocken. (Original work published 1966)

Survivors of Suicide Loss Task Force. (2015). *Responding to grief, trauma, and distress after a suicide: U.S. national guidelines*. Washington, DC: Action Alliance for Suicide Prevention. Retrieved from: http://actionallianceforsuicideprevention.org/sites/actionallianceforsuicideprevention.org/files/NationalGuidelines.pdf

Swanson, L. W., & Lichtman, J. W. (2016). From Cajal to connectome and beyond. *Annual Review of Neuroscience, 39*(1), 197–216. https://doi.org/10.1146/annurev-neuro-071714-033954

Szasz, T. (1974). *The myth of mental illness: Foundations of a theory of personal conduct* (Rev. ed.). New York, NY: Harper.

Takarae, Y., & Sweeney, J. (2017). Neural hyperexcitability in autism spectrum disorders. *Brain Sciences, 7*(10), 129. https://doi.org/10.3390/brainsci7100129

Tangney, J. P., Stuewig, J., & Mashek, D. J. (2007). Moral emotions and moral behavior. *Annual Review of Psychology, 58*, 345–72. https://doi.org/10.1146/annurev.psych.56.091103.070145

Tart, C. (1987). *Waking up: Overcoming the obstacles to human potential*. Boston, MA: Shambala.

Tatti, R., Haley, M. S., Swanson, O. K., Tselha, T., & Maffei, A. (2017). Neurophysiology and regulation of the balance between excitation and inhibition in neocortical circuits. *Biological Psychiatry, 81*(10), 821–831. https://doi.org/10.1016/j.biopsych.2016.09.017

Tavernise, S. (2016, April 22). Sweeping pain as suicides hit a 30-year high. *NY Times.* A1.

Tavris, C. (2014). The negative side of positive psychology. *Skeptic Magazine, 19*(3), 8–9.

Taylor, C. (1989). *Sources of the self: The making of the modern identity.* Cambridge, MA: Harvard University Press.

Taylor, E. (1984). *William James on exceptional mental states: The 1896 Lowell lectures.* Amherst, MA: The University of Massachusetts.

Taylor, E. (2009). *The mystery of personality: A history of psychodynamic theories.* New York, NY: Springer.

Taylor, J. (Ed.). (1958). *Selected writings of John Hughlings Jackson.* (2 Vols.). New York, NY: Basic.

Tedeschi, R. G., Blevins, C. L., & Riffle, O. M. (2017). Posttraumatic growth: A brief history and evaluation. In M. A. Warren & S. I. Donaldson, (Eds.), *Scientific advances in positive psychology* (pp. 131–167). Santa Barbara, CA: Praeger.

Tedeschi, R. G., & Calhoun, L. G. (1995). *Trauma and transformation: Growing in the aftermath of suffering.* Thousand Oaks, CA: Sage.

Tedeschi, R. G., & Calhoun, L. G. (1996). Posttraumatic growth inventory: Measuring the positive legacy of trauma. *Journal of Traumatic Stress, 9*(3), 455–471. https://doi.org/10.1002/jts.2490090305

Tedeschi, R. G., & Calhoun, L. G. (2004a). A clinical approach to posttraumatic growth. In P. Alex Linley & S. Joseph (Eds.), *Positive Psychology in Practice* (pp. 405–419). Hoboken, NJ, USA: John Wiley & Sons, Inc. https://doi.org/10.1002/9780470939338.ch25

Tedeschi, R. G., & Calhoun, L. G. (2004b). Posttraumatic growth: conceptual foundations and empirical evidence. *Psychological Inquiry, 15*(1), 1–18. https://doi.org/10.1207/s15327965pli1501_01

Tedeschi, R. G., & Moore, B. A. (2016). *The posttraumatic growth workbook: Coming through trauma wiser, stronger, and more resilient.* Oakland, CA: New Harbinger.

Teloh, H. (1976). Human nature, psychic energy, and self-actualization in Plato's Republic. *The Southern Journal of Philosophy, 14*(3), 345–358. https://doi.org/10.1111/j.2041-6962.1976.tb01291.x

Terman, L. M. (1938). *Psychological factors in marital happiness.* New York, NY: McGraw-Hill.

Thagard, P. (2010). *The brain and the meaning of life.* Princeton, NJ: Princeton University Press.

The 10 leading causes of death, 2012. (2015, December 10). Retrieved September 17, 2016, from http://www.statcan.gc.ca/pub/82-625-x/2015001/article/14296-eng.htm

Thesleff, H. (2002). An introduction to studies in Plato's two-level model. *Journal of the International Plato Society,* http://positivedisintegration.com/THESLEFF2002.pdf

Thomson, P., & Jaque, S. V. (2016a). Overexcitability and optimal flow in talented dancers, singers, and athletes. *Roeper Review, 38*(2), 32–39. https://doi.org/10.1080/02783193.2015.1112865

Thomson, P., & Jaque, S. V. (2016b). Overexcitability: A psychological comparison between dancers, opera singers, and athletes. *Roeper Review, 38*(2), 84–92. https://doi.org/10.1080/02783193.2016.1150373

Thorne, F. C. (1976). A new approach to psychopathology. *Journal of Clinical Psychology, 32*(4), 751–761. https://doi.org/10.1002/1097-4679(197610)32:4<751::AID-JCLP2270320402>3.0.CO;2-II

Thorpe, L. P. (1938). *Psychological foundations of personality.* New York, NY: McGraw-Hill.

Tibbetts, C. (1979). The anxiety of the gifted. *Roeper Review, 2*(4), 33–34. https://doi.org/10.1080/02783198009552479

Tickle, J. J., Heatherton, T. F., & Wittenberg, L. G. (2001). Can personality change? In W. J. Livesley (Ed.), *Handbook of personality disorders* (pp. 242–258). New York: Guilford Press.

Tieso C. L. (2009). Overexcitabilities. In B. Kerr (Ed.), *Encyclopedia of giftedness, creativity and talent* Volume 2 (pp. 662–664). Thousand Oaks CA: Sage.

Tieso, C. L. (2007a). Overexcitabilities: A new way to think about talent. *Roeper Review, 29*(4), 232–239. https://doi.org/10.1080/02783190709554417

Tieso, C. L. (2007b). Patterns of overexcitabilities in identified gifted students and their parents: A hierarchical model. *Gifted Child Quarterly, 51*(1), 11–22. https://doi.org/10.1177/0016986206296657

Tillier, W. (2008a). Kazimierz Dąbrowski: The man. In S. Mendaglio (Ed.), *Dąbrowski's Theory of Positive Disintegration* (pp. 3–11). Scottsdale, AZ: Great Potential Press.

Tillier, W. (2008b). Philosophical aspects of Dąbrowski's theory of positive disintegration. In S. Mendaglio (Ed.), *Dąbrowski's theory of positive disintegration* (pp. 101–121). Scottsdale, AZ: Great Potential Press.

Tillier, W. (2009). Dąbrowski without the theory of positive disintegration just isn't Dąbrowski. *Roeper Review, 31*(2), 123–126. https://doi.org/10.1080/02783190902737699

Tillier, W. (2016). Foreword. In K. Dąbrowski, *Positive Disintegration* (ix-xxi). Anna Maria, FL: Bassett.

Tillier, W. (2017). Surviving authentic development: Suicide risk in psychoneuroses and positive disintegration. *Advanced Development, 16*, 31–53.

Tillotson, C. (November 20, 2010). *Universality from the perspective of Miguel de Unamuno.* Institute of World Culture. Retrieved from http://www.worldculture.org/articles/Unamuno Philosophy.pdf

Toga, A. W., & Thompson, P. M. (2005). Genetics of brain structure and intelligence. *Annual Review of Neuroscience, 28*(1), 1–23. https://doi.org/10.1146/annurev.neuro.28.061604.135655

Torges, C. M., Stewart, A. J., Duncan, L. E. (2008). Achieving ego integrity: Personality development in late midlife. *Journal of Research in Personality, 42*(4), 1004–1019. https://doi.org/10.1016/j.jrp.2008.02.006

Townsend, J. S., & Martin, J. A. (1983). Whatever happened to neurosis? An overview. *Professional Psychology: Research and Practice, 14*(3), 323–329. https://doi.org/10.1037/0735-7028.14.3.323

Treat, A. R. (2006). Overexcitability in gifted sexually diverse populations. *Journal of Secondary Gifted Education, 17*(4), 244–257. https://doi.org/10.4219/jsge-2006-413

Turrigiano, G. G. (2008). The self-tuning neuron: Synaptic scaling of excitatory synapses. *Cell, 135*(3), 422–435. https://doi.org/10.1016/j.cell.2008.10.008

Turrigiano, G. G. (2011). Too many cooks? Intrinsic and synaptic homeostatic mechanisms in cortical circuit refinement. *Annual Review of Neuroscience, 34*(1), 89–103. https://doi.org/10.1146/annurev-neuro-060909-153238

Turrigiano, G. G. (2012). Homeostatic synaptic plasticity: Local and global mechanisms for stabilizing neuronal function. *Cold Spring Harbor Perspectives in Biology, 4*(1), a005736. https://doi.org/10.1101/cshperspect.a005736

Turrigiano, G. G., & Nelson, S. B. (2000). Hebb and homeostasis in neuronal plasticity. *Current Opinion in Neurobiology, 10*(3), 358–64. https://doi.org/10.1016/S0959-4388(00)00091-X

Turrigiano, G. G., & Nelson, S. B. (2004). Homeostatic plasticity in the developing nervous system. *Nature Reviews Neuroscience, 5*(2), 97–107. https://doi.org/10.1038/nrn1327

Twenge, J. M., Joiner, T. E., Rogers, M. L., & Martin, G. N. (2017). Increases in depressive symptoms, suicide-related outcomes, and suicide rates among U.S. adolescents after 2010 and links to increased new media screen time. *Clinical Psychological Science, 6*(1), 3–17. https://doi.org/10.1177/2167702617723376

Ugochukwu, K. (2012). The notion of spheres in Soren Kierkegaard: A philosophical insight. *Research on Humanities and Social Sciences, 2*(5), 121–128.

Uhlhaas, P. (2009). Neural synchrony in cortical networks: History, concept and current status. *Frontiers in Integrative Neuroscience, 3*(13), 3662–9. https://doi.org/10.3389/neuro.07.017.2009

Unamuno, M. de (1921). *The tragic sense of life in men and nations* (J. E. Crawford Flitch, Trans.). London, England: Macmillan.

Ustun, B., Adler, L. A., Rudin, C., Faraone, S. V., Spencer, T. J., Berglund, P., . . . Kessler, R. C. (2017). The World Health Organization adult attention-deficit/hyperactivity disorder self-report screening scale for DSM-5. *JAMA Psychiatry, 74*(5), 520–526. https://doi.org/10.1001/jamapsychiatry.2017.0298

Van den Broeck, W., Hofmans, J., Cooremans, S., & Staels, E. (2014). Factorial validity and measurement invariance across intelligence levels and gender of the Overexcitabilities Questionnaire-II (OEQ-II). *Psychological Assessment, 26*(1), 55–68. https://doi.org/10.1037/a0034475

van der Hart, O., & Friedman, B. (1989). A reader's guide to Pierre Janet on dissociation: A neglected intellectual heritage. *Dissociation, 2*, 3–16.

van der Kolk, B. A. (2014). *The body keeps the score: Brain, mind, and body in the healing of trauma.* New York, NY: Viking.

van der Kolk, B. A., Brown, P., & van der Hart, O. (1989). Pierre Janet on post-traumatic stress. *J. Traum. Stress 2*(4), 365–378. https://doi.org/10.1002/jts.2490020403

van Nierop, M., Viechtbauer, W., Gunther, N., van Zelst, C., de Graaf, R., ten Have, M., . . . van Winkel, R. (2015). Childhood trauma is associated with a specific admixture of affective, anxiety, and psychosis symptoms cutting across traditional diagnostic boundaries. *Psychological Medicine, 45*(6), 1277–1288. https://doi.org/10.1017/S0033291714002372

Viscott, D. (1996). *Emotional resilience: Simple truths for dealing with the unfinished business of your past.* New York, NY: Crown.

Voyer, B. J., & Tarantola, T. (Eds.). (2017). *Moral psychology: A multidisciplinary guide.* New York, NY: Springer.

Vuyk, M. A., Kerr, B. A., & Krieshok, T. S. (2016). From overexcitabilities to openness: Informing gifted education with psychological science. *Gifted and Talented International, 31*(1), 59–71. https://doi.org/10.1080/15332276.2016.1220796

Vuyk, M. A., Krieshok, T. S., & Kerr, B. A. (2016). Openness to experience rather than overexcitabilities: Call it like it is. *Gifted Child Quarterly, 60*(3), 192–211. https://doi.org/10.1177/0016986216645407

Walker, B. R., & Jackson, C. J. (2016). Moral emotions and corporate psychopathy: A review. *Journal of Business Ethics, 141*(4), 797–810. https://doi.org/10.1007/s10551-016-3038-5

Walker, B. R., & Jackson, C. J. (2017). Examining the validity of the revised Reinforcement Sensitivity Theory scales. *Personality and Individual Differences, 106*, 90–94. https://doi.org/10.1016/j.paid.2016.10.035

Walker, B. R., Jackson, C. J., & Frost, R. (2017). A comparison of revised reinforcement sensitivity theory with other contemporary personality models. *Personality and Individual Differences, 109*, 232–236. https://doi.org/10.1016/j.paid.2016.12.053

Walsh, R. L., Kemp, C. R., Hodge, K., & Bowes, J. M. (2012). Searching for evidence-based practice: A review of the research on educational interventions for intellectually gifted children in the early childhood years. *Journal for the Education of the Gifted, 35*(2), 103–128. https://doi.org/10.1177/0162353212440610

Warne, R. T. (2011a). An investigation of measurement invariance across genders on the Overexcitability Questionnaire-Two. *Journal of Advanced Academics, 22*(4), 578–593. https://doi.org/10.1177/1932202X11414821

Warne, R. T. (2011b). A reliability generalization of the Overexcitability Questionnaire-Two. *Journal of Advanced Academics, 22*(5), 671–692. https://doi.org/10.1177/1932202X11424881

Wasserman, D. (Ed.). (2016). *Suicide: An unnecessary death*. Oxford, UK: Oxford University Press.

Waterman, A. S. (2008). Reconsidering happiness: A eudaimonist's perspective. *The Journal of Positive Psychology, 3*(4), 234–252. https://doi.org/10.1080/17439760802303002

Waterman, A. S. (2013). The humanistic psychology–positive psychology divide: Contrasts in philosophical foundations. *American Psychologist, 68*(3), 124–133. https://doi.org/10.1037/a0032168

Watson, D., Clark, L. A., & Tellegen, A. (1988). Development and validation of brief measures of positive and negative affect: The PANAS scales. *Journal of Personality and Social*

Psychology, 54(6), 1063–1070.
http://dx.doi.org/10.1037/0022-3514.54.6.1063

Watson, J. B. (1913). Psychology as a behaviorist views it. *Psychological Review, 20*(2), 158–177. https://doi.org/10.1037/h0074428

Webb, J. T., & Latimer, D. (1993). ADHD and children who are gifted. *Exceptional Children, 60*(2), 183–184. https://doi.org/10.1177/001440299306000213

Webb, J. T., Amend, E. R., Webb, N. E., Goerss, J., Beljan, P., & Olenchak, F. R. (2004). *Misdiagnosis and dual diagnoses of gifted children and adults: ADHD, bipolar, OCD, Asperger's, depression and other disorders.* Scottsdale, AZ: Great Potential Press.

Weiner, E. S. C., & Simpson, J. A. (Eds.). (1991). *The compact oxford English dictionary.* New York, NY: Oxford University Press.

Weiss, T. (2014). Personal transformation: Posttraumatic growth and gerotranscendence. *Journal of Humanistic Psychology, 54*(2), 203–226. https://doi.org/10.1177/0022167813492388

Welsh, R., & Knabb, J. (2009). Renunciation of the self in psychotherapy. *Mental Health, Religion & Culture, 12*(4), 401–414. https://doi.org/10.1080/13674670902752946

Werdel, M. B., & Wicks, R. J. (2012). *Primer on posttraumatic growth: An introduction and guide.* Hoboken, NJ: Wiley.

White, A. (1996). *Going mad to stay sane: The psychology of self-destructive behavior.* London, England: Duckworth.

White, B. A. (2014). Who cares when nobody is watching? Psychopathic traits and empathy in prosocial behaviors. *Personality and Individual Differences, 56*(1), 116–121. https://doi.org/10.1016/j.paid.2013.08.033

White, S. (2014). The intensities and high sensitivity of a gifted creative genius: Sylvia Ashton-Warner. *Gifted Education International, 30*(2), 106–116. https://doi.org/10.1177/0261429413481121

Whitehead, P. M. (2017). Goldstein's self-actualization: A biosemiotic view. *The Humanistic Psychologist, 45*(1), 71–83. https://doi.org/10.1037/hum0000047

Widiger, T. A. (2016). An integrative model of personality strengths and weaknesses. In A. M. Wood & J. Johnson (Eds.), *The Wiley handbook of positive clinical psychology* (pp. 261–277). Chichester, UK: Wiley/Blackwell.

Widiger, T. A. (2017). (Ed.). *The Oxford handbook of the five-factor model*. New York, NY: Oxford University Press.

Widiger, T. A., & Costa, P. T. (Eds.). (2013). *Personality disorders and the five-factor model of personality* (3rd ed.). Washington, DC: American Psychological Association.

Wiegmann, A., & Osman, M. (Eds.). (2017). Factors guiding moral judgment, reason, decision, and action [Special issue]. *Experimental Psychology, 64*(2), 65–67. https://doi.org/10.1027/1618-3169/a000360

Wilber, K. (1996). *A brief history of everything*. Boston, MA: Shambala.

Wilde, D. J. (2011). *Jung's personality theory quantified.* London, England: Springer.

Wiles, L., Gu, S., Pasqualetti, F., Parvesse, B., Gabrieli, D., Bassett, D. S., & Meaney, D. F. (2017). Autaptic connections shift network excitability and bursting. *Scientific Reports, 7*, 44006. https://doi.org/10.1038/srep44006

Wilkinson, P., Kelvin, R., Roberts, C., Dubicka, B., & Goodyer, I. (2011). Clinical and psychosocial predictors of suicide attempts and nonsuicidal self-injury in the Adolescent Depression Antidepressants and Psychotherapy Trial (ADAPT). *American Journal of Psychiatry, 168*(5), 495–501. https://doi.org/10.1176/appi.ajp.2010.10050718

William Calley. (2017, January 18). In Wikipedia, The Free Encyclopedia. Retrieved February 5, 2017, from https://en.wikipedia.org/wiki/William_Calley

Willings, D., & Arseneault, M. (1986). Attempted suicide and creative promise. *Gifted Education International, 4*(1), 10–13. https://doi.org/10.1177/026142948600400103

Wilson, C. (1971). *The occult: A history.* New York, NY: Random House.

Wilson, C. (1972). *New pathways in psychology: Maslow & the post-Freudian revolution*. London, England: Gollancz.

Winkler, D. L. (2014). Giftedness and overexcitability: Investigating the evidence (Doctoral dissertation). Available from https://digitalcommons.lsu.edu/cgi/viewcontent.cgi?referer=htt ps://www.google.ca/&httpsredir=1&article=4542&context=gr adschool_dissertations

Winkler, D., & Voight, A. (2016). Giftedness and overexcitability: Investigating the relationship using meta-analysis. *Gifted Child Quarterly, 60*(4), 243–257. https://doi.org/10.1177/0016986216657588

Winston, C. N. (2017). To Be and Not to Be: A Paradoxical Narrative of Self-Actualization. *The Humanistic Psychologist.* https://doi.org/10.1037/hum0000082

Winter, D., Bradshaw, S., Bunn, F., & Wellsted, D. (2013). A systematic review of the literature on counselling and psychotherapy for the prevention of suicide: 1. Quantitative outcome and process studies. *Counselling and Psychotherapy Research, 13*(3), 164–183. https://doi.org/10.1080/14733145.2012.761717

Wirthwein, L., Becker, C., & Loehr, E. (2011). Overexcitabilities in gifted and non-gifted adults: Does sex matter? *High Ability Studies, 22*(2), 145–153. https://doi.org/10.1080/13598139.2011.622944

Wirthwein, L., & Rost, D. H. (2011). Focusing on overexcitabilities: Studies with intellectually gifted and academically talented adults. *Personality and Individual Differences, 51*(3), 337–342. https://doi.org/10.1016/j.paid.2011.03.041

Wong, P. T. P. (2017). Meaning-centered approach to research and therapy, second wave positive psychology, and the future of humanistic psychology. *The Humanistic Psychologist, 45*(3), 207-216. https://doi.org/10.1037/hum0000062

Wong, P. T. P., & Roy, S. (2017). Critique of positive psychology and positive interventions. In N. J. L. Brown, T. Lomas, & F. J. Eiroa-Orosa (Eds.), *The Routledge international handbook of critical positive psychology* (pp. 142–160). London, UK: Routledge.

Wood, A. M., & Johnson, J. (Eds.). (2016). *The Wiley handbook of positive clinical psychology*. Chichester, West Sussex, England: John Wiley.

Wood, S. M., & Craigen, L. M. (2011). Self-injurious behavior in gifted and talented youth: What every educator should know. *Journal for the Education of the Gifted, 34*(6), 839–859. https://doi.org/10.1177/0162353211424989

Woods, S. A., & Anderson, N. R. (2016). Toward a periodic table of personality: Mapping personality scales between the five-factor model and the circumplex model. *Journal of Applied Psychology, 101*(4), 582–604. https://doi.org/10.1037/apl0000062

Worchel, D., & Gearing, R. E. (2010). *Suicide assessment and treatment: Empirical and evidence-based practices.* New York, NY: Springer.

Worchel, P., & Byrne, D. (Eds.) (1964). *Personality change.* New York, NY: Wiley.

World Health Organization. (2010). *Towards evidence-based suicide prevention programmes.* Geneva, Switzerland: World Health Organization. Retrieved from http://www.wpro.who.int/mnh/TowardsEvidencebasedSPP.pdf

World Health Organization. (2014). *Preventing suicide: A global imperative.* Geneva, Switzerland: World Health Organization. Retrieved from http://apps.who.int/iris/bitstream/10665/131056/1/9789241564 779_eng.pdf?ua

Wright, J. H. (1906). The origin of Plato's Cave. *Harvard Studies in Classical Philology, 17*(1906), 131. https://doi.org/10.2307/310313

Yablonsky, L. (1972). *Robopaths.* New York, NY: Bobbs-Merrill.

Yakmaci-Guzel, B. & Akarsu, F. (2006). Comparing overexcitabilities of gifted and non-gifted 10th grade students in Turkey. *High Ability Studies, 17*(1), 43–56. https://doi.org/10.1080/13598130600947002

Yankov, G. P. (2017). Between "is" and "ought:" A philosophical investigation of personal values and their application in managerial practice. *Journal of Theoretical and Philosophical Psychology, 37*(3), 164–182. https://doi.org/10.1037/teo0000063

Yin, J., & Yuan, Q. (2015). Structural homeostasis in the nervous system: A balancing act for wiring plasticity and stability.

Frontiers in Cellular Neuroscience, 8(January), 439.
https://doi.org/10.3389/fncel.2014.00439

Yoshor, D., & Mizrahi, E. M. (2012). *Clinical brain mapping.* New York, NY: McGraw-Hill.

Young-Eisendrath, P. (1996). *The resilient spirit: Transforming suffering into insight and renewal.* Cambridge, MA: Perseus.

Young, L., & Koenigs, M. (2007). Investigating emotion in moral cognition: A review of evidence from functional neuroimaging and neuropsychology. *British medical bulletin, 84*(1), 69–79. https://doi.org/10.1093/bmb/ldm031

Zafeiris, A., & Vicsek, T. (2018). *Why we live in hierarchies? A quantitative treatise.* New York, NY: Springer. https://doi.org/10.1007/978-3-319-70483-8

Zalesky, A., Keilholz, S. D., & van den Heuvel, M. P. (Eds.). (2017). Functional architecture of the human brain [Special issue]. *NeuroImage, 160,* 1. https://doi.org/10.1016/j.neuroimage.2017.10.018

Zalsman, G., Hawton, K., Wasserman, D., van Heeringen, K., Arensman, E., Sarchiapone, M., . . . Zohar, J. (2016). Suicide prevention strategies revisited: 10-year systematic review. *The Lancet. Psychiatry, 3*(7), 646–59. https://doi.org/10.1016/S2215-0366(16)30030-X

Zhang, J., Cheng, W., Liu, Z., Zhang, K., Lei, X., Yao, Y., . . . Feng, J. (2016). Neural, electrophysiological and anatomical basis of brain-network variability and its characteristic changes in mental disorders. *Brain, 139*(8), 2307–2321. https://doi.org/10.1093/brain/aww143

Zizek, B., Garz, D., & Nowak, E. (Eds.). (2015). *Kohlberg revisited.* Rotterdam, The Netherlands: Sense.

Zoellner, L. A., & Feeny, N. C. (Eds.). (2014). *Facilitating resilience and recovery following trauma.* New York, NY: The Guilford Press.

Zoellner, T., & Maercker, A. (2006). Posttraumatic growth in clinical psychology: A critical review and introduction of a two-component model. *Clinical Psychology Review, 26*(5), 626–653. https://doi.org/10.1016/j.cpr.2006.01.008

Zuriff, G. E. (1985). *Behaviorism: A conceptual reconstruction.* New York, NY: Columbia University Press.

NOTES

[1] Psychologist, Ministry of Justice and Solicitor General, Alberta (on long-term disability leave).

[2] For more biographical information, see Appendix 1.

[3] See Slaney (2017) and Slaney and Racine (2013) for discussions of constructs in psychology.

[4] Ontogeny is generally used to describe the development of a single organism. Ontogeny is contrasted with phylogeny, that is, the sequence of developments that occur during the evolution of a species.

[5] For a discussion of structures and processes in individual personality, see Cervone (2005).

[6] See Dąbrowski (1970b, p. 118). This viewpoint echoes the Indian theosophist philosopher, Jiddu Krishnamurti: "It is no measure of health to be well adjusted to a profoundly sick society."

[7] It is tempting to speculate whether the experiences described by Richard Maurice Bucke (1837-1902) that he referred to as cosmic consciousness, might be an example of a higher level of reality function (Bucke, 1901/1905).

[8] Grant applications where submitted for the years 1970-1975.

[9] This is contrasted with traditional approaches where diagnosis is made early in the therapeutic relationship.

[10] As a student of Dąbrowski's, I saw him criticized for using the term psychopath, a criticism that I think was largely based on the general understanding of the term in the contemporary American context, a usage that usually carries a criminal context.

[11] Mailer was a prototypic psychopath, for example, he stabbed his second (of six) wife almost to death in a drunken stupor (Lennon, 2013).

[12] This is reminiscent of Freud's (1961, p. 22) observation: "Life, as we find it, is too hard for us; it brings us too many pains, disappointments and

impossible tasks. In order to bear it we cannot dispense with palliative measures . . . There are perhaps three such measures: powerful deflections, which cause us to make light of our misery; substitutive satisfactions, which diminish it; and intoxicating substances, which make us insensible to it."
[13] Dąbrowski occasionally used the pseudonym "Paweł Cienin," which literally translates to "shadow man." I do not know why he used this pseudonym.
[14] I would note that openness to experience has its own challenges as a construct (e.g., Christensen, Cotter, & Silvia, 2018).
[15] This number is contradicted by other authors; for example, Loevinger (1976, p. 140) suggested that self-actualization only occurred in one in a thousand college students, and Sheldon (2004, p. 9) stated: "Maslow claimed that fewer than one person in one thousand achieved self-actualization."
[16] For an excellent introduction to Wilson see Lachman (2016).
[17] Be greeted psychoneurotics!
For you see sensitivity in the insensitivity of the world, uncertainty among the world's certainties.
For you often feel others as you feel yourselves.
For you feel the anxiety of the world, and its bottomless narrowness and self-assurance.
For your phobia of washing your hands from the dirt of the world,
for your fear of being locked in the world's limitations,
for your fear of the absurdity of existence.
For your subtlety in not telling others what you see in them.
For your awkwardness in dealing with practical things, and
for your practicalness in dealing with unknown things,
for your transcendental realism and lack of everyday realism,
for your exclusiveness and fear of losing close friends,
for your creativity and ecstasy
for your maladjustment to that "which is" and adjustment to that which "ought to be,"
for your great but unutilized abilities.
For the belated appreciation of the real value of your greatness
which never allows the appreciation of the greatness of those who will come after you.
For your being treated instead of treating others,
for your heavenly power being forever pushed down by brutal force;
for that which is prescient, unsaid, infinite in you.

For the loneliness and strangeness of your ways.
Be greeted! (Dąbrowski, 1972b, p. xvi)
[18] Butcher, Hass, Greene, and Nelson (2015) described the Pt scale: The Pt scale assesses psychasthenia, a disorder that was prominently assessed when the MMPI was developed. This disorder is characterized by the person's inability to resist specific actions or thoughts regardless of their maladaptive nature (i.e., the person has weak ideational control that cannot resist these negative thoughts). This diagnostic label is no longer used, and such persons are now typically diagnosed as having obsessive–compulsive disorders. In addition to assessing obsessive-compulsive features, the Pt scale addresses the content areas of abnormal fears, self-criticism, difficulties in concentration, and guilt feelings.
[19] It is important to keep in mind that when developmental potential is weak, Dąbrowski considered the environment as the determining factor as to whether there would be a positive development through nervousness and psychoneuroses or a reintegration on a lower level, or a negative disintegration culminating in psychosis or suicide.
[20] In Dąbrowski (1970a) the term is "conjoined."
[21] Mechanisms related to the acquisition of spiritual knowledge.
[22] The authors went on to map individual differences in responsivity of the approach system to extraversion, and differences in responsivity of the withdrawal system to neuroticism.
[23] This chapter is based upon an earlier work (Tillier, 2008b).
[24] Platon Cave Sanraedam 1604.jpg. (2014, July 6). *Wikimedia Commons, the free media repository.* Retrieved 07:45, November 19, 2017 from https://commons.wikimedia.org/w/index.php?title=File:Platon_Cave_S anraedam_1604.jpg&oldid=128275077.
[25] Maslow (1962) explained his construct of instinctoid: "psychoanalysis and other uncovering therapies simply reveal or expose an inner, more biological, more instinctoid core of human nature. Part of this core are certain preferences and yearnings that may be considered to be intrinsic, biologically based values, even though weak ones. All the basic needs fall into this category and so do all the inborn capacities and talents of the individual" (p. 166). The "instinctoid impulses or urges" are not "predetermined instrumental behaviors, abilities or mode of gratification, i.e., not [of] instincts" (Maslow, 1954, p. 341).
[26] Maslow (1968) suggested that the third force is "transitional, a preparation for a still 'higher' Fourth Psychology, transpersonal, transhuman, centered

in the cosmos rather than in human needs and interest, going beyond humanness, identity, self-actualization and the like" (pp. iii–iv).

[27] In the early 1960s, Karl Ludwig von Bertalanffy (1901-1972) and Joseph R. Royce (1921-1989) established the Center for Advanced Study in Theoretical Psychology at the University of Alberta, Edmonton. Royce was involved in securing Dąbrowski's position at the University, and Dąbrowski gave lectures at the Center during his sessions at the University. I completed a graduate level course taught by Dąbrowski; during the course, we discussed Bertalanffy's general systems theory and the factor analytic approach to personality, developed by Royce. See Mos and Kuiken (1998).

[28] It is beyond the scope of this work to fully explore Kierkegaard's framework of the self; the reader interested in more detail is referred to: Bernier, 2015; Nielsen, 2017; Obsieger, 2017; Stokes, 2015.

[29] The word *Übermensch* can be broken down as *über*, German adjective for great example (from the Latin for super; ὑπερ, Greek for hyper), and *Mensch*, German for human being.

[30] For reasons lost to history, the authorship on this publication from the University of Geneva is given as Casimir Dombrowski.

[31] A quotation from a suicide note.

[32] Previous research has described therapy as a daunting process. For example, "seventy-five percent of patients were predicted to improve only after receiving more than 40 treatment sessions in conjunction with other routine contacts, including medication in some cases" (Lambert, Hansen, & Finch, 2001, p. 159). Another study found that clinicians believe that CBT takes six months before successful results are seen but several factors complicate therapy, including the fact that virtually all patients are poly-symptomatic and patterns of comorbidity can double the number of sessions required for success (Morrison, Bradley, & Westen, 2003).

[33] "'Highway'" is often seen translated as "'herd.'"

[34] For biographical information on Maslow, see Hoffman, (1988, 1992).

[35] Unamuno (1921) anticipated that as basic needs are satisfied, existential questions will arise:
"Whence do I come and whence comes the world in which and by which I live? Whither do I go and whither goes everything that environs me? What does it all mean? Such are the questions that man asks as soon as he frees himself from the brutalizing necessity of laboring for his material sustenance." (p. 32)

[36] It is beyond the focus of this book to fully consider Maslow's propositions. As he developed his theories, Maslow's ideas became more

and more challenging and contradictory. For example, Maslow (1971) differentiated the following groups:
– Non-transcending self-actualizers (Theory-Y people): those with little or no experiences of transcendence.
– Transcending self-actualizers (Theory-Z people): those in whom transcendent experiencing was important and even central.
– Transcending nonhealthy people, non-self-actualizers, who have important transcendent experiences. (pp. 270–286)
– Transcenders: peakers, Yea-sayers, eager for life. Aware of and living at, the level of Being (B-realm and B-cognition), metamotivated. Peak and plateau experiences become the most important things in life. Often characterized by the discovery and development of one's own private core religious experiences (Maslow, 1964).
– Non-transcenders: nonpeakers, Nay-sayers, "nauseated or irritated by life; they are more essentially practical, realistic, mundane, capable and secular people, living more in the here-and-now world; i.e., what I have called the D-realm for short, the world of deficiency-needs and of deficiency-cognitions." Tend to be "doers." Do not have personal religious experiences or if they do, repress or suppress them and therefore cannot utilize them in their personal growth, often active in institutional religious activities (Maslow, 1964).
Maslow was criticized for these theoretical elaborations: "This distinction between transcending and nontranscending self-actualizers threw Maslow's theory into comparative disorder" (Daniels, 1982, p. 70).
[37] Maslow did not number the characteristics he described. Some authors close the list at item 15. In Maslow (1970) the section following was entitled "the imperfections of self-actualizing people," and some authors include it as a 16th characteristic. Self-actualizing people show "many of the lesser human failings" (Maslow, 1970, p. 175).
[38] This phrase was represented in a recruitment slogan of the United States Army, "Be all that you can be" (1980-2001).
[39] This situation is certainly not uncommon; psychology has yet to agree on a definition of emotion (Mulligan & Scherer, 2012).
[40] The verbal stimuli were an informal list of words given to subjects to elicit responses. Here are the instructions: Please describe freely in relation to each word listed below your emotional associations and experiences. Use as much space as you need. Here are the words: great sadness, great joy, death, solitude and loneliness, suicide, inner conflict, ideal and success.

[41] Naville later became one of the independent experts investigating the Katyń Massacre.

[42] Dąbrowski's curriculum vitae is available to us as he submitted it as part of his supporting documentation to several Canada Council grant applications: 1970, 1971-1972, 1972-1975 and 1973-1975.

[43] There is some confusion over this degree; Aronson (1964, p. x) indicates it was in "experimental psychology" and was granted by the University of Poznań in 1932.

[44] Dąbrowski's curriculum vitae indicates "Certificate of psychoanalytic studies, Vienna (under Wilhelm Stekel), 1931." Aronson (1964) indicates this was in 1930.

[45] Dąbrowski's curriculum vitae indicates a "Certificate of school of public health," Harvard University, 1934." However, Battaglia (2002, p. 67) indicates that Dąbrowski did not meet the criteria, and no certificate was given.

[46] Translation by Google translation services. Original: "Zaczęły się wówczas wyraźnie krystalizować moje poglądy na zakres i ujęcia wielopłaszczyźniane i wielopoziomowe higieny psychicznej, którą zacząłem widzieć jako naukę niezbędną na terenie każdego działu psychologii, psychoterapii, psychiatrii i autentycznego wychowania. Zdawałem sobie sprawę coraz bardziej z tego, że podejście psychopatologiczne nie jest sprawą prostą, że nie wyraża statycznej i statystycznej anormalności, że na tym terenie stykają się wysokie normalności w sensie przyspieszonego rozwoju, twórczości, wzmożonej pobudliwości, która jest ściśle związana z przyspieszonym rozwojem i twórczością."

[47] Dąbrowski was a logical choice for extortion as he and his family of origin were well-off (Amend, personal communication, 2013).

[48] Dąbrowski's curriculum vitae indicates: "Habilitation in psychiatry," University of Wroclaw, 1948."

[49] Dąbrowski's curriculum vitae indicates: "Professorship in Experimental Psychology, Academy of Catholic Theology, Warsaw, 1956" and "Professorship in the Polish Academy of Sciences since 1958."

[50] See Dąbrowski, K. (1964a).

[51] Universidad Femenina del Sagrado Corazón, Lima, Peru.

[52] Dąbrowski also declined an offer of a position to work with Maslow because he refused to renounce his Polish citizenship, a requirement for American citizenship (a stipulation of the offer).

[53] This bibliography varies slightly from APA format, for example, including issue numbers where available (I find this information helpful in doing research). All links are live as of the date of publication.

[54] The text is a translation of selected fragments from Kazimierz Dąbrowski's book, *Nervousness of Children and Youth* ("Nerwowosc u dzieci i mlodziezy"), Warsaw, 1958, pp. 253–259. In 1932 Dąbrowski received a two-year research scholarship from the National Culture Fund to study in Vienna and Paris. In Vienna, he studied at the Institute of Active Psychoanalysis under fellow Pole, Wilhelm Stekel (1868-1940) and on September 13, 1934, was given a diploma by Stekel authorizing him to conduct psychoanalysis practice.

[55] The published text is an excerpt from Kazimierz Dąbrowski's "Multi-theme Mystery of Development." The text is published for the first time in this version in *Heksis, 1*, 2010, Warsaw.

[56] The text is an excerpt from Kazimierz Dąbrowski's book, *Socio-educational Child Psychiatry*, PZWS, Warszawa, 1959, pp. 110–114, pp. 95–101.

[57] See note 30.

INDEX

Cervone, 455n
channel, and overexcitability, 86
character, emergence of, 31
characteristic adaptations, 250
Charcot, J.-M., 117
childhood trauma, 235
Christensen, Cotter, and Silvia,
  456n
Christie, A. (and disintegration),
  114
chronically disintegrated type,
  180
Churchill, W. (and
  disintegration), 114
Churchland, P., 169-70
Cienin (1972), 70, 191, 228, 237,
  321
Cienin, Pawel, 456n
circumplex models, 179
civilized libido, 119
Claparède, É., xxi, 41, 352, 354
*Clinical Lectures on Mental
  Diseases* (Clouston), 124
Clouston, T. S., 81, 124
Coconut Grove nightclub, fire,
  243
cognitive behavior therapy
  (CBT), 225, 458n
cognitive restructuring, 225
coherent heterogeneity, 102
College of Mental Hygiene, 357-
  58
College of Mental Hygiene and
  Applied Psychology, 358
communion with others, 79
compassion, 67
compulsions, 130, 131
computerized CBT (cCBT), 235
*Conditions Psycholopique du
  Suicide, Les* (Dombrowski), 355
conflicts with horizontal focus,
  63, 115-116

conformity, 3, 13, 16, 58
connectome, 295
Conrad, J. (and disintegration),
  114
conscience, 57
  and the third factor, 147
conscientiousness, 250
conscious choice, 72
consciousness, 20
  and overexcitability, 86
consensus trance, 198-99
constitutional endowment, 56, 79
constructs, 11
contemporary approaches, other,
  305
contemporary personality theory,
  279-81
continuous variable, 338
continuum of excitability, 297
contraception, 224
conventional (developmental
  category), 279
conversion hysteria, 124
coping repertoire, 244-45
corporate psychopathy, 59
Corporation des Psychologues,
  364
cortex, 20
cortical excitation, 292
cosmic consciousness, 455n
cosmic self, 269
  and reintegration, 269-70
counseling the gifted, 333
courage, birth of, 131
creative dynamisms, 284
creative instinct/instincts, 75, 190,
  284
creative self-efficacy (CSE), 290
creativeness, 315
creativity, xxiii, 66, 144, 284-87
crises
  optimal levels of, 23

ABOUT THE AUTHOR

William (Bill) Tillier, received a Bachelor of Science Degree from the University of Calgary and a Master of Science Degree from the University of Alberta. It was there he met Dr. Dąbrowski and became his student. Bill worked as a forensic psychologist for over 20 years before developing a neuromuscular disorder. Dąbrowski and his work remained a passion for Bill, who created a Dąbrowski website and promoted and distributed Dąbrowski's original works. He has also been involved with many Dąbrowski conferences and written an introduction to the republication of Dąbrowski's seminal work, *Positive Disintegration*. Bill is on disability leave and spends his time doing research and volunteering.

Publisher's Catalogue

The Prosperous Series

#1 The Prosperous Coach: Increase Income and Impact for You and Your Clients (Steve Chandler and Rich Litvin)

#2 The Prosperous Hip Hop Producer: My Beat-Making Journey from My Grandma's Patio to a Six-Figure Business (Curtiss King)

* * *

Devon Bandison

Fatherhood Is Leadership: Your Playbook for Success, Self-Leadership, and a Richer Life

Sir Fairfax L. Cartwright

The Mystic Rose from the Garden of the King

Steve Chandler

37 Ways to BOOST Your Coaching Practice: PLUS: the 17 Lies That Hold Coaches Back and the Truth That Sets Them Free

50 Ways to Create Great Relationships

Business Coaching (Steve Chandler and Sam Beckford)

Crazy Good: A Book of CHOICES

Death Wish: The Path through Addiction to a Glorious Life

Fearless: Creating the Courage to Change the Things You Can

RIGHT NOW: Mastering the Beauty of the Present Moment

The Prosperous Coach: Increase Income and Impact for You and Your Clients (The Prosperous Series #1) (Steve Chandler and Rich Litvin)

Shift Your Mind Shift The World (Revised Edition)

Time Warrior: How to defeat procrastination, people-pleasing, self-doubt, over-commitment, broken promises and chaos

Wealth Warrior: The Personal Prosperity Revolution

Kazimierz Dąbrowski

Positive Disintegration

The Philosophy of Essence: A Developmental Philosophy Based on the Theory of Positive Disintegration

Charles Dickens

A Christmas Carol: A Special Full-Color, Fully-Illustrated Edition

James F. Gesualdi

Excellence Beyond Compliance: Enhancing Animal Welfare Through the Constructive Use of the Animal Welfare Act

Janice Goldman

Let's Talk About Money: The Girlfriends' Guide to Protecting Her ASSets

Sylvia Hall

This Is Real Life: Love Notes to Wake You Up

Christy Harden

Guided by Your Own Stars: Connect with the Inner Voice and Discover Your Dreams

I Heart Raw: Reconnection and Rejuvenation Through the Transformative Power of Raw Foods

Curtiss King

The Prosperous Hip Hop Producer: My Beat-Making Journey from My Grandma's Patio to a Six-Figure Business (The Prosperous Series #2)

David Lindsay

A Blade for Sale: The Adventures of Monsieur de Mailly

Abraham H. Maslow

The Psychology of Science: A Reconnaissance

Being Abraham Maslow (DVD)

Maslow and Self-Actualization (DVD)

Albert Schweitzer

Reverence for Life: The Words of Albert Schweitzer

William Tillier

Personality Development Through Positive Disintegration: The Work of Kazimierz Dąbrowski

Margery Williams

The Velveteen Rabbit: or How Toys Become Real

Colin Wilson

New Pathways in Psychology: Maslow and the Post-Freudian Revolution

Join our Mailing List:

www.MauriceBassett.com

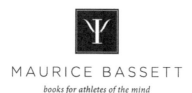

MAURICE BASSETT
books for athletes of the mind

Made in United States
Troutdale, OR
12/16/2023

16012782R10296